AF784711

Pituitary Surgery – A Modern Approach

Frontiers of Hormone Research

Vol. 34

Series Editor

Ashley B. Grossman *London*

KARGER

Pituitary Surgery – A Modern Approach

Volume Editors

Edward R. Laws, Jr. *Charlottesville, Va.*
Jason P. Sheehan *Charlottesville, Va.*

99 figures, 11 in color, and 34 tables, 2006

KARGER

Basel · Freiburg · Paris · London · New York ·
Bangalore · Bangkok · Singapore · Tokyo · Sydney

Edward R. Laws, Jr., MD, FACS
Department of Neurological Surgery
Health Sciences Center
University of Virginia
Charlottesville, Va., USA

Jason P. Sheehan, MD, PhD
Department of Neurological Surgery
Health Sciences Center
University of Virginia
Charlottesville, Va., USA

Library of Congress Cataloging-in-Publication Data

Pituitary surgery : a modern approach / volume editors, Edward R. Laws, Jr.,
Jason P. Sheehan.
p. ; cm. – (Frontiers of hormone research, ISSN 0301-3073 ; v. 34)
Includes bibliographical references and index.
ISBN 3-8055-8051-7 (hard cover : alk. paper)
1. Pituitary gland–Surgery. I. Laws, Edward R. II. Sheehan, Jason
P. III. Series.
[DNLM: 1. Pituitary Neoplasms–surgery. 2. Central Nervous System
Neoplasms–surgery. 3. Endocrine Surgical Procedures–methods.
4. Neurosurgical Procedures–methods. 5. Pituitary Diseases–surgery.
W1 FR946F v.34 2006 / WK 585 P6934 2006]
RD599.5.P58P58 2006
617.4′4059–dc22

2005035999

Bibliographic Indices. This publication is listed in bibliographic services, including Current Contents® and Index Medicus.

Disclaimer. The statements, options and data contained in this publication are solely those of the individual authors and contributors and not of the publisher and the editor(s). The appearance of advertisements in the book is not a warranty, endorsement, or approval of the products or services advertised or of their effectiveness, quality or safety. The publisher and the editor(s) disclaim responsibility for any injury to persons or property resulting from any ideas, methods, instructions or products referred to in the content or advertisements.

Drug Dosage. The authors and the publisher have exerted every effort to ensure that drug selection and dosage set forth in this text are in accord with current recommendations and practice at the time of publication. However, in view of ongoing research, changes in government regulations, and the constant flow of information relating to drug therapy and drug reactions, the reader is urged to check the package insert for each drug for any change in indications and dosage and for added warnings and precautions. This is particularly important when the recommended agent is a new and/or infrequently employed drug.

All rights reserved. No part of this publication may be translated into other languages, reproduced or utilized in any form or by any means electronic or mechanical, including photocopying, recording, microcopying, or by any information storage and retrieval system, without permission in writing from the publisher.

© Copyright 2006 by S. Karger AG, P.O. Box, CH–4009 Basel (Switzerland)
www.karger.com
Printed in Switzerland on acid-free paper by Reinhardt Druck, Basel
ISSN 0301–3073
ISBN 3–8055–8051–7

Contents

Foreword

In the time that I have been practising clinical endocrinology, transsphenoidal surgery has gone from being an innovative approach to pituitary adenomas to having become the standard procedure for a whole variety of sellar and parasellar lesions. However, while many practising clinicians refer patients for this procedure on a regular basis, there have been few texts able to explain the details of the technique, its indications and indeed limitations, as well as the newer extensions such as image guidance and endoscopy. I am therefore delighted to welcome this short volume, where Ed Laws and his colleagues at Charlottesville, one of the leading international centers in transsphenoidal surgery, offer an overview of this whole area, including sections on perioperative management and surgical pathology. Together with other international contributors, they also identify the complementary roles of radiosurgery and transcranial surgery in the approach to sellar and suprasellar tumors. I am sure this will be of great value for all who have to deal with these fascinating and ever-challenging lesions.

Ashley B. Grossman, London

Preface

The management of pituitary adenomas and other sellar tumors is one of the most difficult tasks for neurosurgeons and endocrinologists. The profound systemic sequelae of hypersecretory adenomas and the deleterious effects of local tumor growth must be halted. Medical management, surgical resection, and adjuvant treatment with radiosurgery are just a few of the tools employed by physicians to achieve these goals. The tendency for recurrence, either early or late, demonstrates the need for vigilant follow-up. Optimal treatment requires a multidisciplinary approach; neurological, ophthalmological, and endocrinological testing are all required.

Fortunately, the past decade has seen rapid improvements in the management of patients with pituitary adenomas and other sellar tumors. Technological advances including a better understanding of tumor biology, discovery of molecular events at the basis of tumor development, and development of new equipment to treat the tumors have all been made. The wide range of such advances speaks to the fact that a variety of skills and techniques are typically employed to diagnosis, treat, and follow patients with sellar tumors. The technical and personnel resources of a state-of-the-art medical center are ideally utilized throughout this treatment.

This book aims to provide a comprehensive understanding of the standard of care for treating sellar tumors. The text includes detailed discussions about operative approaches, perioperative management, and adjuvant treatment. In addition, it gives a glimpse of what the future may hold for the treatment of such tumors. In general, the contributing authors have chosen references based upon scientific significance, ease of access, and historical interest.

The fruition of this project was the result of hard work by many people. Unfortunately, it is not possible to adequately acknowledge all those who have helped. However, we wish to call attention to the assistance of several people. First and foremost, we thank the contributing authors for their effort. In addition, Prof. Grossman provided a great deal of stimulation and guidance in this endeavor. The work of Juliane Sättler and Gunhild Hinderling at Karger Publishing proved invaluable.

Finally, we are grateful for the patience and support of our wives, Peggy and Diane.

Edward R. Laws, Jr.
Jason P. Sheehan
Charlottesville, Va.

Laws ER Jr, Sheehan JP (eds): Pituitary Surgery – A Modern Approach.
Front Horm Res. Basel, Karger, 2006, vol 34, pp 1–28

Role of Transcranial Approaches in the Treatment of Sellar and Suprasellar Lesions

Nicholas F. Maartens, Andrew H. Kaye

Department of Neurosurgery, Royal Melbourne Hospital and Department of Surgery, University of Melbourne, Melbourne, Australia

Abstract

The principles in the surgical management of sellar and suprasellar tumors are to relieve mass effect, normalize pituitary hypersecretion, preserve or restore normal pituitary function, prevent tumor recurrence and to provide tissue for pathological and scientific study. Over the past century, the transsphenoidal approach has evolved as the approach of choice for pituitary surgeons. Despite the limitations of transcranial approaches in accessing the intrasellar component of pituitary adenomas and historically their increased morbidity and mortality, there are situations where transcranial procedures have considerable advantages over transsphenoidal approaches. As a consequence, transcranial approaches retain an essential role in the treatment of certain sellar and suprasellar tumors and it remains necessary for all pituitary surgeons to master this approach.

Copyright © 2006 S. Karger AG, Basel

> '. . . the hemisphere can be readily compressed upwards by inserting a flat spatula cautiously beneath it. . . . With this procedure properly applied to the temporal lobe it is remarkable how much can be seen and correctly examined. With good illumination the crura cerebri, the circle of Willis, the pituitary body and internal carotid, the second and third cranial nerves come into view.'
>
> *Sir Victor Horsley* (1906) [1]

Introduction

The principles in surgical management of sellar and suprasellar tumors are to relieve mass effect – particularly on the visual apparatus, normalize pituitary

Table 1. An overview of mortality after transcranial surgery

Author	Year	Patients	Mortality, %
Henderson	1939	205	2.4
Bakay	1950	232	1.4
Elkington and McKissock	1967	260	10
Svien and Colby	1967	117	6.8
Ray and Patterson	1971	146	1.4
McCarty et al.	1973	100	3
Wirth et al.	1974	157	8.9
Symon and Jakubowski	1979	117	2.5
Symon	1979	16	18.7
Fahlbusch	1994	146	2

Table 2. An overview of mortality after transsphenoidal surgery

Author	Year	Patients	Mortality, %
Guiot and Derome	1976	613	1.4
Fahlbusch and Stass	1981	601	1.2
Hardy and Mohr	1985	1,102	0.9
Laws	1982	810	0.5
Landolt	1985	496	0.8
Tindall and Barrow	1985	709	0.3
Fahlbusch	1994	1,688	0.2
Zada	2003	100	0

hypersecretion, preserve or restore normal pituitary function, prevent tumor recurrence and to provide tissue for pathological and scientific study. In order to achieve this, one requires a surgical approach that ideally provides the shortest route to the lesion, confers minimal trauma to surrounding structures, provides adequate exposure and will permit the manipulation necessary to resect the lesion. Over the past century, the transsphenoidal approach, first successfully performed in 1907 by Hermann Schloffer [2, 3], has evolved as the approach of choice by virtually all pituitary surgeons. Recent advances with regard to endoscopic [4] and extended transsphenoidal techniques [5] have served to further consolidate the advantages of this approach over traditional transcranial procedures. Despite the limitations of transcranial approaches in accessing and removing the intrasellar component of pituitary adenomas and historically their increased morbidity and mortality (tables 1, 2) [6], there are, however, situations where transsphenoidal procedures may either be limited or contraindicated and clinical settings where transcranial procedures have considerable advantages over the transsphenoidal approach. As a consequence, transcranial approaches retain an essential role in the treatment of sellar and very large suprasellar tumors and it is a requirement of all pituitary surgeons to master this time-honored approach [7].

History

> 'The endonasal technique is entirely foreign to the surgeon's experience. From beginning to end the field of operation is cramped, one must depend on artificial illumination, and at no time has one what might be called a satisfactory view. It is quite natural that it should fall to the lot of a nasal specialist, Hirsch, to originate the endonasal method.'
>
> *Charles Frazier* (1919) [8]

Until the 18th century, our understanding of the pituitary gland was based largely on primitive, archaic theories regarding its function. By the 19th century, however, there had been a resurgence of interest in the pituitary precipitated by Pierre Marie's observations with regard to acromegaly [9]. Simultaneously, the effect of canine hypophysectomy had begun to be investigated [10] and visual failure being related to pituitary enlargement and certain systemic changes became appreciated. Eventually in 1889, Sir Victor Horsley (1857–1916; fig. 1) became the first surgeon to operate on a pituitary tumor. He used a bifrontal craniotomy approach and a technique he described as 'cerebral dislocation' encountering a cystic adenosarcoma which he described as inoperable [11].

The first actual recorded attempt to resect a pituitary tumor surgically was by Frank Thomas Paul (1851–1941), honorary surgeon to the Royal Infirmary, Liverpool. In 1893 he operated on a patient of Richard Caton's, his physician colleague [12]. He consulted Horsley who recommended a subtemporal approach. Horsley's suggestion was influenced by his laboratory work on sheep in which the pituitary is very accessible subtemporally. The patient was a young woman with acromegaly. She had presented with headaches, facial pain – usually a poor prognostic sign to the old surgeons indicating inoperability, and visual failure. The surgery entailed a two-stage lateral subtemporal decompression. Unfortunately the tumor could not be accessed and the patient, blind as a consequence but with her facial pain having resolved, died 3 months later. In 1903, Otto George Theobald Kiliani, a New York surgeon, began practicing a bifrontal intradural approach to the pituitary region on cadavers [13]. His first clinical procedure was on a patient presenting with severe pituitary apoplexy

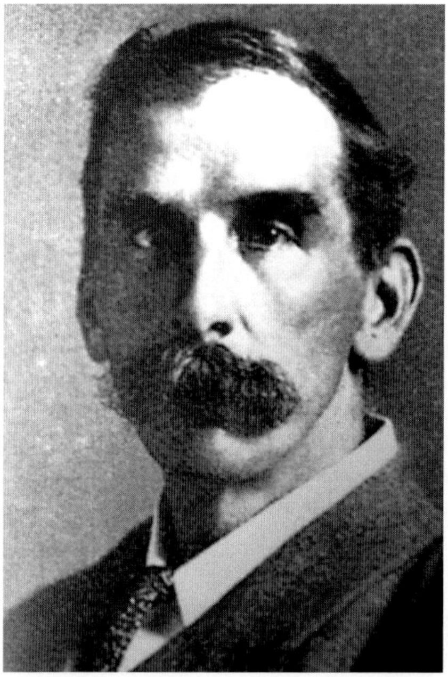

Fig. 1. Sir Victor Horsley (1857– 1916). From the personal collection of E.R. Laws – with permission.

complicated by subdural extension of the hemorrhage. After encountering blood over the convexity and failing in the placement of a ventriculostomy drain to help contain brain swelling, he abandoned the procedure and the patient died 8 h later. In 1900, in Berlin, Fedor Victor Krause (1857–1937) undertook an extradural right frontal approach to access and remove a bullet lodged in the region of the right optic foramen of a patient who had attempted suicide [14]. The patient did remarkably well and Krause was quick to appreciate the significance of the view he had obtained of the sella turcica. In 1905 he performed the first successful transfrontal pituitary surgery choosing an extradural approach to avoid retraction injury to the brain [15]. This procedure provided the basis on which the majority of subsequent variations of the transcranial approach were developed [16].

Between 1904 and 1906, Horsley operated on 10 pituitary tumors utilizing both subfrontal and lateral middle fossa approaches with a mortality rate of 20%, improving on the results of colleagues who hitherto had experienced prohibitive mortality rates ranging between 50 and 80% [1, 17]. He advocated surgical intervention for pituitary region lesions, emphasizing the importance of relieving mechanical pressure on the chiasm exerted by the tumor in order to avoid blindness – considerations that are still pertinent today [18]. Horsley's approach, however, did not gain universal popularity and Cushing also found it impracticable [19]. In 1907, after performing a number of cadaver studies, Braun was convinced that the pituitary should be accessible via a transtemporal approach through the cavernous sinus but this necessitated division of the maxillary branch of the trigeminal nerve as well as ligation of the carotid artery in the neck. In 1908, in order to access a pituitary adenoma, Louis Linn McArthur (1858–1934) turned a right frontal osteoplastic flap and resected the supraorbital rim together with part of the orbital roof. This approach allowed access to lesions with high suprasellar extension. The entire approach was extradural until 5 mm proximal to the chiasmatic sulcus [20, 21]. Charles Frazier (1870–1936) initially adopted this approach but later changed to an intradural frontobasal approach [22]. Upon experiencing unexpected hypertension, even in patients who had not experienced significant bleeding, he changed to a two-stage procedure [23]. He later concluded that the transnasal operation, with which he had accrued some experience, should not be used for patients with visual symptoms, a view later shared by Cushing.

In 1910, after a number of experimental hypophysectomies in dogs, Silbermark suggested an approach to the hypophysis through the Sylvian fissure [11, 24]. In May 1914, George Heuer (1882–1950) of Baltimore, Md., utilized Silbermark's proposal by performing an intracranial intradural approach to the chiasm [25, 26]. He was followed shortly afterwards by Alfred Adson (1887–1951) of the Mayo Clinic [27]. After being conscripted to France in 1917, Heuer's experience of 20 cases was presented by Walter Dandy before the Johns Hopkins Medical Society on February 4, 1918, on the insistence of Halstead.

In March 1907 in Vienna, Schloffer performed the first successful transsphenoidal removal of a pituitary tumor. The technique subsequently underwent a number of modifications culminating in the description by Halstead of the oronasal rhinoseptal submucosal approach with a sublabial gingival incision subsequently adopted by Cushing [28]. After initial disappointments with transcranial procedures, Cushing adopted this approach. Combining suggestions from other surgeons and using the submucosal dissection technique advocated by Eisenberg and Kocher, Cushing went on to perform 231 such procedures between 1910 and 1925 with a reported mortality of 5.6% [16]. Cushing later, in fact, abandoned the transsphenoidal approach, reverting back to the transcranial approach, believing that it enabled the optic apparatus to be more readily decompressed. Due to Cushing's enormous influence at the time, transsphenoidal procedures subsequently became largely neglected. Norman McOmish Dott of Edinburgh (1897–1973), however, who had worked under Cushing, remained committed to the transsphenoidal approach. Probably out of deference to his mentor, he never publicized his preference, eventually passing on his skills to Gérard Guiot (1912–1996) [29] and Jules Hardy [30], respectively. They in turn then introduced fluoroscopy and the operating microscope to the procedure with Hardy advancing to pioneer selective adenomectomy as we know it today. Although this transsphenoidal approach has been universally adopted as the standard approach for almost all sellar tumors, a role for transcranial approaches has, nevertheless, persisted.

The advantages of the pterional approach to lesions in the suprasellar area or inferior third ventricle region, using the natural tissue planes along the sphenoid wing at the frontotemporal junction, eventually and rapidly became apparent. This is now the most frequently used transcranial approach to the sellar region [31]. The pterional approach as we know it today was then refined and described in detail by Gazi Yasargil who advocated minimizing brain retraction by splitting the Sylvian fissure and opening the basal arachnoid [32].

Anatomy

The microsurgical anatomy of the sellar region is complex and a detailed description besides important pertinent surgical points is beyond the scope of this chapter. It has been reviewed and described in detail by Albert L. Rhoton Jr. [33, 34]. Both the referenced works analyze the microsurgical sellar region anatomy firstly from the point of view of the relationships important in performing the various transcranial and subcranial approaches to pituitary region tumors, and secondly from the point of view of the various neural, arterial and venous relationships in the sellar and third ventricular regions that are important in planning surgery for tumors extending from the pituitary gland into these regions. In 1975, Rhoton, together with Renn dissected and analyzed the microsurgical anatomy of 50 adult sellar regions removed en bloc. The particular emphasis of their study was to investigate the implications the variations in the anatomy held for different surgical approaches and the incidence of each variation [35]. Their findings considered factors disadvantageous to transsphenoidal surgery were: (a) large anterior intercavernous sinuses extending anterior to the gland just posterior to the anterior sellar wall (10%); (b) a thin diaphragm (62%) and a diaphragm with a large opening (56%); (c) carotid arteries exposed in the sphenoid sinus with no bone covering (4%); (d) carotid arteries that approach within 4 mm of the midline within the sella (10%; fig. 2); (e) optic canals with bone defects exposing the optic nerves in the sphenoid sinus (4%); (f) a thick sellar floor (18%); (g) sphenoid sinuses with no major septum (28%) or a sinus with the major septum well off midline (47%), and (h) a presellar type of sphenoid sinus with no obvious bulge of the sellar floor into the sphenoid sinus (20%).

Findings considered disadvantageous to the transfrontal approach were: (a) a prefixed chiasm (10%) and a normal chiasm with 2 mm or less between the

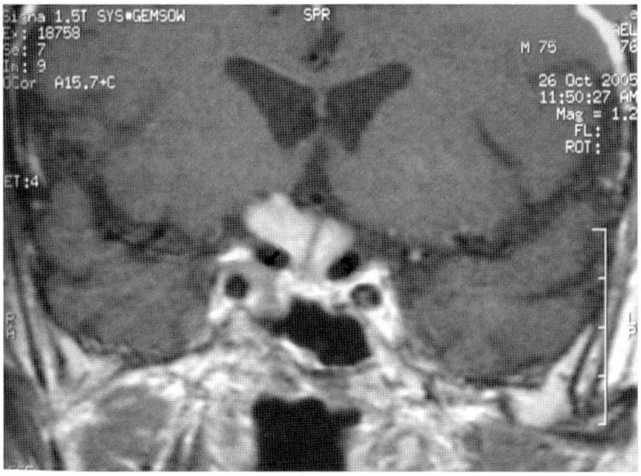

Fig. 2. Coronal T1 MRI gadolinium-enhanced MRI scan illustrating 'kissing carotids' – a relative contraindication for the transsphenoidal resection of a sellar lesion. The narrow access between the cavernous sinuses predisposes the patient to an iatrogenic carotid artery injury during the approach.

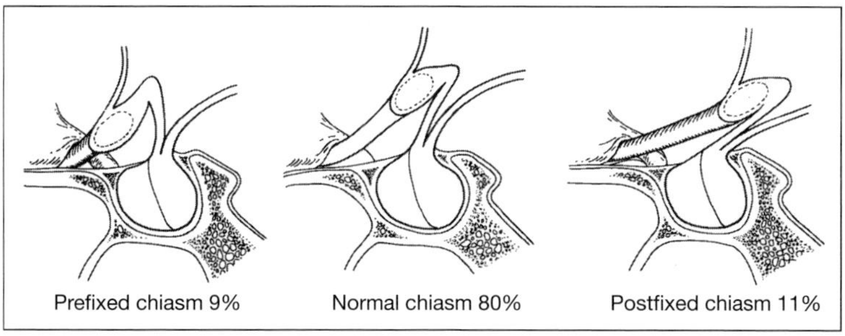

Fig. 3. Diagram illustrating the various anatomical positions of the optic chiasm relative to the tuberculum sellae. In 9% of cases the chiasm is prefixed, 11% being postfixed. The former configuration obscures transcranial access to sellar and suprasellar lesions. The position of the chiasm is regarded as 'normal' in 80%.

chiasm and tuberculum sella (14%; figs 3, 4); (b) an acute angle between the optic nerves as they entered the chiasm (25%); (c) a prominent tuberculum sella protruding above a line connecting the optic nerves as they entered the optic canals (44%), and (d) carotid arteries approaching within 4 mm of the midline within or above the sella turcica (12%) – 'kissing carotids' (fig. 2).

The introduction of modern high-speed micro-drills has largely facilitated being able to approach the pituitary gland through very thick sella floors or in

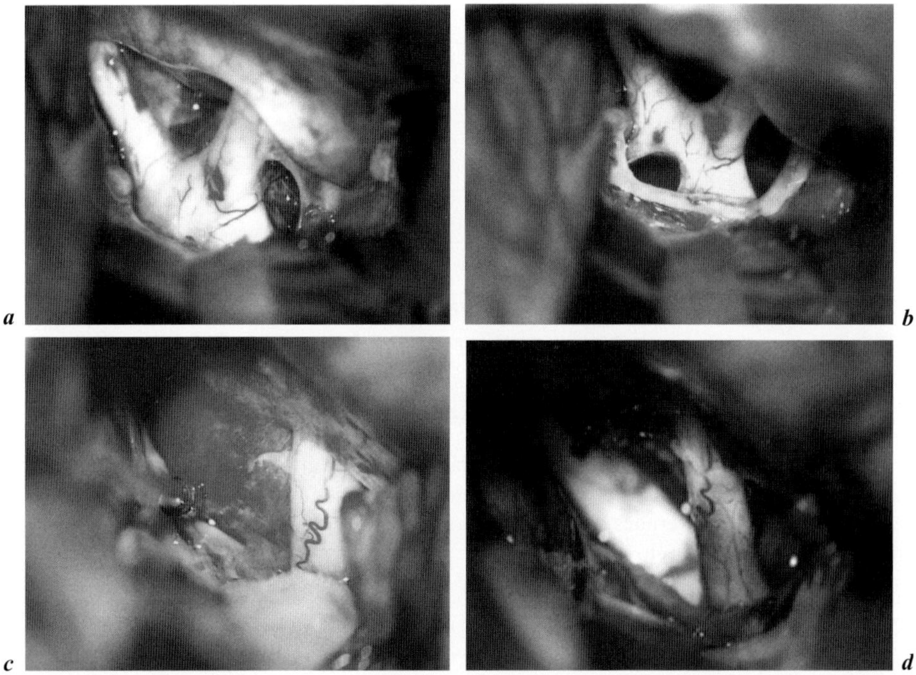

Fig. 4. Intraoperative photomicrographs illustrating the various anatomical positions of the optic chiasm relative to the tuberculum sellae. ***a*** The chiasm is 'prefixed' obscuring the ACTH-secreting macroadenoma with suprasellar extension as illustrated in figure 5. ***b*** After an initial very limited transsphenoidal resection the large residuum was resected transcranially. Access was obtained predominantly via the optico-carotid triangle and the lamina terminalis. ***c*** The intraoperative exposure of the suprasellar/tuberculum meningioma shown in figure 9. In this case the chiasm was very 'postfixed' permitting a large prechiasmal exposure. ***d*** The postoperative view showing complete resection.

children with poorly aerated sphenoid sinuses. Uncertainty generated by aberrant sphenoid sinus and septal anatomy is overcome by preoperative planning using coronal bone window CT scans and intraoperative frameless stereotaxy [36, 37].

The relationship of the optic chiasm to the tuberculum sellae was first determined by the criteria of Bergland et al. [38] who demonstrated that 9% of optic chiasms were prefixed, 11% postfixed and 80% 'normal' in position (figs 3, 4). Modern MRI is frequently able to indicate the position of the optic chiasm preoperatively (fig. 5). This has important implications in the choice of which transcranial or transsphenoidal approach is indicated and in predicting how difficult the surgery will be. A postfixed chiasm facilitates a considerably easier approach and resection as the tumor is accessible between the tuberculum

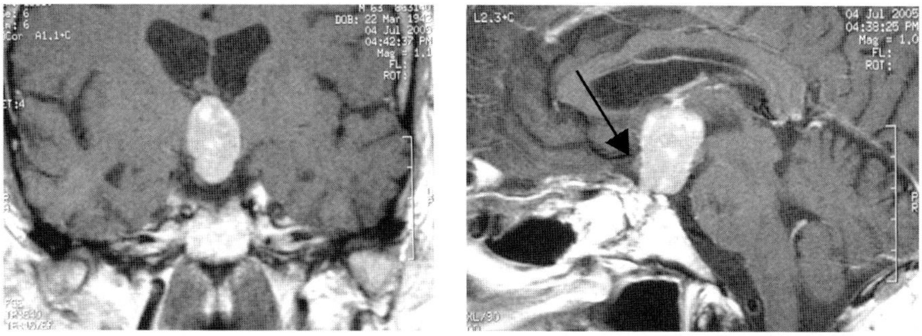

a b

Fig. 5. Coronal (***a***) and sagittal (***b***) T1-weighted contrasted MRI scan illustrating a recurrent ACTH-secreting macroadenoma with dramatic suprasellar extension. A prefixed optic chiasm can be seen (arrow) anterior to the tumor (***b***). The position of the anterior communicator as a landmark for the optic chiasm can also be appreciated just above the chiasm.

sellae and the front of the chiasm, negating having to work across and between the long axis of the optic apparatus and the internal carotid artery risking iatrogenic visual failure.

During the course of transcranial surgery, the most significant complicating anatomical feature is the microvascular supply to the hypothalamus and optic chiasm, the position of the optic apparatus itself. The pituitary tumor pseudocapsule is usually situated below an arachnoid layer intervening between these vessels and the surface of the tumor. Despite this these small vessels are still exposed and even at risk from the tips of coated bipolar forceps.

Indications for the Transcranial Approach

The low morbidity and mortality associated with transsphenoidal surgery (tables 1 and 2) has encouraged many pituitary surgeons to adopt this approach as standard for virtually all sellar and suprasellar tumors [39]. There remain, nevertheless, a few indications for transcranial approaches to lesions in these anatomical locations (table 3). These indications have, however, continued to diminish with the recent introduction of extended transsphenoidal approaches [5, 40], endoscope-assisted pituitary surgery and the readiness of some surgeons to widely open the subarachnoid space transsphenoidally [41]. The operative mortality rate for transsphenoidal procedures is now less than 1% with a morbidity of less than 10% [39]. These mortality and morbidity rates vary in relation to different pathologies and increase in proportion to the size of the tumor. Most giant pituitary adenomas still remain amenable to transsphenoidal

Table 3. Indications for transcranial surgery

1	Tumor with extension into middle, anterior or posterior cranial fossa
2	Dumbell configuration
3	Indurated pituitary adenoma
4	Ectatic 'kissing' carotids
5	Sphenoid sinusitis
6	Dural tail of suprasellar/tubercular meningiomas

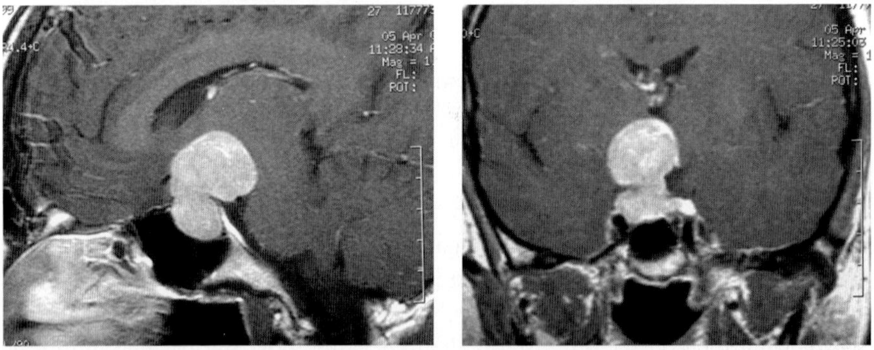

a ***b***

Fig. 6. Sagittal (***a***) and coronal (***b***) T1-weighted contrasted MRI scans demonstrating a non-functioning pituitary macroadenoma with a bi-lobed configuration due to a narrow 'waist' in the suprasellar membrane. In order to resect such a tumor transsphenoidally, the arachnoid layer would have to be widely transgressed risking a postoperative CSF fistula.

surgery [7]. Ideally such tumors need to be situated directly above the sella turcica, along the axis of the transsphenoidal approach and should not be excessively lobulated or fibrous. However, some large tumors do not meet these specifications and in these cases transcranial approaches assume an important role. The indications for craniotomy are: (a) a dumbbell configuration to the tumor with an hourglass constriction at the level of the diaphragma sella (fig. 6); (b) a tumor with extension in the anterior, middle or posterior cranial fossa (fig. 7); (c) sphenoid sinusitis that may delay surgery until adequately treated;

Fig. 7. Preoperative sagittal (***a***), coronal (***b***) T1-weighted gadolinium-enhanced MRI scans and axial contrasted CT scan (***c***) demonstrating a giant nonfunctioning pituitary macroadenoma extending out into the right cavernous sinus and temporal lobe regions. The majority of the tumor was resected transcranially via a right pterional trans-Sylvian craniotomy. The postoperative axial CT (***d***) and coronal (***e***) and sagittal (***f***) MRI scans demonstrate subtotal resection of the lesion – namely the intrasellar portion of the adenoma. The residuum was totally resected transsphenoidally at a second operation.

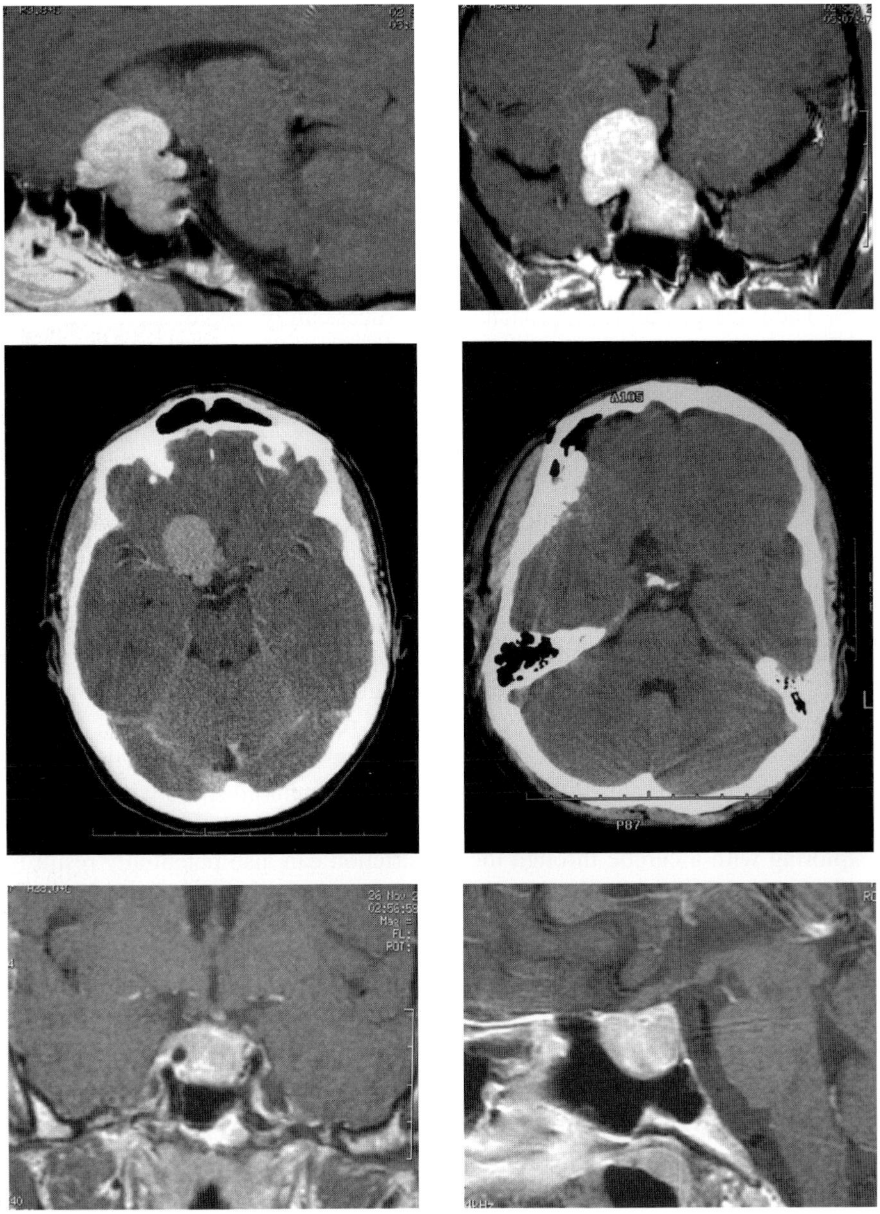
a
b
A105
P87
c
d
e
f

(d) the presence of ectatic carotid arteries projecting towards the midline – 'kissing carotid arteries' (fig. 2); (e) tumors with an indurated or fibrous consistency (reviews of reported surgical series have confirmed that such tumors are difficult and potentially hazardous to manage via the transsphenoidal approach, fig. 8) [42]; (f) normal size sella with a substantial component in the suprasellar cistern (if the chiasm is clearly postfixed a transcranial approach becomes considerably easier, fig. 4); (g) inaccessible dural 'tails' of a suprasellar/tuberculum meningioma (figs 4, 9); (h) uncertainty regarding the diagnosis, and (i) the transsphenoidal pituitary surgeon not being available.

The transsphenoidal approach can be successfully employed, not only for lesions confined to the sella, but also for lesions with significant suprasellar extension where the extension has remained fairly central and the tumor has maintained a symmetrical configuration. In these cases the suprasellar extension has gradually stretched the diaphragma above as it has grown out of the sella and into the suprasellar cistern (fig. 10). By gradual initial resection of the inferolateral components of such tumors and frequently with the aid of either a Valsalva maneuver and/or the intrathecal injection of gas or saline [43], descent of the diaphragma into the surgical field, with the attached residual tumor can be achieved for complete resection. Occasionally (12%) the diaphragma sella is partially incompetent around the pituitary stalk [35]. In such cases the adenoma may extend through the hiatus in the diaphragma before expanding asymmetrically in the suprasellar region (figs 6, 7). The resultant tumor shape is 'dumbbell' or 'hourglass' in configuration. Dealing with lesions of this shape transsphenoidally requires transgressing the subarachnoid space widely exposing the patient to the risk of postoperative CSF fistula and meningitis. Blindly exploring with a curette through the constriction can also potentially result in iatrogenic injury to the optic chiasm. In such instances the options are either to perform an extended transsellar transdiaphragmatic transsphenoidal approach or to perform staged transsphenoidal then transcranial approaches.

Size is not a contraindication to the transsphenoidal approach but an indurated tumor certainly is. If one encounters a very hard tumor transsphenoidally, it is best to obtain an adequate biopsy (debulking if possible) using countertraction with a microsucker and then pack off the sphenoid sinus in preparation for a transcranial approach so that one does not end up with a defect into an empty sphenoid sinus through a patent anterior wall of the pituitary fossa. Traction on and manipulation of fibrous tumors from below may result in serious morbidity and mortality [44]. Injudicious traction on a fibrous tumor may result in occult hemorrhage or damage to important structures to which the tumor may unknowingly be adherent. Fortunately these are not common and only about 5–7.5% of large pituitary tumors have an indurated consistency [45, 46]. These tumors are difficult to remove from below (fig. 8) because the

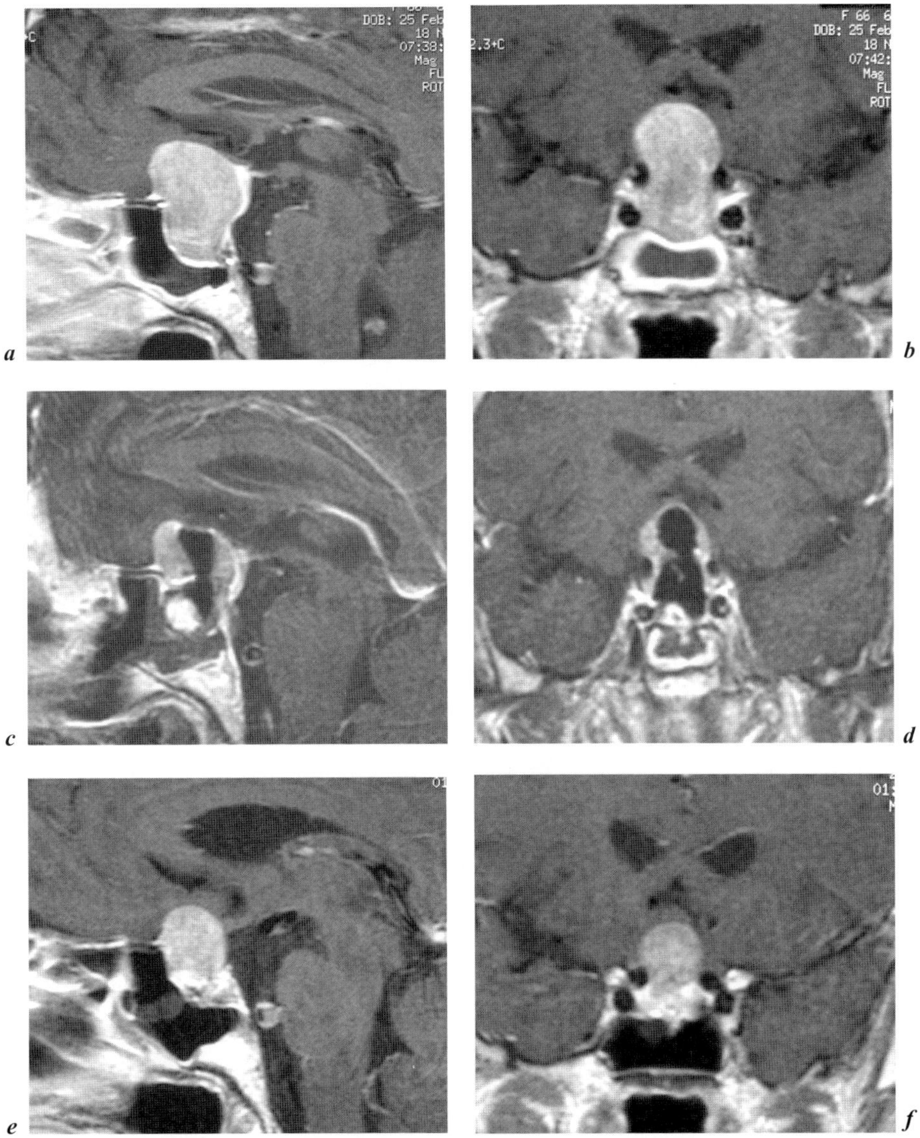

Fig. 8. Sequential sagittal and coronal T1-weighted MRI sections of a nonfunctioning pituitary macroadenoma. The preoperative sections (***a, b***) demonstrate the bulbous suprasellar extension. Due to the fibrous consistency of the tumor a very limited transsphenoidal resection was achieved (***c, d***). However, after anticipating that a transcranial resection was required, a delayed MRI scan 3 months postoperatively demonstrated that the tumor had spontaneously reduced into the pituitary fossa (***e, f***) enabling complete resection via a second transsphenoidal approach.

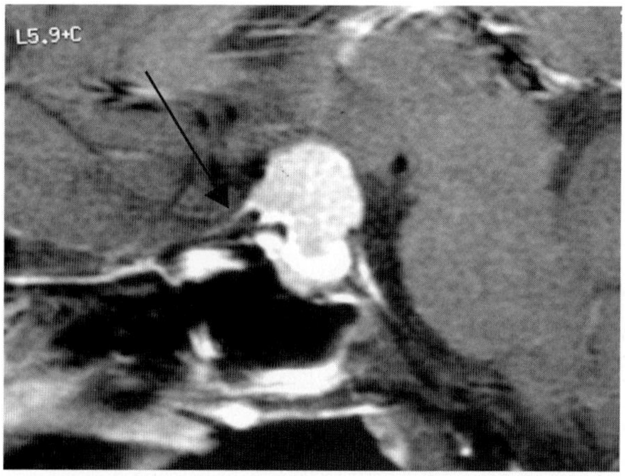

Fig. 9. Midline sagittal T1-weighted gadolinium-enhanced MRI scan demonstrating a lesion based on the suprasellar membrane and tuberculum with a typical dural tail (arrow) extending over the planum sphenoidale – very suggestive of a meningioma.

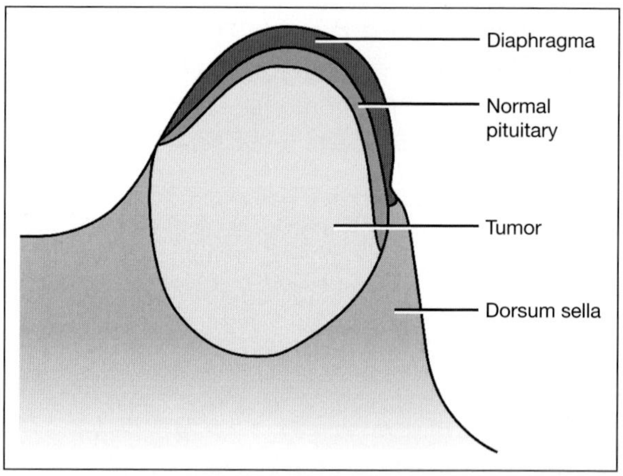

Fig. 10. Sagittal section diagram illustrating a pituitary macroadenoma arising within the pituitary fossa showing the normal effaced pituitary tissue draped over the superior aspect and obscuring an approach from above. This explains why transcranial procedures often have a higher incidence of hypopituitarism than transsphenoidal approaches from below. From Adams CBT: A Neurosurgeon's Notebook (Oxford, Blackwell Science, 1998, p 149) – with permission.

suprasellar component will not descend, even if the sella has been adequately decompressed, leaving a rind of tumor with identical and persistent mass effect. Occasionally, however, with time such residual tumors can spontaneously reduce into the sella where they may be accessed via a redo transsphenoidal procedure (fig. 8). The alternatives in such instances are to approach the lesion transcranially or to consider an extracapsular transtubercular extended transsphenoidal approach [40].

In a retrospective review by Snow and Patterson [47] of 300 consecutive patients who underwent surgery for pituitary adenomas, only 18 (6%) of the patients underwent craniotomy, the rest being managed transsphenoidally. The indications for craniotomy in their series were: (a) the indurated consistency of the tumors making transsphenoidal reduction and resection hazardous; (b) giant macroadenomas deemed to be more safely resected transcranially; (c) a dumbbell shape, and (d) uncertainty regarding the diagnosis. The dilemma with regard to indurated tumors is that this is a finding that is usually only appreciated at the time of surgery. In order to address this Snow et al. [42, 48] analyzed the MRI appearances of 42 patients with large pituitary tumors in which 7 were found to be indurated or fibrous at surgery. The remaining 35 had the typical soft 'cold mushroom soup' consistency. All 7 in the indurated group had an isointense signal on long TR MRI sequences and only 3 in the second 'soft consistency' group.

The options to be considered with large lesions that are anticipated to require both transsphenoidal and transcranial approaches is to either perform the procedure simultaneously as advocated by Barrow et al. [49] and Alleyne et al. [50] or to stage the procedure performing the transsphenoidal procedure first. Performing the transsphenoidal procedure first invariably permits adequate decompression of the optic apparatus, the principal reason for the surgery, and may in fact, with tumor descent, permit resection of sufficient tumor, making a subsequent craniotomy superfluous. Performing the transcranial approach first increases the risk of a postoperative CSF fistula after the subsequent transsphenoidal operation. If transcranial surgery is performed first and transsphenoidal surgery delayed, residual tumor beyond the narrow exposure of the transsphenoidal approach will then not descend into the operative field of the subsequent transsphenoidal procedure due to the development of fibrosis and adhesions. One can usually, during a transcranial approach, even detect a previous transsphenoidal procedure with intracapsular resection and preservation of the arachnoid layer by the increased amount of adhesions present in the suprasellar cistern.

Suprasellar meningiomas have traditionally been approached transcranially (figs 4, 9). This approach has the considerable advantage of facilitating complete resection of dural tails which frequently track anteriorly over the planum sphenoidale, thereby preventing recurrence. Recently, there have been reports on series of extended transsphenoidal, endoscope-assisted procedures for suprasellar meningiomas [40, 41, 51] and recordings of very elegant endoscopic resections demonstrated at conferences. Such procedures, however,

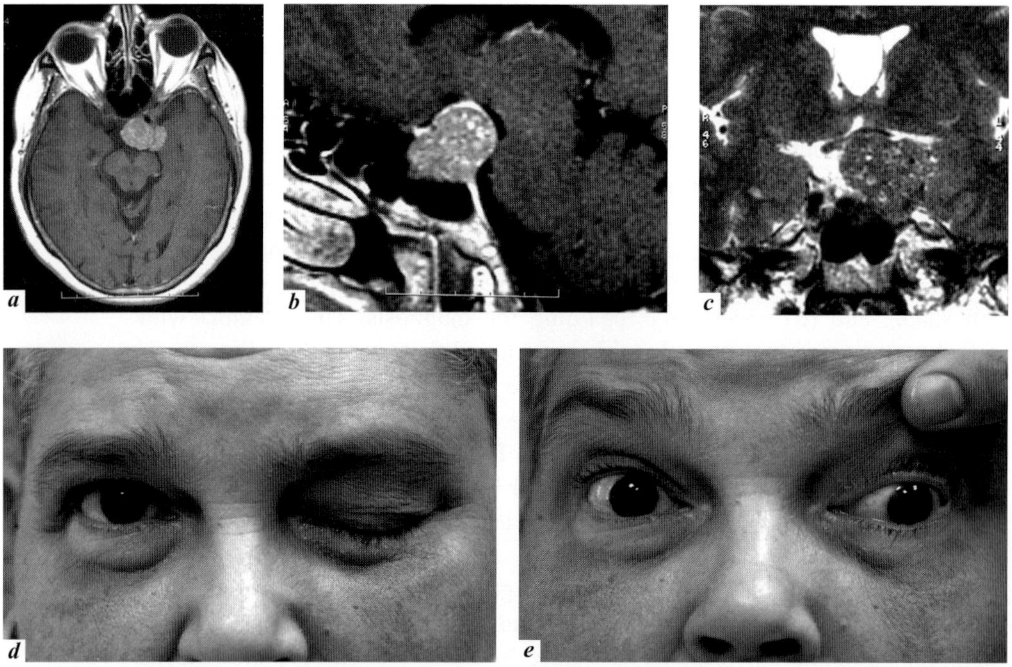

Fig. 11. Axial (***a***), sagittal (***b***) T1-weighted gadolinium-enhanced and coronal (***c***) T2-weighted MRI scans demonstrating a sellar-based tumor extending into the left cavernous sinus and temporal lobe regions. This was initially approached transcranially via the optico-carotid triangle and from between the internal carotid and the tentorium inadvertently injuring the oculomotor nerve. Histopathology confirmed a nonfunctioning macroadenoma. Immediate postoperative photographs (***d***, ***e***) of the patient demonstrate a complete third nerve palsy that later incompletely resolved.

should only be undertaken by experienced pituitary surgeons and on midline lesions with minimal lateral, anterior or posterior dural extensions. The long-term recurrence rates for such surgery is still subject to scrutiny.

While a pituitary surgeon, familiar with the transsphenoidal approach, not being available in a unit, is not really a regular indication for a transcranial procedure, this is a scenario that is occasionally encountered – particularly with apoplexy. Under these circumstances transcranial debulking is often performed. Frequently the optic chiasm is inadequately decompressed, the tumor insufficiently resected, and the patient left with a neurological deficit. Not infrequently, in such a setting, surgery is associated with damage to the oculomotor nerve on the side of the approach (see section 'Complications'; fig. 11). Residual tumor, obscured from view within the fossa, also tends to hemorrhage postoperatively. Ideally every pituitary service should have a second surgeon capable of debulking a macroadenoma transsphenoidally to provide continuity of emergency cover. Occasionally an apoplectic pituitary hemorrhage may rupture into the brain. This can be a desperate situation but need not be, and here a transcranial approach may be preferable.

Preoperative Considerations

Minor complications associated with pituitary surgery can usually be managed without difficulty. However, the anatomical location of the pituitary fossa may result in more major complications with potentially disastrous consequences. Meticulous preoperative planning and preparation are therefore critical and patients should undergo thorough clinical, neurological, neuro-ophthalmological and endocrinological evaluation preoperatively. All antiplatelet or anticoagulant drugs should be discontinued preoperatively. Patients should be assessed and if necessary treated by an endocrinologist in order to avoid intraoperative catastrophe due to inadequate pituitary reserve. Particular attention must be paid to cortisol and thyroxine levels and to the possibility of disturbances of sodium homeostasis. Patients with prolactinomas, particularly large macroprolactinomas, should be commenced on a trial of dopamine agonists in order to ascertain whether the lesion responds, thereby potentially avoiding surgery. Although we do not recommend universal administration of glucocorticoids for transsphenoidal procedures [52], we frequently administer dexamethasone for transcranial procedures where dissection across the long axis of the optic apparatus, with possible consequent trauma, is necessary.

Parenteral hydrocortisone is administered preoperatively, as required, based on the results of early morning cortisol levels in combination with a short tetracosactrin (Synacthen 250 μg) test for pituitary procedures. For very large lesions with brain swelling or progressive visual failure, dexamethasone 4 mg q.i.d. is given empirically. Dilantin (loading 15 mg/kg and maintenance 5 mg/kg/day) is used for seizure prophylaxis. Brain relaxation, if necessary, can be augmented by using mannitol (1 g/kg) in combination with 10–20 mg furosemide but we find that gradual drainage of basal cisternal CSF usually suffices.

Preoperative radiological examination usually consists of full diagnostic MRI in three planes together with the application of fiducials for frameless stereotaxy co-registration. Additional information about the bony anatomy from CT using bone windows may be invaluable in planning the approach and in managing difficulties expectantly. It is still our policy to always obtain plain skull X-rays in all patients to delineate the size of the frontal sinus. A team approach, with close consultation between surgeon, endocrinologist, ophthalmologist, radiologist and pathologist, cannot be overemphasized and should be initiated preoperatively.

Pterional Trans-Sylvian Approach

This approach, first proposed by Silbermark [24], and then pioneered by Heuer [25] and Adson [27] provides the shortest distance to the sellar and is the approach most frequently used. In the craniopharyngioma series of Fahlbusch et al. [31] it was used exclusively in 58 of 148 (39.2%) procedures. It is ideal for situations where the optic chiasm is postfixed but, if required, the pterional approach also allows access to the inferior anterior third ventricle through the lamina terminalis.

The patient is positioned supine with the head of the table raised 25° bringing the operative site above the level of the heart. The patient's neck is slightly extended and the head rotated 25° to the side opposite to that of the incision. This positions the ipsilateral malar prominence uppermost in the surgical field with the medial sphenoid ridge vertical avoiding awkward tilting of the operating microscope eyepiece. This position also allows the semisolid brain to fall backwards, creating a vital few extra millimeters of exposure which simultaneously helps to minimize brain retraction. The head is secured in a 3-point Mayfield clamp positioned horizontally. Rotating the head any further will incrementally obscure the surgeon's intraoperative view of the contralateral optic nerve. The side of entry is initially determined by the laterality of the tumor's projection. When possible the tumor is approached from the non-dominant side which is usually the right-hand side. This facilitates a comfortable approach for right-handed surgeons. In the event of severe unilateral visual failure, preservation of vision in the good eye can be optimized by approaching from the side of the most compromised optic nerve. Dissection across the long axis of the optic apparatus and injudicious use of bipolar diathermy can exacerbate visual failure, particularly in already compromised optic nerves. It is also easier to decompress an optic nerve by being able to remove the tumor from below as one is able to do for the optic nerve opposite to the side of the approach. Cushing exploited the development of unilateral blindness by sectioning the affected optic nerve to improve access. He later abandoned this practice after appreciating the delayed potential for reversal of visual failure – even in severely compressed and affected optic nerves.

After marking out the midline and the zygomatic process, a curvilinear skin incision is placed within the hairline from a point 0.5 cm in front of the tragus, just above the zygomatic process to a point near the midsagittal plane.

The scalp and temporalis muscle and fascia are then reflected antero-inferiorly using diathermy to release the temporalis muscle from its insertion into the temporal bone. Different techniques are described for adequately exposing the pterion and determined largely by the bulk of the temporalis muscle. The important consideration is the preservation of the frontalis branch of the facial nerve. Three standard burr holes are then marked out; one just behind the zygomatic process of the frontal bone – the 'keyhole', a second on the floor of the middle fossa, and a third along the superior temporal line off the forehead. The burr holes are then linked using a craniotome, taking care not to lacerate the dura and removing the footplate in order to complete the craniotomy over the pterion. A large craniotomy exposure is seldom necessary. The medial extension of the craniotomy exposure above the supraorbital ridge can be increased for tumors with significant suprasellar extension, particularly those projecting up between the optic nerves with a postfixed chiasm. In order to do so a burr hole is placed just above the glabella. This facilitates an additional more medial subfrontal approach. It becomes very useful when planning the craniotomy flap to be able to utilize frameless stereotaxy in order to map out the superior extent of the frontal sinus.

Using a diamond burr the sphenoid ridge is then drilled down medially as far as the lateral aspect of the superior orbital fissure. The frontal bone is drilled down flush with the floor of the anterior cranial fossa, once again in order minimize retraction and increase exposure (fig. 4). If necessary the frontal sinus may need to be opened as the risk of excessive frontal lobe retraction usually far outweighs the risk of exposing the frontal sinus. It is, however, best to avoid opening the sinus if at all possible, being guided by either frameless stereotaxy or the skull X-ray. If the sinus is transgressed it requires formal cranialization with removal of all frontal sinus mucosa and obliteration and watertight sealing of the frontonasal duct. The dura is then incised in an elliptical fashion around the Sylvian fissure based on the cranial floor and hitched under tension. Relieving incisions in the dura may be made posteriorly. The operating microscope and brain retractors are then introduced and positioned.

Attention is first turned to the Sylvian fissure which is opened using the technique described in detail by Yasargil [53]. The larger the tumor, the more important this step becomes. Initial entry is facilitated by very gentle retraction on the frontal lobe putting mild tension on the arachnoid overlying the fissure and incising this layer anterior to the Sylvian veins. This allows identification of the interpial plane on either side of an M2 branch of the middle cerebral artery. By following an artery into the fissure, this plane is then gradually developed down onto the M1 segment. The fissure is then gently opened both proximally and distally by using deep to superficial dissection. Dissecting medially eventually exposes the carotid bifurcation allowing identification of the A1 and M1 segments and their relationship to the tumor. Splitting the Sylvian fissure allows the temporal lobe to disengage from the frontal lobe posteriorly and for the frontal lobe to fall backwards with gravity creating a 90° exposure. Using Teflon-coated brain retractors the frontal lobe is then elevated to allow subfrontal exploration of the basal cisterns with a microsucker. The olfactory tract is identified next. Care must be taken to prevent anosmia, a CSF fistula or hemorrhage due to avulsion of the olfactory bulb from the cribriform plate. This is dissected free from the arachnoid adhesions holding it to the undersurface of the frontal lobes. The carotid and chiasmal cisterns are then opened allowing gradual egression of CSF. Patient, slow microsuction allows gradual brain relaxation and identification of the chiasm and the internal carotid artery with minimal brain retraction. By this stage the tumor should have come in to view (fig. 4).

The primary concern should be the blood supply to the hypothalamus and optic chiasm as well as the position of the optic apparatus. Virtually all pituitary tumors are situated beneath an arachnoid layer. Access is usually obtained via the optico-carotid triangle if not obscured by perforators. By opening the arachnoid and then developing a plane beneath this layer, potential compromise to the vasculature of the optic chiasm and hypothalamus is prevented. At this stage tumor specimens are taken and sent for frozen section analysis together with specimens for formal paraffin sections and specimens to be snap-frozen and banked for research. Priority is then given to decompressing the optic nerves and chiasm (fig. 4). If the lesion has a cystic component or is of soft consistency, then the tumor can be debulked via one of the various anatomical windows for access. Depending on the consistency of the lesion, debulking can be achieved using the precision nosepiece of the CUSA or curettes of variable lengths and rotations. Fine bipolar diathermy should henceforth be used very cautiously in order to prevent coagulating microvasculature responsible for perfusing the chiasm.

If the tumor is very fibrous or calcified, the falciform ligament over the optic nerve is released and if necessary the optic canal opened using a microdiamond drill bit. Lateral extension of the tumor may also be obscured by the ipsilateral optic nerve (fig. 11). Initial extensive decompression medial to the optic nerve followed by subsequent mobilization of the tumor from the lateral compartment beneath the optic nerve from lateral to medial facilitates mobilization of this remnant. At this stage it is very easy to injure an attenuated oculomotor nerve resulting in a permanent palsy. This occurs when access via the optico-carotid triangle is inadequate and exploration posterolateral to the internal carotid artery is undertaken (fig. 4). The pituitary stalk and the basilar artery are displaced posteriorly and separated by an intact Liliequist membrane. Care must also be taken to define the internal carotid artery and its ophthalmic branch. Perforating vessels from the internal carotid to the posterior aspect of the chiasm and optic nerve must be preserved. As the tumor is being debulked the position of the contralateral optic nerve must be anticipated. The rotation of the head away from the side of the incision alters the position of the optic nerves and their relationship to the trajectory of the approach. It is critical to have a clear idea of this relationship during the resection in order to prevent iatrogenic damage to the optic apparatus and optic nerves. While normal optic nerves may tolerate some degree of manipulation, this should be avoided. Stretched, attenuated optic nerves have very little reserve. A very useful anatomical feature is Liliequist's membrane which, because left intact by suprasellar extension, protects the underlying basilar artery.

It is important to remember that the primary aim of the operation is to decompress the optic nerves. It is very unlikely that every last fragment of tumor will be able to be removed. If the tumor capsule is adherent to the optic nerves it is best left attached if a good plane of cleavage cannot be identified. Attempting to dissect it from the optic chiasm may damage the vasa vasorum of the optic nerves and lead to infarction and visual loss or else injury to the midline neuraxis. Ultimate tumor control invariably requires delayed adjuvant radiotherapy. For large tumors, a real concern is postoperative ooze from the tumor bed – particularly from residual tumor. It is thus important to remove as much tumor as possible. After irrigating liberally with saline warmed to 37°C, the use of the microfibrillar collagen hemostatic agent Avitene® via the endoscopic applicator in combination with patience, pressure and cottonoid patties, is usually effective in obtaining good hemostasis before covering the tumor bed with a single carpet of the oxidized regenerated cellulose hemostat Surgicel®.

The dura is closed in a water-tight fashion using an absorbable 5/0 monofilament suture before being hitched up to the edges of the craniotomy defect. The bone flap is secured with titanium miniplates and any significant bone defect filled in with Bonesource® or acrylic cement.

Other Transcranial Approaches

Frontobasal Interhemispheric Approach

In this approach it is critical to extend the frontal exposure low down onto the anterior fossa floor in order to minimize brain retraction, if necessary cranializing the frontal sinus. In this approach it is critical to open the subarachnoid space as early as possible and drain CSF slowly to allow brain relaxation. The main risk of this approach is postoperative seizures as a consequence of frontal lobe retraction in combination with sacrifice of bridging venous structures. The aim is to expose the optic nerves, optic chiasm, A_2 segments and anterior communicating artery by opening up the chiasmatic and interhemispheric cisterns. Access is obtained through the lamina terminalis for large tumors and the approach therefore carries less risk to the fornix. It is considered the best transcranial approach for large retrochiasmatic and suprasellar craniopharyngiomas which can be exposed through the lamina terminalis giving you a midline view into the interpeduncular cistern [31, 54, 55]. Care must be taken to protect the optic apparatus during retrochiasmatic removal and the olfactory tracts require mobilization from the gyrus rectus in order to preserve smell. The midline approach always confers an advantage in permitting earlier identification of important midline structures which may be less easily identified via a pterional approach.

Orbitozygomatic Approach

Technically, this is a more difficult exposure with marginally increased morbidity. It does, however, provide the versatility of both lateral and anterior access with absolutely minimal brain retraction. Care must be taken to preserve the supraorbital and supratrochlear nerves which, if sacrificed, can be a source of considerable postoperative discomfort. The distance to the tumor from an anterior approach is approximately 2 cm further than the pterional approach [47].

Combined Transsphenoidal Transcranial Approach

These can be done during the same or at separate sittings. The transcranial portion is frequently performed first in order to alleviate hydrocephalus by decompressing the foramina of Monroe or in order to preserve vision by decompressing the optic apparatus. Exceptional care must be taken with regard to effecting a watertight dural seal and skull base reconstruction.

Interhemispheric Transcallosal Approach

This approach is usually only necessary for large septated craniopharyngiomas [56], for tumors exclusively in the third ventricle or for tumors extending up to the foramen of Monro (fig. 12). Dilatation of the lateral ventricles becomes advantageous in the exposure. Care must be taken to avoid excessive manipulation of the fornix and to preserve both the thalamostriate and internal cerebral veins. In order to prevent the development of complex hydrocephalus, the septum pellucidum should be fenestrated and postoperatively a ventriculostomy drain placed under direct vision and left in situ, closed, to be used if required. Frameless stereotaxy is very useful for precise placement and minimizing the size of the corpus callosum fenestration.

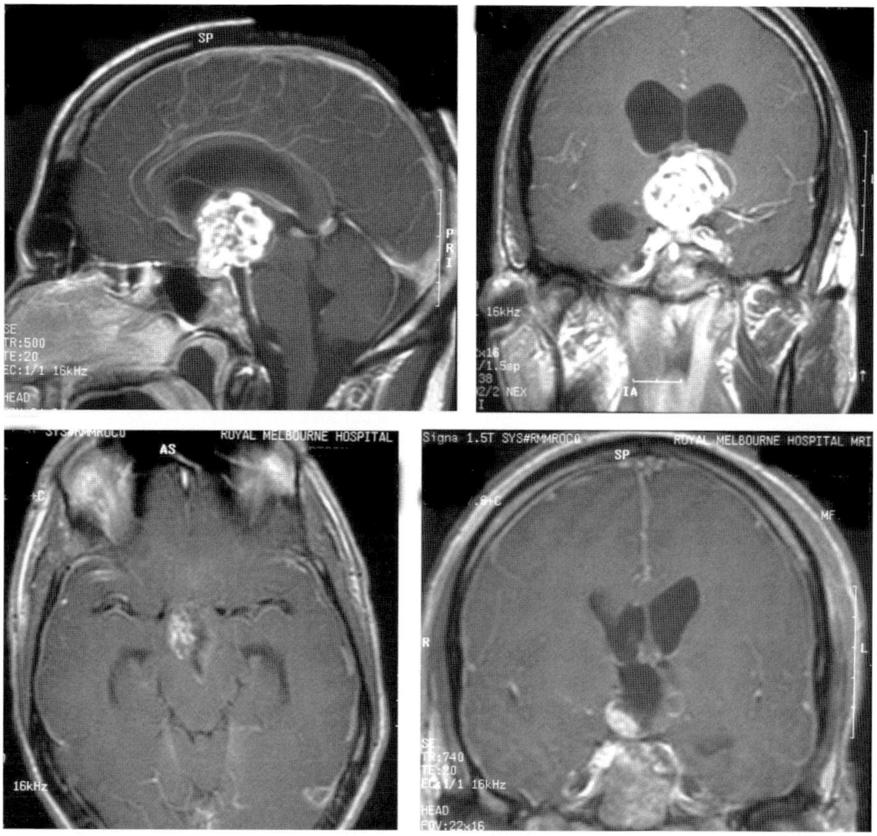

a *b* *c* *d*

Fig. 12. Preoperative sagittal and coronal (***a, b***) and postoperative axial and coronal (***c, d***) T1-weighted gadolinium-enhanced MRI scans illustrating a large third ventricle craniopharyngioma resected transcallosally. A small residuum is visible beneath the anterior commissure laterally on the right. Despite being aware of this intraoperatively, exposure was inadequate to permit safe resection of this residuum.

Complications

The most common complications associated with the transcranial approach (table 4) are no different from those encountered during other transcranial neurosurgical procedures [7]. Although pituitary surgery with all its modern day adjuncts has evolved to the point at which the associated morbidity and mortality is extremely low (tables 1, 2), the location of the sella at the base of the brain with its intimate and important anatomical associations is a potential source for serious morbidity and even mortality [57]. Morbidity and mortality rates also

Table 4. Operative complications of pituitary surgery

Parasellar
CSF rhinorrhea
Hypopituitirism
Diabetes insipidus
Cavernous sinus injury
Hemorrhage
Cranial nerve injury
Carotico-cavernous fistula
False aneurysm
Intracranial
Hemorrhage
Hypothalamic damage
Meningitis
Visual loss
Cerebral ischemia

increase as the size of the sellar tumor increases. Surgery for large macroadenomas is thus more risky than surgery for smaller lesions and microadenomas [39].

Hypopituitarism is more common after transcranial surgery for pituitary adenomas than transsphenoidal resections. Pituitary adenomas arise in the adenohypophysis and as they enlarge they push the normal pituitary tissue posterosuperiorly leaving a thinned out mantle of gland beneath the diaphragma (fig. 10). One is thus able to understand the considerable advantages for preventing hypopituitarism of being able to gently reduce and resect a pituitary adenoma from below. With experience a normal gland can be distinguished from neoplastic tissue by its red/orange color, striated by a fine capillary network. The consistency of the normal gland also distinguishes it from adenoma as it tends to resist removal by microsuction and gentle curettage more.

Diabetes insipidus, either transient or permanent, is common with manipulation of the pituitary stalk. Once again it is less common after transsphenoidal surgery for the reasons outlined above and most common after surgery for craniopharyngiomas that frequently arise in the stalk. It is, therefore, best to avoid diuretics and Mannitol during pituitary surgery. It is also useful to restrict fluids to 2 liters/day for 48 h postoperatively and not to give unnecessary, excessive steroids. This will prevent a physiological diuresis confusing the diagnosis of diabetes insipidus. If a patient's urine output has been in excess of 250 ml/h for more than 3 h consecutively then urgent electrolyte analysis together with both plasma and urine osmolality should be arranged. If the serum sodium is raised and the plasma osmolality is $>$295 mosm/kg, then a diagnosis of diabetes insipidus is likely. Vigilance for and proactive management of diabetes insipidus is important before more severe hyponatremia supervenes compromising the patient's clinical state. It is important to remember that postoperative diuresis is normal in patients with acromegaly [44] and that excessive glucocorticoids cause diabetes insipidus.

Visual deterioration is not uncommon after transcranial surgery for sellar and parasellar tumors, particularly calcified craniopharyngiomas. This is a consequence of having to resect the tumor across the long axis of the optic nerve and chiasm and may occur in an immediate or delayed manner. As already emphasized, normal optic nerves tolerate manipulation to a greater extent than compromised nerves. This tolerance is a function of the degree and chronicity of the mechanical compression. Factors associated with postoperative visual loss are prior irradiation, previous surgery, preexisting deficit, technical difficulties with surgery and diabetes mellitus [58–60]. The most common cause of visual loss is disruption of the blood supply to the optic chiasm or nerves – even if the anatomic continuity of these structures is preserved and they are minimally manipulated. A detailed understanding of the microvascular anatomy of the optic nerves and chiasm as well as meticulous microdissection techniques are the most important factors in preventing postoperative visual deterioration [7]. Perioperative steroid cover with 4 mg q.i.d. of dexamethasone prophylactically is also recommended.

Hypothalamic injury may occur as a result of direct surgical injury, hemorrhage or ischemia. It is rare and frequently lethal. It is more commonly encountered in patients having undergone previous surgery or radiation therapy. Clinically it manifests acutely with diabetes insipidus, somnolence or autonomic dysfunction – specifically difficulties with temperature regulation or chronically with morbid obesity, memory loss, insatiable hunger or thirst. If severe it manifests with a depressed level of consciousness [61, 62]. Gentle surgical technique, avoidance of traction on the tumor capsule and pituitary stalk, and retracting on the tumor and not the brain minimizes the occurrence of such injury. Extensive experience with deformed and pathologic anatomy encountered with tumors involving the suprasellar and inferior third ventricle region is very advantageous [7].

Another frequent complication of transcranially resecting the lateral extension of a pituitary adenoma is not appreciating the presence and position of the third nerve splayed over the surface of the tumor (fig. 11), particularly when exploring the lesion posterolateral to the internal carotid artery.

Conclusion

For the majority of large pituitary macroadenomas, an attempt should be made to resect the tumor via a transsphenoidal route due to the safety of this approach, its efficacy with regard to tumor resection, preservation of pituitary function and resolution of visual failure. There are, however, certain situations where a transcranial procedure is indicated, either de novo or as a secondary procedure to complete the resection in order to adequately decompress the optic nerves and in some instances the hypothalamus, frontal or temporal lobes. As with the surgeons of old, the pterional route with all its variations provides an ideal approach to lesions extending into the suprasellar cistern and parasellar regions and should be mastered by all specialist pituitary surgeons.

References

1 Horsley V: On the technique of operations on the central nervous system. BMJ 1906;ii:411–423.
2 Schloffer H: Zur Frage der Operationen an der Hypophyse. Beitr Klin Chir 1906;50:767–817.
3 Schloffer H: Erfolgreiche Operation eines Hypophysentumors auf nasalem Wege. Wien Klin Wochenschr 1907;20:621–624.
4 de Divitiis E, Cappabianca P (eds): Endoscopic Endonasal Transsphenoidal Surgery. New York, Springer, 2003.
5 Couldwell WT, Weiss MH, Rabb C, Liu JK, Apfelbaum RI, Fukushima T: Variations on the standard transsphenoidal approach to the sellar region, with emphasis on the extended approaches and parasellar approaches: surgical experience in 105 cases. Neurosurgery 2004;55:539–550.
6 Black PM, Zervas NT, Candia GL: Incidence and management of complications of transsphenoidal pituitary surgery. Neurosurgery 1987;20:920–924.
7 Krisht AF: The pterional approach; in Krisht AF, Tindall GT (eds): Pituitary Disorders: Comprehensive Management. Baltimore, Lippincott Williams and Wilkins, 1999, pp 361–368.
8 Frazier C: Choice of method in operations upon the pituitary body. Surg Gynecol Obstet 1919;29:9–16.
9 Marie P: Sur deux cas d'acromégalie: hypertrophie singulière non congénitale, des extrémités supérieures, et céphalique. Rev Med Liege 1886;6:297–333.
10 Horsely V: Functional nervous disorders due to loss of the thyroid gland and pituitary body. Lancet 1886;ii:5.
11 Landolt A: History of pituitary surgery; in Greenblatt A (ed): A History of Neurosurgery. Park Ridge, American Association of Neurological Surgeons, 1997, pp 373–400.
12 Caton R, Paul FT: Notes of a case of acromegaly treated by operation. BMJ 1893;ii:1421–1423.
13 Kiliani O: Some remarks on tumours of the chiasm, with a proposal how to reach the same by operation. Ann Surg 1904;40:35–43.
14 Krause F: Hirnchirurgie. Dtsch Klin 1905;8:953–1024.
15 Krause F: Bemerkungen zur Operation der Hypophysen-geschwulste. Dtsch Med Wochenschr 1927;53:691–694.
16 Liu JK, Das K, Weiss MH, Laws ER Jr, Couldwell WT: The history and evolution of transsphenoidal surgery. J Neurosurg 2001;95:1083–1096.
17 Cope V: The pituitary fossa and the methods of the surgical approach thereto. Br J Surg 1916;4: 107–144.
18 Pollock JR, Akinwunmi J, Scaravilli F, Powell MP: Transcranial surgery for pituitary tumours performed by Sir Victor Horsley. Neurosurgery 2003;52:914–926.
19 Cushing H: Surgical experiences with pituitary disorders. JAMA 1914;63:1515–1525.
20 McArthur L: An aseptic approach to the pituitary body and its neighbourhood. JAMA 1912;58: 2009–2011.
21 McArthur L: Tumor of the pituitary gland: technique of operative approach. Surg Clin Chicago 1918;2:691–699.
22 Frazier C: Lesions of the hypophysis from the viewpoint of the surgeon. Surg Gynecol Obstet 1913;17:724–736.

23 Frazier C: Surgery of the pituitary lesion. Ann Surg 1928;88:1–5.
24 Silbermark M: Die intrakranielle Extirpation der Hypophyse. Wien Klin Wochenschr 1910;23: 467–468.
25 Heuer G: Surgical experiences with intracranial approach to chiasmal lesions. Arch Surg 1920;1:368–381.
26 Heuer G: The surgical approach and the treatment of tumors and other lesions about the optic chiasm. Surg Gynecol Obstet 1931;53:489–518.
27 Adson A: Hypophysial tumors through the intradural approach. JAMA 1918;71:721–726.
28 Halstead A: Remarks on the operative treatment of tumours of the hypophysis (two cases operated on by an oronasal route). Surg Gynecol Obstet 1910;10:494–502.
29 Guiot G: Considerations on the surgical treatment of pituitary adenomas; in Fahlbusch R, Werder KV (eds): European Workshop on the Treatment of Pituitary Adenomas. Stuttgart, Thieme, 1978, pp 202–218.
30 Hardy J: Transsphenoidal microsurgery of the normal and pathological pituitary. Clin Neurosurg 1969;16:185–217.
31 Fahlbusch R, Honegger J, Paulus W, Huk W, Buchfelder M: Surgical treatment of craniopharyngiomas: experience with 168 patients. J Neurosurg 1999;90:237–250.
32 Guidetti B, Fraioli B, Cantore GP: Results of surgical management of 319 pituitary adenomas. Acta Neurochir (Wien) 1987;85:117–124.
33 Rhoton AL Jr, Natori Y: The Orbit and Sellar Region. Microsurgical Anatomy and Operative Approaches. New York, Thieme, 1996, p 311.
34 Rhoton AL Jr: The sellar region. Neurosurgery 2002;51(suppl):S335–S374.
35 Renn WH, Rhoton AL Jr: Microsurgical anatomy of the sellar region. J Neurosurg 1975;43: 288–298.
36 Jane JA Jr, Thapar K, Alden TD, Laws ER Jr: Fluoroscopic frameless stereotaxy for transsphenoidal surgery. Neurosurgery 2001;48:1302–1308.
37 Elias WJ, Chadduck JB, Alden TD, Laws ER Jr: Frameless stereotaxy for transsphenoidal surgery. Neurosurgery 1999;45:271–277.
38 Bergland RM, Ray BS, Torack M: Anatomical variations in the pituitary gland and adjacent structures in 225 human autopsy cases. J Neurosurg 1968;28:93–99.
39 Zervas N: Surgical results in pituitary adenomas: results of an international survey; in Zervas N, Black PM, Ridgeway EC (eds): Secretory Tumours of the Pituitary Gland. New York, Raven Press, 1984, pp 377–385.
40 Kaptain GJ, Vincent DA, Sheehan JP, Laws ER Jr: Transsphenoidal approaches for the extracapsular resection of midline suprasellar and anterior cranial base lesions. Neurosurgery 2001;49: 94–101.
41 Jho HD, Alfieri A: Endoscopic endonasal pituitary surgery: evolution of surgical technique and equipment in 150 operations. Minim Invasive Neurosurg 2001;44:1–12.
42 Snow RB, Lavyne MH, Lee BCP, Morgello S, Patterson RH Jr: Craniotomy versus transsphenoidal excision of large pituitary tumors: the usefulness of magnetic resonance imaging in guiding the operative approach. Neurosurgery 1986;19:59–64.
43 Kaye AH, Rosewarne F: Forced subarachnoid air for transsphenoidal surgery. J Neurosurg 1990;73:311–312.
44 Adams CBT: A Neurosurgeon's Notebook. 1998, Oxford: Blackwell Science.
45 Laws ER: Comment. Neurosurgery 1984;14:488.
46 Wilson C: Neurosurgical management of large and invasive pituitary tumours; in Wilson C, Tindall G (eds): Clinical Management of Pituitary Disorders. New York, Raven Press, 1979, pp 335–342.
47 Snow RB, Patterson RH Jr: Craniotomy for pituitary tumours; in Kaye AH, Black P (eds): Operative Neurosurgery. London, Churchill Livingstone, 2000, pp 709–714.
48 Snow RB, Johnson CE, Morgello S, Lavyne MH, Patterson RH Jr: Is magnetic resonance imaging useful in guiding the operative approach to large pituitary tumors? Neurosurgery 1990;26: 801–803.
49 Barrow DL, Tindall G, Tindall SC: Combined simultaneous transsphenoidal transcranial operative approach to selected sellar tumours. Perspect Neurol Surg 1992;3:49–57.

50 Alleyne CH Jr, Barrow DL, Oyesiku NM: Combined transsphenoidal and pterional craniotomy approach to giant pituitary tumours. Surg Neurol 2002;57:380–390.
51 Cooke SW, Smith Z, Kelly DF: Endonasal transsphenoidal removal of tuberculum sellae meningiomas: technical note. Neurosurgery 2004;55:239–244.
52 Inder WJ, Hunt P: Glucocorticoid replacement in pituitary surgery: guidelines for perioperative assessment and management. J Clin Endocrinol Metab 2002;87:2745–2750.
53 Yasargil MG: Microneurosurgery. Stuttgart, Thieme, 1984, vol 2.
54 Hoffman HJ, De Silva M, Humphreys RP, Drake JM, Smith ML, Blaser SI: Aggressive surgical management of craniopharyngiomas in children. J Neurosurg 1992;76:47–52.
55 Patterson RH Jr, Danylevich A: Surgical removal of craniopharyngiomas by a transcranial approach through the lamina terminalis and sphenoid sinus. Neurosurgery 1980;7:111–117.
56 Steno J, Malacek M, Bizik I: Tumor-third ventricular relationships in supradiaphragmatic craniopharyngiomas: correlation of morphological, magnetic resonance imaging, and operative findings. Neurosurgery 2004;54:1051–1060.
57 Zada G, Kelly D, Cohan P, Wang C, Swerdloff R: The endonasal transsphenoidal approach for pituitary adenomas and other sellar lesions: an assessment of efficacy, safety and patient impressions. J Neurosurg 2003;98:350–358.
58 Barrow DL, Tindall G: Loss of vision after transsphenoidal surgery. Neurosurgery 1990;27:60–68.
59 Adams C: The management of pituitary tumours and post-operative visual deterioration. Acta Neurochir (Wien) 1988;94:103–116.
60 Martins A: Pituitary tumors and intrasellar cysts; in Vonken PJ, Bruyn GW (eds): Handbook of Clinical Neurology. Amsterdam, North Holland Publishing, 1974, p 431.
61 Tindall CT, Barrow D: Disorders of the Pituitary. St Louis, Mosby, 1986, pp 349–400.
62 Landolt A: Transsphenoidal surgery of pituitary tumors: its pitfalls and complications; in de Villiers JC (ed): Some Pitfalls and Problems in Neurosurgery. Prog Neurol Surg. Basel, Karger, 1990, vol 13, p 1.

Nicholas F. Maartens, MD
Department of Neurosurgery, Royal Melbourne Hospital
University of Melbourne
Parkville, VIC 3050 (Australia)
Tel. +61 3 93427000, Fax +61 3 93427273, E-Mail niki.maartens@mh.org.au

Laws ER Jr, Sheehan JP (eds): Pituitary Surgery – A Modern Approach.
Front Horm Res. Basel, Karger, 2006, vol 34, pp 29–45

Extended Transsphenoidal Approach

Aaron S. Dumont, Adam S. Kanter, John A. Jane, Jr., Edward R. Laws, Jr.

Department of Neurological Surgery, Health Sciences Center, University of Virginia, Charlottesville, Va., USA

Abstract

Transsphenoidal surgery is well established as an effective primary treatment for tumors of the sellar region. The technique of transsphenoidal surgery has evolved over the years with many prominent surgeons contributing to its present state of refinement. The transsphenoidal approach can be modified in various ways to permit resection of parasellar tumors that otherwise would require a transcranial or transbasal operation. Our experience with these 'extended' techniques has primarily involved the transtuberculum sella approach in which bone is removed from the tuberculum sellae and the posterior portion of the planum sphenoidale. Experience with this technique continues to burgeon, and offers an excellent alternative to transcranial surgery in dealing with a difficult constellation of tumors. Meticulous attention to detail, particularly with respect to reconstruction and closure of the sellar floor, is necessary for its effective application.

Copyright © 2006 S. Karger AG, Basel

Introduction

The transsphenoidal approach provides safe and effective access to tumors arising within the sella. Transsphenoidal adenomectomy preserves pituitary function and decompresses the optic apparatus in the majority of patients. The approach provides direct access to the sella and pituitary gland without brain retraction and is generally well tolerated with rare major morbidity.

Extirpation of pituitary adenomas with significant suprasellar extension is often possible via the standard transsphenoidal approach. Intrasellar tumor growth expands the sella turcica and creates an adequate surgical corridor for resection of suprasellar tumor extensions. Without sellar expansion, however, access to suprasellar and extrasellar components is greatly restricted. Tumors that do not arise from within the sella are thereby difficult to resect using the standard transsphenoidal approach. Certain primary suprasellar tumors and other tumors with suprasellar and/or anterior cranial base extension pose unique management challenges. These lesions have been traditionally approached through various transcranial corridors. Although several different transcranial approaches can be employed, most require some degree of brain retraction. Transbasal approaches require less brain manipulation but morbidity is not insignificant. Particularly in the setting of a pre-fixed chiasm, the surgical window provided by these transcranial approaches is often limited to dissection between the optic nerves and carotid arteries. More recent modifications to the standard transsphenoidal approach have brought a portion of these tumors into the purview of the transsphenoidal corridor. Transsphenoidal removal of the tuberculum sellae and a portion of the planum sphenoidale along with the anterior wall of the sella provides surgical access to lesions in the suprasellar region and along the anterior cranial base.

Historical Considerations

The frontal transcranial approach to the sella turcica was introduced by Krause [1] in 1905. Subsequently, other pioneering neurosurgeons including Dandy [2], Heuer [3], Frazier [4, 5] and Cushing [6, 7] improved upon this initial work providing the basis for contemporary transcranial approaches. The initial difficulties and high complication rates of early transcranial approaches provided impetus for the development of extracranial approaches to sellar lesions.

Based upon initial work of Giordano, who proposed a transfacial approach to the pituitary gland [8], Schloffer [9, 10] reported the first successful resection of a pituitary tumor via a transsphenoidal approach in March 1907. This approach was modified by Theodor Kocher [11] in 1909 who resected the septum submucosally, expanding the visualization of sellar anatomy, and by Oskar Hirsch [12–14] in 1910 who advocated an endonasal transseptal transsphenoidal approach based on the approach to the sphenoid sinus used by his mentor, Hajek, for the treatment of sphenoid sinusitis [12]. Hirsch performed his first transsphenoidal tumor resection in a multi-staged fashion over a 5-week period, with each session done under local anesthesia (fig. 1). The patient's visual symptoms dramatically improved following which Hirsch subsequently developed more effective and efficient techniques, including the introduction of the nasal speculum.

Later in 1910, Albert Halstead [15] described his sublabial gingival incision which remains popular today. Harvey Cushing [6, 7, 16] helped to further refine the transsphenoidal sublabial approach to the sella (figs 2, 3) although he would

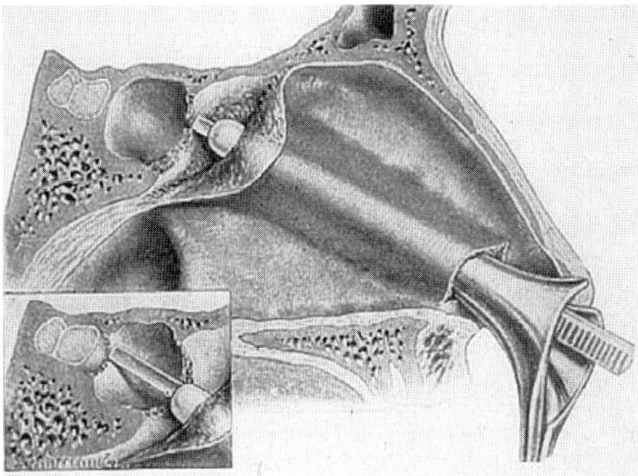

Fig. 1. Hirsch's endonasal, submucosal, transseptal approach to the sella turcica. A speculum is used to laterally retract the mucosal flaps and to maintain exposure. Courtesy of Dr. Edward Laws' personal slide collection.

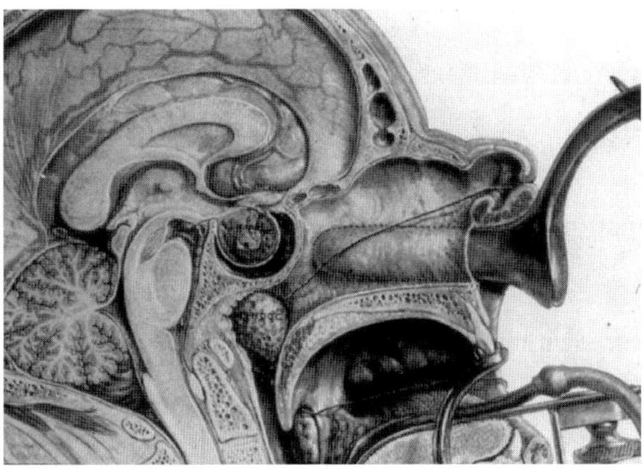

Fig. 2. Midline sagittal illustration with the nasal speculum in place demonstrating Cushing's sublabial approach. From Cushing H: Disorders of the pituitary gland, retrospective and prophetic. JAMA 1921;76:1721–1726.

abandon it completely from 1929–1932 in favor of the transcranial approach. The reason for Cushing's return to the transcranial approach are not entirely known although it is thought that he felt that intraoperative complications were more easily dealt with from above. Despite Cushing's lack of enthusiasm, Hirsch

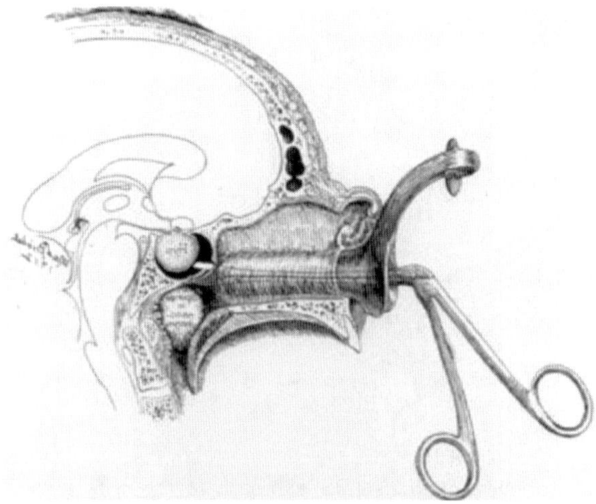

Fig. 3. Cushing's sublabial approach. Removal of the anterior wall of the sphenoid sinus. From Cushing H: Disorders of the pituitary gland, retrospective and prophetic. JAMA 1921;76:1721–1726.

continued to perform the procedure, traveling from Vienna to Boston, thus remaining an 'obscure voice in the wilderness' [17].

Although the majority of the neurosurgical community followed Cushing's lead, Norman Dott, who studied Cushing's transsphenoidal approach at the Peter Bent Brigham Hospital from 1923–1924, continued to use and modify the transsphenoidal approach upon his return to the Royal Infirmary in Edinburgh [18]. Dott subsequently designed instruments specifically for the transsphenoidal procedure, such as a speculum with an attached lighting apparatus [19]. Gerard Guiot, a French neurosurgeon, learned the technique from Dott and also contributed to its resurgence with the introduction of intraoperative radiological guidance [20] (fig. 4). Jules Hardy from Montreal subsequently learned the technique from Guiot and further refined it by adopting the operating microscope with its superior illumination and magnification (fig. 5) [21–23]. Utilizing microscopic dissection techniques, Hardy introduced the concept of microadenomectomy and demonstrated the possibility of surgical cure in these small hyperfunctioning lesions. Equally significant advances in the fields of endocrinology and radiology during this period indisputably contributed to the transsphenoidal renaissance which occurred in the late 1960s. Fluoroscopy was introduced, hormones were isolated, their physiologic roles elucidated, and radioimmunoassays developed for both diagnosis and post-treatment surveillance [14]. These and other innovations provided the foundation for the modern transsphenoidal approach practiced by neurosurgeons throughout the world today.

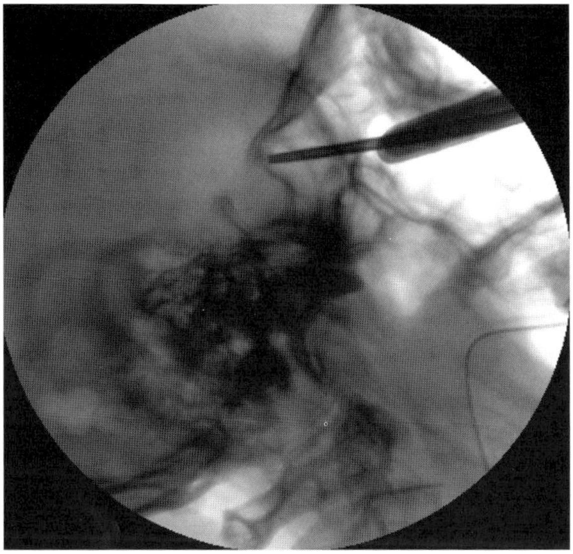

Fig. 4. The addition of mobile fluoroscopic imaging techniques dramatically improved operative accuracy and efficiency.

a 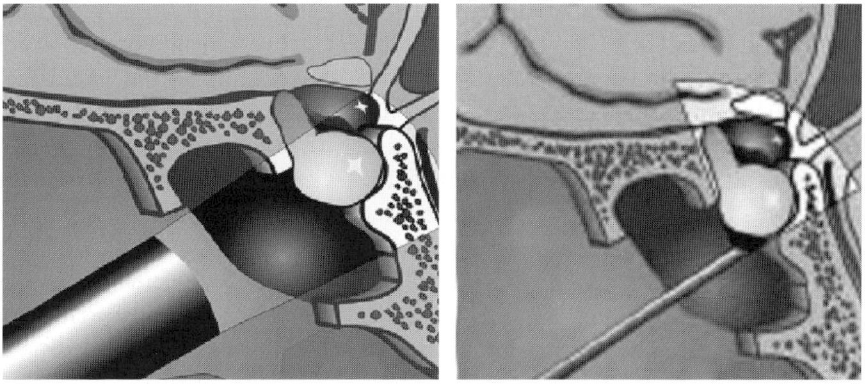 b

Fig. 5. Innovations such as the microscope (***a***) and later the endoscope (***b***) further contributed to the evolution of the transsphenoidal approach allowing improved illumination, magnification, and visualization.

Further refinements have occurred including the introduction of the endoscope as a primary or adjunctive tool (fig. 5), use of frameless stereotactic guidance, and aggressive resection of the cranial base; each innovation providing corridors to previously unreachable tumors while preserving anatomic structures [24–47].

The transsphenoidal transtuberculum sellae approach was originally described by Weiss [47] in 1987. Contemporary neurosurgical pioneers including Oldfield, Kato, Laws, Jho, Frank, de Divitiis, and Cappabianca have subsequently adopted and refined the technique for resection of various tumors with suprasellar, parasellar, and/or anterior cranial base extension including, but not limited to, craniopharyngiomas, tuberculum sellae meningiomas and Rathke's cleft cysts [35, 36, 38–43, 48–50].

Patient Selection

Patients with midline tumors involving an anatomical region extending from the planum sphenoidale to the lower clivus, who are fit candidates for a surgical procedure, may potentially be considered candidates for this approach. Patients with primarily suprasellar tumors without sellar enlargement may also be considered potential candidates for this approach. However, not every patient harboring a midline tumor confined to these anatomical boundaries is a candidate. The normal pituitary is often displaced ventrally and inferiorly and can be easily injured during the approach as it is encountered before the tumor. Thus the transsphenoidal approach is sometimes reserved for those patients with preexisting hypopituitarism and is less desirable in children with normal pituitary function [51]. Conversely, several biological considerations combined with modern technologic advances have made operating on the para- and suprasellar compartment via the extended approach a favorable route. For example, adenomas with significant extension often exhibit invasive growth patterns such that radical resection in lieu of vital structure preservation is unwarranted. Additionally, avoiding brain retraction, cranial nerve dissection, and skin incisions cannot be underestimated [17].

Careful evaluation of preoperative high-resolution magnetic resonance (MR) imaging is necessary to guide the decision regarding the appropriateness of this procedure. The relationship of the tumor to the chiasm, hypothalamus, third ventricle and major blood vessels must be determined. This is particularly important when the goal of the surgery is gross total resection. When palliation is the goal, this procedure can usually be applied safely and effectively. The surgical operating times are significantly shorter than for standard craniotomy. The extended transsphenoidal approach has also been applied effectively in the setting of multiple prior surgical procedures and/or radiation. The procedure can also be used to provide a histological diagnosis in lesions not easily amenable to other surgical approaches.

Despite careful preoperative evaluation and patient selection, some tumors will prove to be unsuitable for resection based upon intraoperative inspection.

In the authors' experience, an attempted extended transsphenoidal resection was aborted in 3 cases. For example, in a retroinfundibular meningioma extending to and abutting the midbrain, the extended transsphenoidal approach was abandoned due to a firm tumor consistency, large tumor size and adherence to critical structures, in favor of a later craniotomy.

General Technical Aspects

All patients require a thorough preoperative neurological and endocrinological history and physical examination. Biochemical testing should be performed to screen for pituitary endocrine dysfunction. Formal visual field testing with static perimetry and visual acuity testing is also mandatory. Contrast-enhanced MR imaging should also be performed and the authors' practice has also been to perform sequences for frameless image guidance.

After intubation, a lumbar drain is inserted which allows insufflation of air intraoperatively as well as cerebrospinal fluid (CSF) diversion during the postoperative period. The lumbar drain usually remains in place for 48 h postoperatively. In a semirecumbent position, patients are placed in a horseshoe headrest with the head in slight extension. In contradistinction to our traditional sellar approach in which the head is positioned such that the bridge of the nose is parallel to the floor, the slight extension allows a more rostral view towards the planum sphenoidale. Although patients are not fixated to the table, a head holder is required to mount the array for frameless stereotaxy.

A direct endonasal or sublabial approach may be used depending upon the amount of room and scope of vision required (fig. 6). The authors preferentially elect the latter approach as the direct endonasal approach often leads to inadequate working space and all too often an unfavorable angle to the lesion for proper surgical manipulation, effective bipolar hemostasis, and instrument maneuverability [17]. Through either approach, a wide anterior sphenoidotomy is performed to expose the bony landmarks of the sellar floor, cavernous sinus, and the optic and carotid protuberances (fig. 7). A high speed air drill and Kerrison punches can be used to open the sellar floor to the limits of the cavernous sinus laterally and the intercavernous sinus superiorly (fig. 8). If the tumor does not extend inferiorly into the sella, the inferior portion of the pituitary gland does not have to be exposed. Nevertheless, some exposure of the pituitary gland is necessary, not only to provide a transdural entry point below the superior intercavernous sinus, but also to allow visualization of the gland and protection thereof during the operation.

Using frameless stereotactic guidance, the tuberculum sellae and planum sphenoidale are removed (fig. 8). Although a high-speed drill is usually

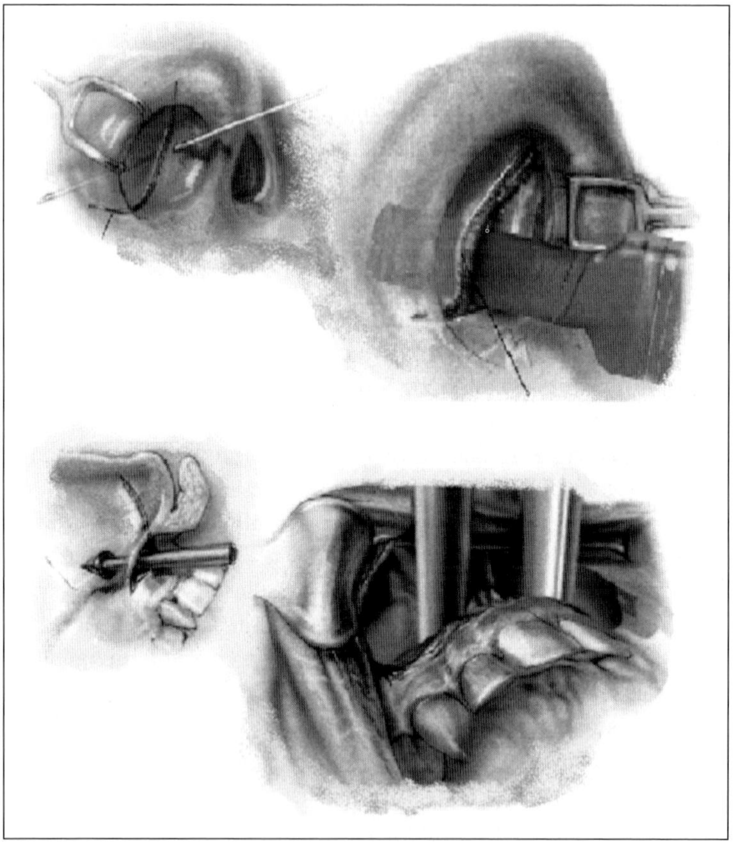

Fig. 6. Endonasal and sublabial transsphenoidal approaches. The endonasal approach avoids resection of the anterior nasal spine of the maxilla but limits the extended superior and lateral visualization afforded by the sublabial approach.

employed, we have also had success using angled punches and curettes. Neuronavigation is a useful adjunct during this stage allowing the rostral bony removal to be tailored to the geometry of the tumor and the lateral bony removal to avoid carotid and optic nerve injury. Generally, the lateral exposure does not exceed 15 mm in diameter. The position of the carotid arteries may also be confirmed through the use of a micro-Doppler probe.

Dural opening requires special attention as the superior intercavernous sinus may be robust and not amenable to simple bipolar cautery. The sellar dura is opened parallel and just inferior to the superior intercavernous sinus which is readily visible through the dura. Surgical clips are then placed across the sinus which can then be incised. The dura of the anterior cranial fossa is

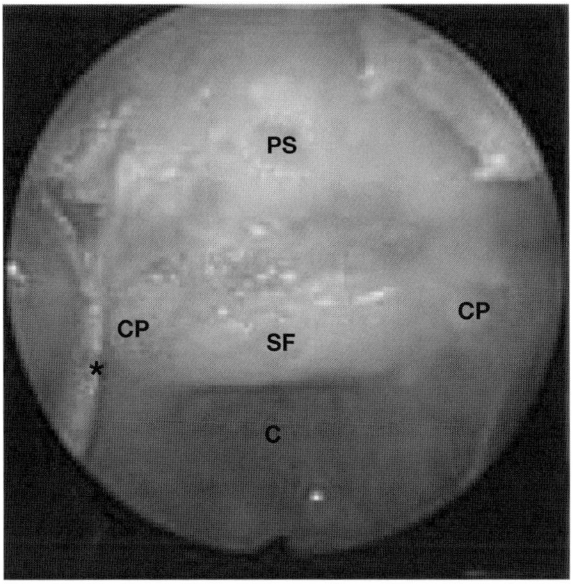

Fig. 7. Typical endoscopic view of the bony landmarks following removal of the anterior wall of the sphenoid. C = Clivus; CP = carotid protuberance; SF = sellar floor; PS = planum sphenoidale; * = sphenoid septation.

then coagulated and opened. Following dural opening, extra-arachnoidal dissection is performed and the pituitary gland is carefully identified and protected. The arachnoid is sharply opened and general principles of microsurgery are implemented. The capsule of the tumor is delineated and cauterized with bipolar electrocoagulation. Capsular feeders can be identified, coagulated and cut sharply. The tumor is subsequently debulked, allowing the capsule to be carefully mobilized. Circumferential dissection of the capsule is undertaken and extracapsular feeders are controlled as they are encountered.

Meningiomas often respect arachnoidal planes, particularly at the tumor-chiasm interface. There are often preserved arachnoidal planes between the tumor and the carotid arteries, although not universally so, and meticulous microsurgical technique is necessary for removal of the lateral portion of suprasellar meningiomas arising from the tuberculum sellae or diaphragm (fig. 9).

The most dorsal and rostral aspects of the tumor can pose a challenge to removal as it is often adherent to the surrounding brain, as is frequently encountered in the resection of craniopharyngiomas [51, 52]. Infradiaphragmatic lesions rarely transgress through the anatomic barrier of the diaphragma sella thus theoretically enabling a 'gross total resection' while those predominantly of

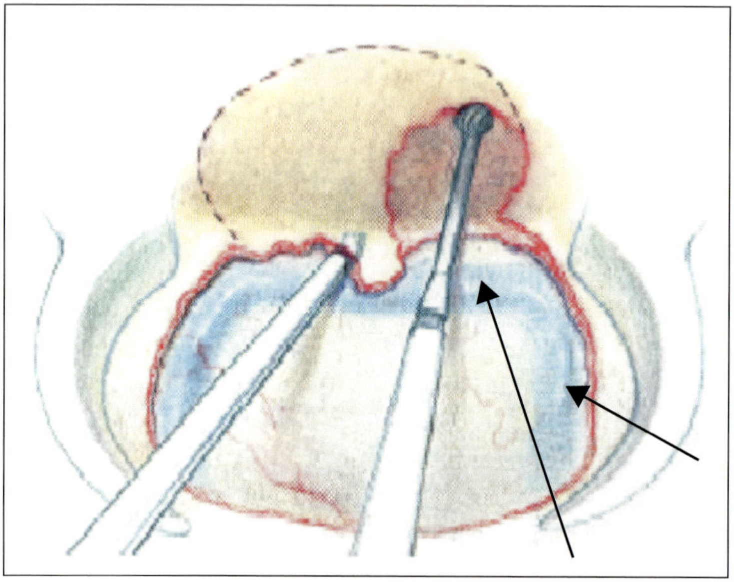

Fig. 8. Following removal of the sellar floor, the cavernous and intercavernous sinuses are visualized (arrows). Further superior bony removal of the planum sphenoidale and tuberculum sellae can then ensue paying particular attention to preserve arachnoidal/tumor planes. From Mason et al. [45].

the suprasellar compartment pose the operative challenges listed above; thereby limiting safe 'total' resection and favoring a palliative goal with subtotal removal and decompression of the optic apparatus and intracranial structures [52]. The endoscope is often useful for the careful dissection and removal of this part of the tumor, either as a primary tool or adjunct. With mobilization of the dorsal tumor capsule the pituitary stalk is observed and can often be preserved.

As tumor removal proceeds, the local anatomy is exposed (fig. 10) including the optic nerves, chiasm, anterior communicating artery complex, and basilar artery. Neuroendoscopy is of particular utility in assessing local anatomy and the extent of tumor resection without the optical limitations imposed by the transsphenoidal retractor and is indispensable during these operations [17].

Absolute hemostasis must be ensured upon completion of the procedure. The endoscope is very useful in this respect, particularly to inspect the resection cavity if the tumor has been removed into the recesses of the third ventricle.

In many cases, such as following resection of planum sphenoidale meningiomas, the dural and cranial base defect can be large. This remains the greatest challenge of this procedure and a perfect means of closure and reconstruction has not yet been identified. We have tended to use harvested fat and synthetic

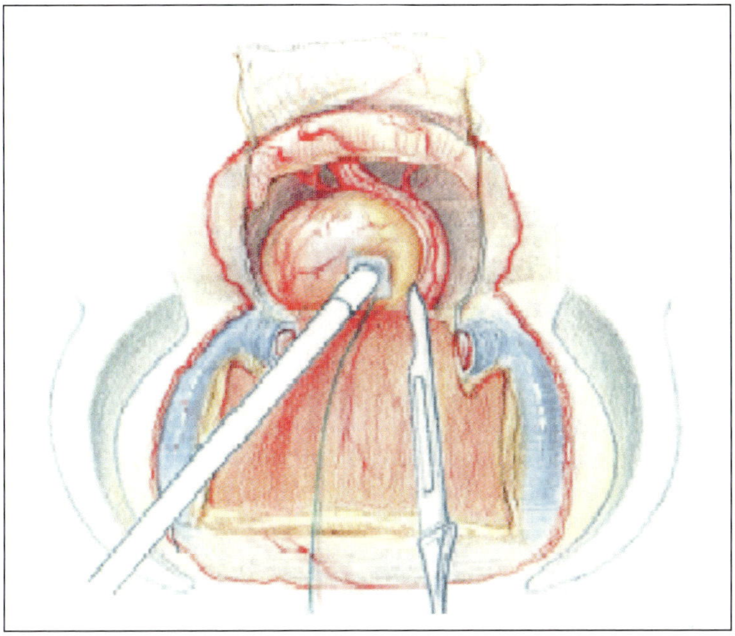

Fig. 9. A meticulous microsurgical technique is necessary for removal of the dorsal and lateral portions of suprasellar lesions arising from the tuberculum sellae or diaphragm. From Mason et al. [45].

dural substitutes to close the dural defect. The bony defect may then be closed with an extradural layer of harvested septal bone or fabricated plates of titanium or bioabsorbable compounds. The intracranial fat graft and dural substitute can be sutured and cinched down onto this bone graft or plate (fig. 11). Fat is also placed within the sphenoid sinus and lumbar drainage is maintained postoperatively for 2 days (fig. 12). Nasal packing is usually maintained for 24–48 h.

Stress dose hydrocortisone is administered for the first 24 h after surgery and morning cortisol levels are drawn on postoperative days 2 and 3 to assess the pituitary-adrenal axis. Patients are monitored closely for diabetes insipidus using daily serum sodium levels, urinary specific gravity every 4 h, fluid intake and output, and daily weight.

Complications and Their Avoidance

Complications are a potential consequence of any surgical procedure, however, there are some unique considerations specific to the transsphenoidal

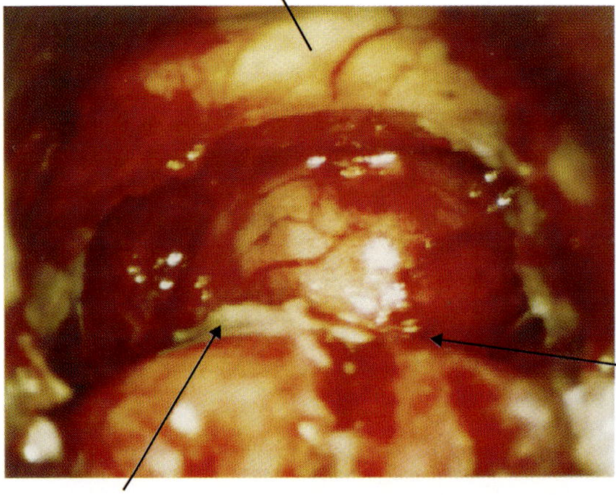

Fig. 10. Intraoperative photograph of a suprasellar mass abutting the optic chiasm superiorly. A portion of the diaphragma sella is visualized along the inferior border of the tumor, abutting the superior surface of the compressed gland. From Mason et al. [45].

approach [54] that are magnified even further when an extended procedure is necessitated. As mentioned above, closure of the dural and cranial base defect remains the most significant ongoing challenge of this procedure. The authors have experienced postoperative CSF leak in 6 of 56 cases (11%). Five of these occurred in patients with craniopharyngiomas that often extended into the third ventricular chamber. Five of these 6 patients developed meningitis, often in a delayed fashion. Much respect must be paid to the closure, as a complicated postoperative course due to CSF fistula and meningitis will mitigate the success of an otherwise uncomplicated complete tumor resection. The authors have traditionally used a fat graft soaked in chloramphenicol and coated in Avitene, secured to a structural support wedged into the epidural space (such as titanium mesh or bioabsorable plate) as a primary means of closure. The fat graft must be large enough to securely span the defect but not so large as to compromise the visual apparatus. This is reinforced by dural substitute, Bioglue, and more fat. Others have employed alternative means of closure with inlay and onlay dural grafts supported by fibrin sealant and fat packing with some success (Kassam, personal communication, 2004) or other ingenious methods (fig. 4) [54, 55].

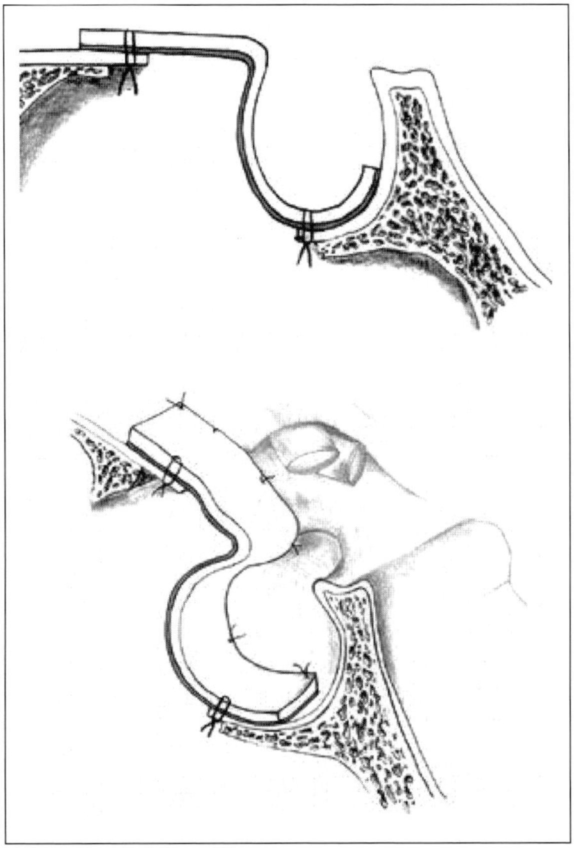

Fig. 11. Schematic representation of a subdural patch graft technique. CSF pressure from above the graft promotes dural adhesion. From Kitano and Taneda [54].

Bleeding at different points during the procedure can occur and may impede or prohibit effective tumor resection. Bleeding from arteries of the nasal mucosa, such as branches of the sphenopalatine artery or posterior nasal artery, can be controlled with surgical clips or bipolar electrocoagulation. For epidural bleeding, the application of FloSeal or Gelfoam followed by gentle compression with a cottonoid patty has proven to be highly effective. Brisk bleeding from the superior intercavernous sinus can be difficult to deal with at times. In fact, in the authors' series, attempted surgical resection of 1 craniopharyngioma was halted prematurely because of profuse bleeding from an elaborate intercavernous sinus. Bipolar electrocoagulation is often effective, however, the combination of electrocautery with surgical clips is sometimes necessary. The sinus must be

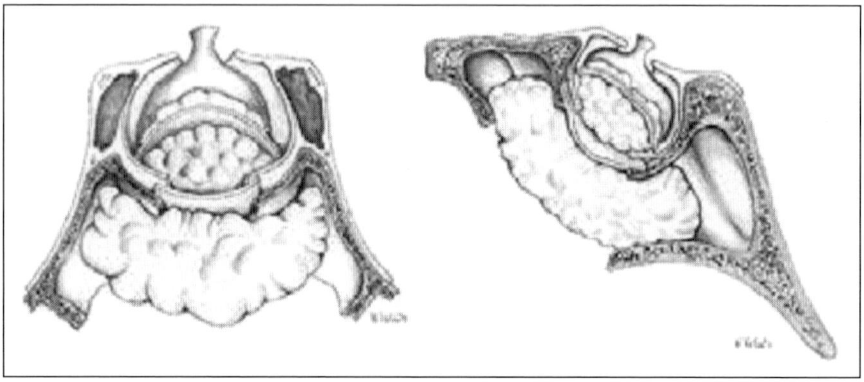

Fig. 12. Schematic drawing of sellar and sphenoid sinus packing with fat. From Cappabianca et al. [55].

thoroughly coagulated prior to sectioning. The transection of the sinus may be performed in steps, with bipolar coagulation performed followed by partial sectioning of the sinus until it is completely divided. Hemostasis in the intracranial compartment must be complete. The authors have encountered 1 case of extensive postoperative intraventricular hemorrhage following resection of a large craniopharyngioma that extended to the roof of the third ventricle.

Visual loss/cranial neuropathies may occur following resection of tumors with the extended transsphenoidal approach. A meticulous microsurgical technique must be maintained throughout tumor resection. Manipulation of the visual apparatus must be minimized and the tumor and its capsule must be mobilized away from the optic apparatus. With careful sharp dissection, perforating vessels can be preserved. Once again, the fat graft packing into the suprasellar compartment must not compromise the visual system.

New endocrine deficits can occur following tumor resection in the suprasellar space. Gentle dissection and anatomic preservation of the stalk can help to prevent these complications. Contemporary series utilizing the endoscopic transsphenoidal approach have revealed encouraging preliminary results [56–58]. Perhaps future technical experience and advanced instrumentation and fiber optics may further reduce the iatrogenic burden thus allowing more radical resections and improved preservation of sellar and suprasellar structures.

Conclusions

Over the years the significant contributions from prominent surgeons have established the transsphenoidal approach as an effective primary treatment for tumors arising within the sella. The transsphenoidal transtubercular approach, in which bone is removed from the tuberculum sellae and the posterior portion of the planum sphenoidale, has emerged as a modification of the standard transsphenoidal approach. This approach, founded upon principles of cranial base surgery, has brought tumors previously amenable only to transcranial approaches into the purview of the transsphenoidal corridor. The approach is the result of an evolutionary process rather than a revolutionary process, involving multiple generations of neurosurgical pioneers, scientific and technologic advances [13]. Experience with this technique continues to grow, and the extended transsphenoidal approach appears to offer an excellent (and sometimes superior) alternative to transcranial surgery in dealing with a difficult group of tumors. Meticulous attention to detail, particularly with respect to preoperative planning and to reconstruction and closure, is necessary for its success.

References

1 Krause F: Hirnchirurgie. Dtsch Klin 1905;8:953–1024.
2 Dandy WE: A new hypophysis operation. Bull Johns Hopkins Hosp 1918;29:154.
3 Heuer GJ: The surgical approach and the treatment of tumors and other lesions about the optic chiasm. Surg Gynecol Obstet 1931;53:489–518.
4 Frazier CH: An approach to the hypophysis through the anterior cranial fossa. Ann Surg 1913;57:145–150.
5 Frazier CH: Choice of method in operations upon the pituitary body. Surg Gynecol Obstet 1919;29:9–16.
6 Cushing H: The Pituitary Body and Its Disorders: Clinical States Produced by Disorders of the Hypophysis Cerebri. Philadelphia, Lippincott, 1912, pp 296–305.
7 Cushing H: The Weir Mitchell Lecture. Surgical experiences with pituitary disorders. JAMA 1914;63:1515–1525.
8 Liu JK, Das K, Weiss MH, Laws ER Jr, Couldwell WT: The history and evolution of transsphenoidal surgery. J Neurosurg 2001;95:1083–1096.
9 Schloffer H: Zur Frage der Operationen an der Hypophyse. Beitr Klin Chir 1906;50:767–817.
10 Schloffer H: Erfolgreiche Operation eines Hypophysentumors auf nasalem Wege. Wien Klin Wchnschr 1907;20:621–624.
11 Kocher T: Ein Fall von Hypophysis Tumor mit operativer Heilung. Dtsch Z Chir 1909;100:13–37.
12 Hirsch O: Endonasal method of removal of hypophyseal tumors. With a report of two successful cases. JAMA 1910;55:772–774.
13 Lanzino G, Laws ER: Key personalities in the development and popularization of the transsphenoidal approach to pituitary tumors: an historical overview. Neurosurg Clin North Am 2003;14:1–10.
14 Jane JA, Thapar K, Laws ER: A history of pituitary surgery. Operative Techniques Neurosurg 2002;5:200–209.
15 Halstead AE: Remarks on the operative treatment of tumors of the hypophysis. With the report of two cases operated on by an oro-nasal method. Surg Gynecol Obstet 1910;10:494–502.
16 Cushing H: Partial hypophysectomy for acromegaly. With remarks on the function of the hypophysis. Ann Surg 1909;50:1002–1017.
17 Zervas NT: Reflections on the surgery of the pituitary. Clin Neurosurg 1980;27:124–132.
18 Dott NM, Bailey P: A consideration of the hypophyseal adenomata. Br J Surg 1925;13:314–366.

19 Lanzino G, Laws ER, Erfan I, White WL: Transsphenoidal approach to lesions of the sella turcica: historical overview. Barrow Q 2002;18:4–8.
20 Guoit G, Thibault B: L'extirpation des adénomes hypophysaires par voie trans-sphénoïdale. Neurochiurgia 1959;1:133–150.
21 Hardy J: Surgery of the pituitary gland, using the trans-sphenoidal approach. Comparative study of 2 technical methods. Union Med Can 1967;96:702–712.
22 Hardy J: Exercision of pituitary adenomas by trans-sphenoidal approach. Union Med Can 1962;91:933–945.
23 Welbourn RB: The evolution of transsphenoidal pituitary microsurgery. Surgery 1986;100: 1185–1190.
24 Jho HD, Carrau RL: Endoscopic endonasal transsphenoidal surgery: experience with 50 patients. J Neurosurg 1997;87:44–51.
25 Jho HD, Carrau RL, Ko Y, Daly MA: Endoscopic pituitary surgery: an early experience. Surg Neurol 1997;47:213–222.
26 Jho HD, Carrau RL: Endoscopy assisted transsphenoidal surgery for pituitary adenoma. Technical note. Acta Neurochir (Wien) 1996;138:1416–1425.
27 Cappabianca P, Buonamassa S, Cavallo LM, Mariniello G, de Divitiis O: Neuroendoscopy: present and future applications. Clin Neurosurg 2004;51:186–190.
28 Cappabianca P, de Divitiis E: Endoscopy and transsphenoidal surgery. Neurosurgery 2004;54: 1043–1050.
29 Cappabianca P, Cavallo LM, Colao A, et al: Endoscopic endonasal transsphenoidal approach: outcome analysis of 100 consecutive procedures. Minim Invasive Neurosurg 2002;45:193–200.
30 Cappabianca P, Alfieri A, Thermes S, Buonamassa S, de Divitiis E: Instruments for endoscopic endonasal transsphenoidal surgery. Neurosurgery 1999;45:392–396.
31 Jane JA Jr, Thapar K, Alden TD, Laws ER Jr: Fluoroscopic frameless stereotaxy for transsphenoidal surgery. Neurosurgery 2001;48:1302–1308.
32 Elias WJ, Chadduck JB, Alden TD, Laws ER Jr: Frameless stereotaxy for transsphenoidal surgery. Neurosurgery 1999;45:271–277.
33 Couldwell WT, Weiss MH, Rabb C, Liu JK, Apfelbaum RI, Fukushima T: Variations on the standard transsphenoidal approach to the sellar region, with emphasis on the extended approaches and parasellar approaches: surgical experience in 105 cases. Neurosurgery 2004;55:539–550.
34 Arai H, Sato K, Okuda O, et al: Transcranial transsphenoidal approach for tuberculum sellae meningiomas. Acta Neurochir (Wien) 2000;142:751–757.
35 De Divitiis E, Cappabianca P, Cavallo LM: Endoscopic transsphenoidal approach: adaptability of the procedure to different sellar lesions. Neurosurgery 2002;51:699–707.
36 Frank G, Pasquini E, Mazzatenta D: Extended transsphenoidal approach. J Neurosurg 2001;95: 917–918.
37 Jane JA Jr, Thapar K, Kaptain GJ, Maartens N, Laws ER Jr: Pituitary surgery: transsphenoidal approach. Neurosurgery 2002;51:434–442.
38 Jane JA Jr, Dumont AS, Vance ML, Laws ER Jr: The transsphenoidal transtuberculum sellae approach for suprasellar meningiomas. Semin Neurosurg 2003;14:211–217.
39 Jho HD, Alfieri A: Endoscopic endonasal pituitary surgery: evolution of surgical technique and equipment in 150 operations. Minim Invasive Neurosurg 2001;44:1–12.
40 Jho HD, Ha HG: Endoscopic endonasal skull base surgery: part 1 – the midline anterior fossa skull base. Minim Invasive Neurosurg 2004;47:1–8.
41 Kaptain GJ, Vincent DA, Sheehan JP, Laws ER Jr: Transsphenoidal approaches for the extracapsular resection of midline suprasellar and anterior cranial base lesions. Neurosurgery 2001;49: 94–101.
42 Kato T, Sawamura Y, Abe H, Nagashima M: Transsphenoidal-transtuberculum sellae approach for supradiaphragmatic tumours: technical note. Acta Neurochir (Wien) 1998;140:715–719.
43 Kim J, Choe I, Bak K, Kim C, Kim N, Jang Y: Transsphenoidal supradiaphragmatic intradural approach: technical note. Minim Invasive Neurosurg 2000;43:33–37.
44 Kitano M, Taneda M: Extended transsphenoidal approach with submucosal posterior ethmoidectomy for parasellar tumors. Technical note. J Neurosurg 2001;94:999–1004.

45 Mason RB, Nieman LK, Doppman JL, Oldfield EH: Selective excision of adenomas originating in or extending into the pituitary stalk with preservation of pituitary function. J Neurosurg 1997;87:343–351.
46 Romano A, Zuccarello M, van Loveren HR, Keller JT: Expanding the boundaries of the transsphenoidal approach: a microanatomic study. Clin 2001;14:1–9.
47 Weiss MH: Transnasal transsphenoidal approach; in Apuzzo MLJ (ed): Surgery of the Third Ventricle. Baltimore, Williams & Wilkins, 1987, pp 476–494.
48 Honegger J, Fahlbusch R, Buchfelder M, Huk WJ, Thierauf P: The role of transsphenoidal microsurgery in the management of sellar and parasellar meningioma. Surg Neurol 1993;39:18–24.
49 Kouri JG, Chen MY, Watson JC, Oldfield EH: Resection of suprasellar tumors by using a modified transsphenoidal approach. Report of four cases. J Neurosurg 2000;92:1028–1035.
50 Laurent JJ, Jane JA Jr, Laws ER: A case of midline suprasellar tumor removal by an extended transsphenoidal skull base technique; in Kobayashi S (ed): Complex Tumors and Vascular Lesions. New York, Thieme, 2004, pp 174–177.
51 Laws ER: Transsphenoidal removal of craniopharyngioma. Pediatr Neurosurg 1994;21:57–63.
52 Laws ER, Weiss MH, White WL: Experts' corner: craniopharyngioma. Skull Base 2003;13:55–58.
53 Laws ER, Kern EB: Complications of trans-sphenoidal surgery. Clin Neurosurg 1976;23: 401–416.
54 Kitano M, Taneda M: Subdural patch graft technique for watertight closure of large dural defects in extended transsphenoidal surgery. Neurosurgery 2004;54:651–660.
55 Cappabianca P, Cavallo LM, Esposito F, Valente V, de Divitiis E: Sellar repair in endoscopic endonasal transsphenoidal surgery: result of 170 cases. Neurosurgery 2002;51:1365–1372.
56 Cappabianca P, Cavallo LM, Colao AM, de Divitiis E: Surgical complications associated with the endoscopic endonasal transsphenoidal approach for pituitary adenomas. J Neurosurg 2002;97: 293–298.
57 Cappabianca P, de Divitiis E: Endoscopy and transsphenoidal surgery. Neurosurgery 2004;54: 1043–1050.
58 De Divitiis E, Cappabianca P, Cavallo LM: Endoscopic transsphenoidal approach: adaptability of the procedure to different sellar lesions. Neurosurgery 2002;51:699–707.

Aaron S. Dumont, MD
Department of Neurological Surgery, Health Sciences Center
University of Virginia, PO Box 800212
Charlottesville, VA 22908 (USA)
Tel. +1 434 982 3244, Fax +1 434 243 2954, E-Mail asd2f@virginia.edu

Laws ER Jr, Sheehan JP (eds): Pituitary Surgery – A Modern Approach.
Front Horm Res. Basel, Karger, 2006, vol 34, pp 46–63

Image Guidance in Pituitary Surgery

Ashok R. Asthagiri, Edward R. Laws, Jr., John A. Jane, Jr.

Department of Neurological Surgery, Health Sciences Center, University of Virginia, Charlottesville, Va., USA

Abstract

Image guidance in pituitary surgery has evolved since diagnostic imaging of the sellar region was first introduced at the turn of the 20th century. These advances have played a key role in the decrease in morbidity and mortality once associated with pituitary surgery. This chapter details the history of sellar imaging as a preoperative diagnostic aide, and then examines the subsequent development of image guidance systems and intraoperative imaging. The utility and limitations of common intraoperative aides including video fluoroscopy, frameless stereotaxy, ultrasound, and magnetic resonance imaging are reviewed.

Copyright © 2006 S. Karger AG, Basel

Introduction

Surgery for pituitary tumors has significantly evolved since 1893 when Caton and Paul [1] of Liverpool first approached the sella turcica. Improvements have been made possible by significant progress in the fields of radiology, endocrinology, neurosurgery, and pathology. This chapter discusses the utility and limits of radiology in the evolution of diagnosis and surgical management of pituitary disorders.

History of Sellar Imaging

The introduction of X-rays was reported by Roentgen [2] in 1895. Cushing [3] recognized its clinical utility and in 1897 described the use of X-ray technology for the diagnosis of a bullet fragment within the spinal cord. In 1899 at a meeting of the Berlin Society of Psychiatry and Nervous Diseases, the neurologist, Hermann Oppenheim, demonstrated that the sella turcica was enlarged in a patient with acromegaly [4]. Schloffer [5] used plain film radiography to confirm the presence of sellar pathology prior to what would be the first transsphenoidal procedure in 1907. By 1912 Schuller [6] of Vienna had published the first textbook of skull radiography which remarked on the radiographic appearance of patients with sellar tumors.

Plain radiographs allowed surgeons to preoperatively confirm what they previously could only speculate about. For the first time, surgeons could see the site of pathology prior to the first incision. This increased surgical confidence and encouraged the pursuit of operative solutions for pituitary tumors. It should be noted, however, that the early equipment was expensive and cumbersome, limiting its applicability to intraoperative image guidance.

Continued advances occurred in the field of radiology during the 20th century. After the plain X-ray, the next major advance in neuroradiology came when Dandy [7, 8] of Baltimore introduced ventriculography (1918) and subsequently pneumoencephalography (1919). Preoperative encephalography more accurately indicated the size and extent of sellar lesions than plain radiographs and was regularly employed [9–11]. Lesions which did not induce radiographic changes to the sella turcica, but rather extended primarily in the suprasellar direction, could now also be diagnosed due to disruption of the suprasellar cisternal anatomy. The principles of air-contrast enhanced imaging brought the ability to conceptualize soft tissue structures indirectly through an understanding of anatomic planes and potential spaces.

More progress in the diagnosis of intracranial pathology came in the late 1920s with the introduction of cerebral angiography by Moniz [12]. The technique of percutaneous carotid angiography, introduced in 1936, allowed the procedure to gain wider acceptance [13]. Although not universally used preoperatively, angiography allowed surgeons to understand the position of the carotid arteries as well as the working distance between them. This represented the first time that information regarding neurovascular structures and their relation to the bony anatomy could be appreciated in a direct manner.

After the introduction of linear tomography in 1931, polytomography was developed in the 1950s and came into increasing use in the early 1960s [14]. Biplanar polytomograms of the sella and sphenoid sinus allowed improved comprehension of bone thickness and asymmetries within the sphenoid sinus that would be encountered intraoperatively [15].

Imaging studies began to be used intraoperatively as well. In 1962 Hardy [10, 11] described his use of intraoperative radiofluoroscopy for image guidance and by 1965 had reported the utility of intraoperative air encephalography to gauge the extent of tumor removal. Intraoperative imaging allowed surgeons to correlate their anatomical findings with imaging in real time, thereby increasing the safety of surgery. This, in addition to significant advances in perioperative care, led to a significant decline in the morbidity and mortality associated with transsphenoidal surgery.

Thus, in the late 1960s and early 1970s, at the time of the renaissance of the transsphenoidal technique for pituitary surgery, the radiologic techniques available to most surgeons included plain radiographs, video fluoroscopy, encephalography, angiography, and polytomography. This armamentarium of imaging modalities represented a significant advance over the plain radiographs available to pioneers of pituitary surgery at the beginning of the 20th century.

Nevertheless, there were limitations. These images did not provide a direct view of the pituitary gland nor of the adjacent brain parenchyma and cranial nerves. Surgeons were still unable to visualize the precise anatomy and intracranial extensions of a neoplasm. The diagnosis of hypersecretory syndromes due to microadenomas relied heavily on the expertise of the endocrinologist. No imaging study could direct the surgeon regarding the laterality of these tumors. Also, none of these imaging modalities was suited for routine postoperative assessment of the extent of tumor removal or surveillance for recurrence.

The introduction of computerized tomography (CT) and magnetic resonance imaging (MRI) into clinical practice in the 1970s and 1980s revolutionized the perioperative management of patients presenting with pituitary-based disease. By this time, Hardy had popularized the use of the operative microscope in transsphenoidal surgery and its utility in selective adenomectomy [16–22]. As these imaging techniques improved in resolution, increasing numbers of hypersecreting microadenomas without mass effect could be identified and lateralized. At the other end of the spectrum, these imaging modalities also allowed a greater understanding of the intimate relationship between large, invasive pituitary tumors and critical neurovascular structures, thereby improving preoperative planning. These imaging modalities in conjunction with biochemical assays also improved the postoperative surveillance of patients with residual and recurrent disease.

Image Guidance

The improvements in diagnostic radiology initially played a significant role in the perioperative management of the patient with pituitary pathology. Although information regarding the working distance between the carotid arteries, position of the optic chiasm and nerves, and exact morphology and extent of disease could be well documented with these diagnostic imaging modalities, the morbidity associated with transsphenoidal surgery remained more or less unchanged [23]. Continuous attempts to reduce the risk of surgery through the improvement in surgical techniques led to the innovative use of existing imaging

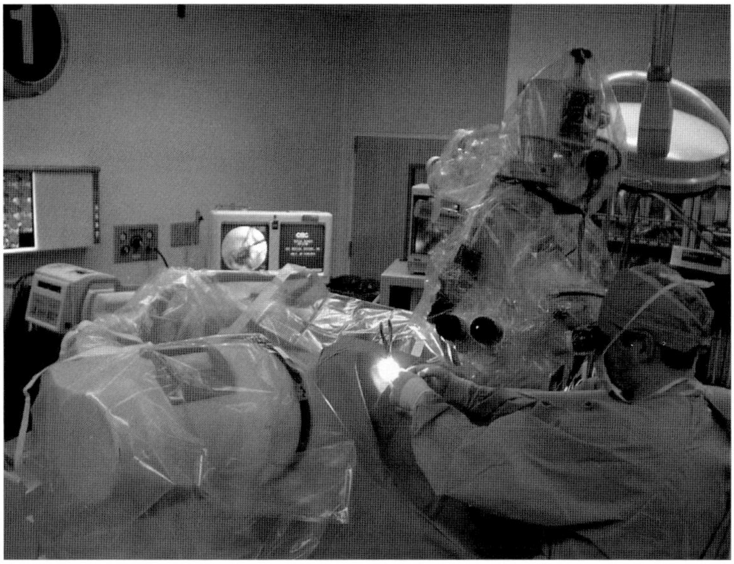

Fig. 1. Use of the c-arm video fluoroscope intraoperatively. Use in routine, initial transsphenoidal approaches to sellar confined lesions remains widespread.

techniques to guide the surgeon intraoperatively. Image guidance in pituitary surgery began with the use of intraoperative air encephalography and c-arm video fluoroscopy [10, 11], and continues to expand with the addition of newer techniques such as intraoperative ultrasound, computer-based neuronavigation, intraoperative MRI, and endoscopic assisted surgery.

Video Fluoroscopy

Although it is possible to rely solely on anatomic landmarks to reach the sphenoid sinus and sella, intraoperative imaging is used by most surgeons as an integral part of the transsphenoidal approach. The most widely used intraoperative imaging device is the c-arm video fluoroscope. Standard positioning for transsphenoidal surgery is employed, with the head placed onto a horseshoe headrest (fig. 1). Most often, the c-arm is positioned such that a lateral image is obtained and confirms the appropriate trajectory to the sella turcica, defining its superior and inferior confines [11] (fig. 2). Knowing the superior and inferior limits of the sella turcica allows the surgeon to confirm adequate exposure and prevents unnecessary opening of the planum sphenoidale and the risk of a cerebrospinal fluid leak and anosmia [24, 25].

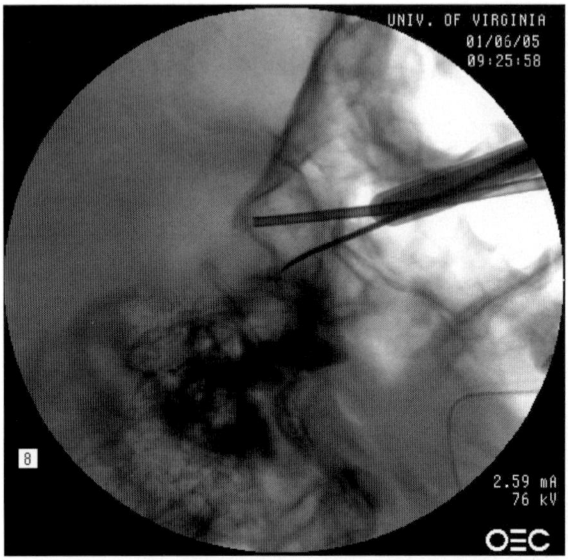

Fig. 2. Lateral video fluoroscopic view defining the superior and inferior margins of the sella turcica. The video fluoroscope is best suited to help with vertical orientation en route to the sella turcica.

The advantage of using a standard fluoroscope is its simplicity and accuracy. Its disadvantages are the radiation exposure and its inability to depict soft tissue anatomy, including the tumor and neurovascular structures. Any intraoperative rotational adjustment of the head for an improved surgical viewpoint requires a concurrent adjustment in the c-arm angle to maintain a true lateral image. It is ineffective in demonstrating the midline in the anteroposterior view, and its use for this intraoperatively is limited due to microscope positioning conflicts and disruption of surgical access to the operative corridor. The ubiquitous presence of c-arm video fluoroscopy has enabled this quick, cost-effective, real-time image guidance technique to find a niche within pituitary surgery. The c-arm video fluoroscope is sufficient for most routine, first-time transsphenoidal operations where tumors confined to the sella can be removed under direct microscopic visualization.

Frameless Stereotaxy

A more recent advance in intraoperative imaging has been frameless stereotaxy. Frameless stereotactic systems were introduced in the 1990s and are

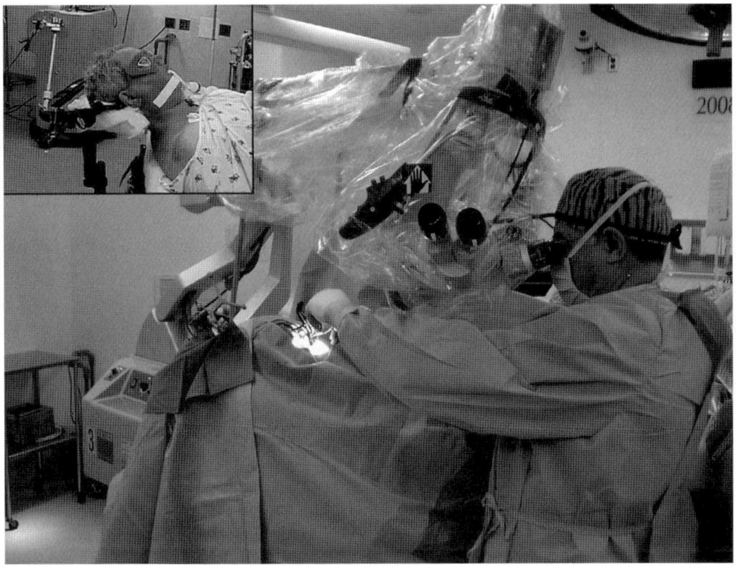

Fig. 3. Intraoperative set-up with frameless neuronavigation techniques requires reference array fixation (inset), but allows removal of the c-arm video fluoroscope (when plain radiograph reference images are utilized) and decreased intraoperative radiation exposure.

widely available at most neurosurgical centers. These systems allow the surgeon to refer intraoperatively to preoperative images (CT, MRI, or radiographs) in several planes of view simultaneously. In the setting of radiographs, the c-arm video fluoroscope is utilized to obtain the images after fixation of the reference array but is removed prior to starting surgery (fig. 3). Preoperative CT and MRI scans are obtained with fiducial markers, and these are calibrated with the affixed reference array at the time of surgery. We have previously published our preliminary experience with the systems as they pertain to transsphenoidal surgery [26, 27]. The sagittal plane view, much like the traditional fluoroscopic image, provides information regarding the trajectory to the sphenoid sinus and sella. The coronal and axial views are most useful in maintaining the midline and thereby preventing errant exposure of the carotid arteries and cavernous sinus (fig. 4). Nevertheless, each system has a small but inescapable degree of inaccuracy, and anatomic markers seen within the surgical field should be used to confirm the data provided by the navigational system [28].

After initially using the system for all transsphenoidal procedures, we have now limited the use of frameless stereotaxy. In our practice we use radiograph-based neuronavigation only in selected settings, such as repeat surgery in which the normal anatomic structures may be disrupted, and we believe that an accurate

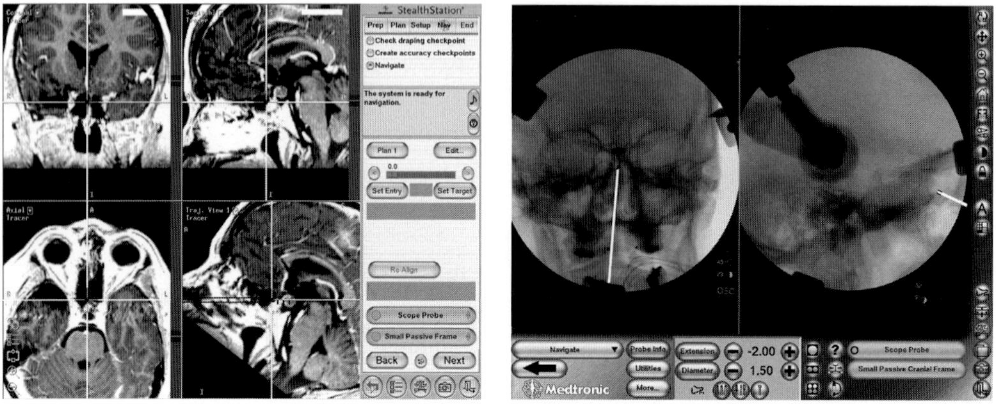

Fig. 4. Screen snapshots depicting the use of preoperative magnetic resonance images and skull X-rays in the approach to sellar-based tumors with frameless neuronavigation techniques.

assessment of the anatomic midline may be difficult to discern. We also use neuronavigation in first-time transsphenoidal surgery when the carotid arteries are closely approximated. Again, in this situation the information regarding the midline helps to safeguard against vascular injury. These indications for the use of neuronavigation have been reported by others [29, 30]. Although we believe that these systems do improve accuracy and safety in second-time surgery, we do not believe that they should be considered the standard of care.

MRI-based neuronavigation is used in the removal of either suprasellar tumors that have not expanded the sella or tumors that extend along the anterior skull base [31]. In these extended transsphenoidal approaches, the planum sphenoidale and the tuberculum sellae are removed to provide increased access to the either the suprasellar region or the anterior cranial fossa. Under guidance by the neuronavigational system, bone is removed to the lateral limits of the carotid arteries and the anterior limit of the cribriform plate, and a direct trajectory to the extrasellar components of lesions can be identified.

At one time, the cost of the neuronavigational systems represented a significant deterrent to their widespread utilization. Currently, most neurosurgical centers have access to frameless stereotaxy, and this is not a major issue. Another small inconvenience is the need to rigidly fixate the reference array to a head holder (fig. 3, inset). Although the skull pins rarely cause major morbidity, they do cause some minor discomfort. Fixation of the reference array with pins does not require skull fixation to the operative table, and thus the head can still be adjusted to improve the surgical vantage point. Evaluation of headset-based fixation of the reference array not requiring skull pins has shown similar accuracy, thereby providing a less invasive option for optical and electromagnetic-based neuronavigation systems [32, 33]. The primary limitation in the systems now is that the setup and registration of the system adds to surgical times.

In routine first-time transsphenoidal surgery, we believe that the benefit of the information regarding soft tissue structures and the anatomic midline is offset by the time added to the procedure to set up the system. Therefore, standard c-arm video fluoroscopy is used for our first-time uncomplicated transsphenoidal operations. In pituitary surgery, frameless stereotaxy cannot be used to gauge the extent of tumor removal. During tumor debulking, the morphology of the tumor necessarily shifts, as do the intracranial neurovascular structures. The surgeon must be aware that the images provided are preoperative.

Intraoperative Imaging

Intraoperatively gauging the extent of tumor removal is a major issue in transsphenoidal surgery. The inherently narrow and deep surgical corridor renders the suprasellar and lateral sellar compartments difficult to visualize. The relation of the tumor to the anterior cerebral circulation often cannot be determined, and an accurate estimation of the extent of tumor resection may not be possible. Because of this limited view, the surgeon must rely on surgical clues that the suprasellar tumor has been removed. The primary visual clue is seeing the diaphragma descend into the sellar compartment and surgical field. This does not, however, ensure that the suprasellar component has actually been completely removed. A lateral fluoroscopic image after air is instilled via a lumbar drain has traditionally allowed the surgeon to indirectly assess the extent and adequacy of surgical resection.

Ultrasonography

To circumvent these difficulties, surgeons have recently described the use of transcranial ultrasonography during resection of these large tumors [34]. By using right frontal trephination, ultrasonography can accurately differentiate tumor from brain and provide a color Doppler depiction of the anterior circulation (fig. 5). Unlike other modalities, ultrasonography provides true real-time feedback to the surgeon as the resection is being performed (fig. 6). The surgeon is able to visualize the dynamic changes in tumor geometry during the excision, in a cost- and time-efficient manner. Importantly, standard surgical instruments can be monitored within the tumor cavity in real time. Although the data published are preliminary, ultrasonography may improve the extent of

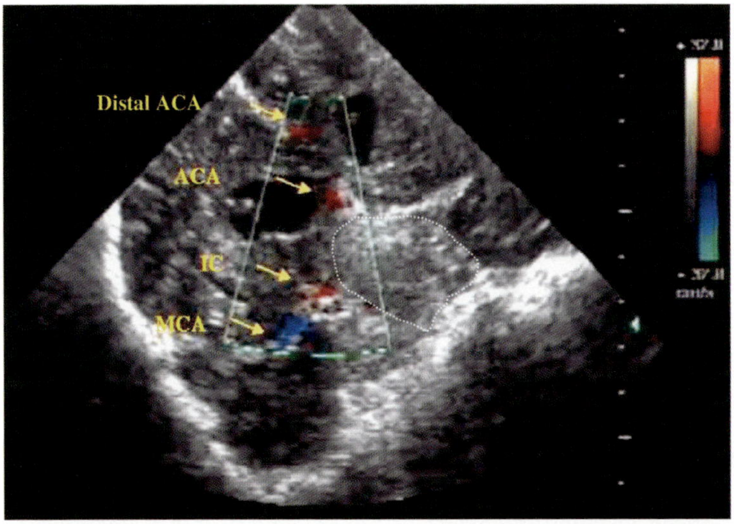

Fig. 5. A Doppler color flow image of the tumor (surrounded by the dotted white line). Major arteries surrounding the lesion are identified. ACA = Anterior cerebral artery; IC = internal carotid artery; MCA = middle cerebral artery. With permission from Suzuki et al. [34].

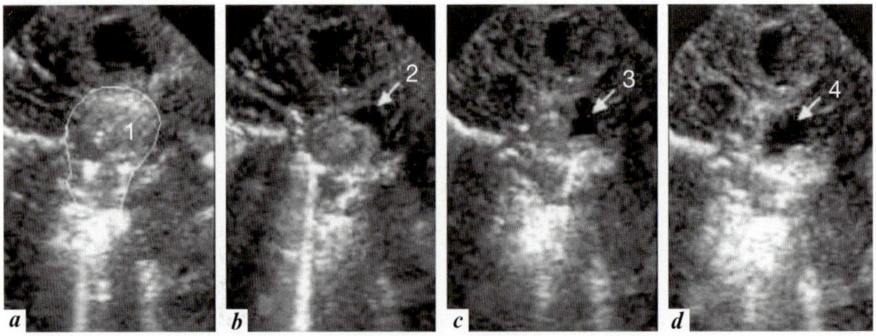

Fig. 6. Serial sagittal B-mode echo images obtained during tumor removal. ***a*** The bulk of the tumor is clearly seen at the start of the operation (1 and dotted white line). ***b*** The visibility of the prepontine cistern (2) has increased due to debulking of the tumor. ***c*** A clearer identification of the cistern (3) is possible. ***d*** The visibility of the suprasellar cistern (4) has increased because of the gross total removal of the suprasellar tumor and the cistern is seen folding into the sella turcica. With permission from Suzuki et al. [34].

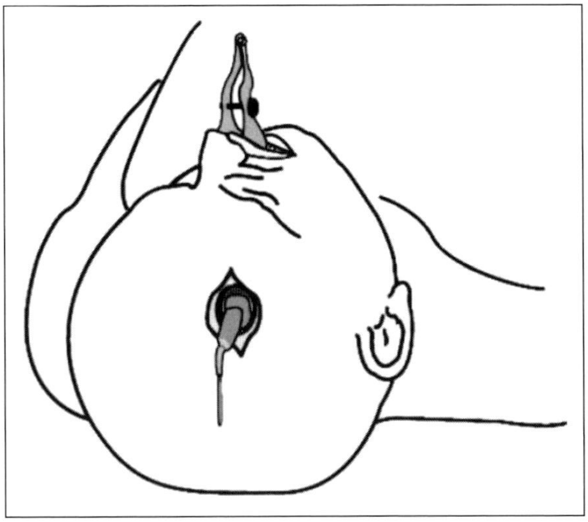

Fig. 7. Schematic drawing showing insertion of the echo probe into the right frontal trephination [34].

surgical resection for massive macroadenomas [34, 35]. The drawback of intraoperative ultrasonography remains, however, the clarity and resolution of the images. Ultrasonography can guide the surgeon during macroscopic tumor removal but its resolution does not allow the surgeon to monitor for small tumor remnants. Additionally, a separate cranial incision and burr hole must be performed, adding minimally to the surgical risk [36] (fig. 7).

Intraoperative Magnetic Resonance Imaging

MRI has become the preferred modality for the preoperative evaluation of brain tumors and epilepsy [37, 38]. With the advent of open MR systems, the applicability of MRI as an intraoperative tool was realized. The first interventional unit was installed in Boston in 1994. Since then, selected centers have used MRI in the interventional and operative forum and reported that the extent of tumor resection can be monitored with significantly improved accuracy [39, 40]. There are several types of intraoperative MRI (iMRI), and they differ based on field strength (low and high), the surgeon's access to the patient, ease of utility, and time efficiency in image acquisition [41].

Among the low-field systems are the GE 0.5 Tesla double doughnut, the Siemens 0.2 Tesla open magnet, the Hitachi 0.3 Tesla shared resource magnet, and the Odin 0.12 Tesla magnet [42–48]. With the exception of the GE double doughnut, surgery is not performed within the magnet. In the other low-field systems, surgery is performed outside the 5-Gauss line where standard operative equipment and microscope can be utilized, except for a specially designed nasal speculum and drill bit [42]. This also allows free access to the patient. The disadvantage is the relative difficulty in obtaining images compared with the double doughnut system. To obtain images using the Siemens and Hitachi systems, surgery is halted and the patient is brought within the magnet for image acquisition. This process tends to lengthen the operative time and disrupts the flow of the operation. The ultra-low-field Odin system resides beneath the operative table and is brought into the surgical field much like a c-arm fluoroscope. The image quality is poor relative to the other systems, but the ease in obtaining images is superior to that of the Siemens and Hitachi magnets.

When the double doughnut is used, surgery is performed within the magnet itself without the need to move either the patient or the magnet and allows the surgeon to acquire images easily (each plane within 60–120 s). Indeed, surgeons who use the double doughnut take images throughout the procedure; those using systems where the patient must be brought into the scanner tend to take images at the end of the resection. The GE double doughnut system, however, creates a somewhat restricted surgical field and requires specific MR-compatible instruments, microscope, and anesthesia equipment. The constrained surgical field limits the application in transsphenoidal surgery.

Also in use are high-field systems made by Phillips (at the University of Minnesota), the 1.5-T Magnex system in use in Calgary, and the Siemens 1.5 Tesla unit. These systems provide superior quality images and allow the surgeons to use MRI-incompatible equipment outside the 5-Gauss line. High-field systems improve the signal-to-noise ratio and provide standard diagnostic MR capabilities including MR spectroscopy, MR angiography, MR venography, diffusion weighted imaging, and functional imaging [49, 50]. The high-field imager allows shorter examination times but its primary drawback is the significant financial and structural investment in comparison to their low-field system counterparts. Each of these systems requires transportation of either patient or magnet to obtain images. Whereas in the Phillips and Siemens systems patients are transported into the scanner, in the Calgary system it is the scanner that is brought around the patient [51].

Transsphenoidal surgery series have been published using the Siemens 0.2 Tesla open magnet [42], the Hitachi 0.3 Tesla shared resource magnet [46, 47], and the Siemens 1.5 Tesla imager [52]. Using the open Siemens magnet, Fahlbusch et al. [42] reported that iMRI led to further tumor resection in 34% (15/44) of patients with large intrasellar and suprasellar macroadenomas (fig. 8). Of course, iMRI does not improve resection of tumors that cannot be removed (i.e., those with cavernous sinus invasion). Indeed, even with iMRI, 30% (13/44)

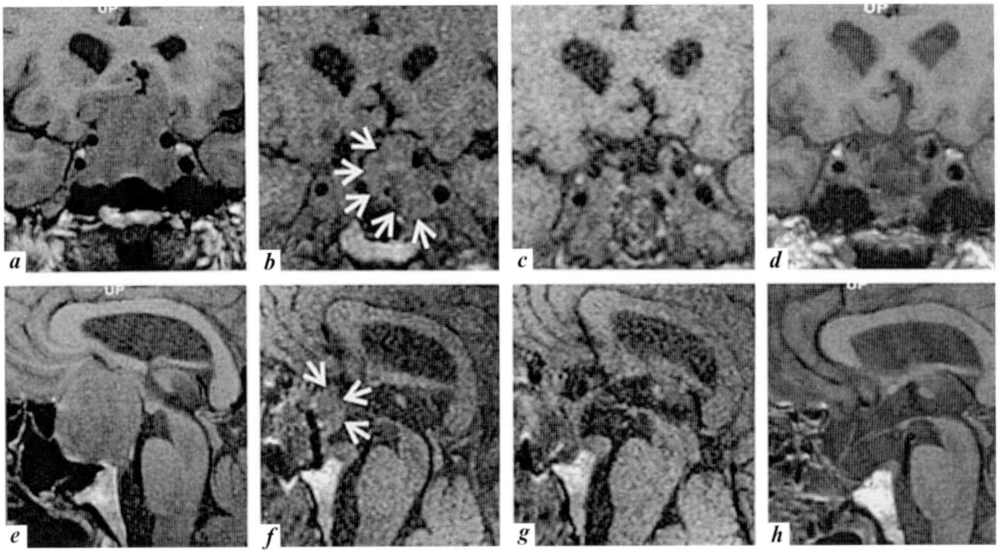

Fig. 8. Coronal (***a–d***) and sagittal (***e–h***) MRIs obtained in a 59-year-old man with a large intra-, para-, and suprasellar, endocrinologically asymptomatic pituitary adenoma. ***a***, ***e*** Preoperative images. ***b***, ***f*** Intraoperative images revealing some remaining tumor (arrows), which led the surgeon to take a second look and remove the remaining portions of tumor. ***c***, ***g*** Additional images obtained at the end of surgery demonstrating that the remaining adenoma has been removed. ***d***, ***h*** Follow-up MRIs confirming that the tumor is no longer present. With permission from Fahlbusch et al. [42].

of tumors with difficult suprasellar and parasellar extension could not be resected. The interpretation of iMRI can be difficult: 27% (12/44) of the iMRI results could not be definitively interpreted. In 20% (9/44) of cases, iMRI was interpreted as revealing residual tumor, but this interpretation was subsequently found to be incorrect upon second look and 3-month postoperative MRI. Nevertheless, false-negative results were not encountered. When the iMRI could be interpreted and was determined to have shown no residual tumor, follow-up study confirmed complete resection.

The application of the Hitachi shared-resource magnet to transsphenoidal surgery has also been assessed [46, 47]. This magnet is also used as diagnostic MRI as well, thus helping to offset the costs of the scanner. iMRIs were obtained at the perceived completion of the operation. In 66% (19/30) of cases, further surgery was performed after complete or optimal resection was thought to have been accomplished. A second MRI was performed in 8 of 19 patients, revealing persistent residual tumor in 3. A third image acquisition was not pursued in any patient. Operative time for a single imaging session was reported to be extended by approximately 20 min. Although the authors noted some difficulty interpreting the intraoperative images secondary to blood products or leakage of contrast material into the operative bed, they reported that adequate images were obtained in 100% of cases. Early postoperative endocrinological results were comparable to those in large surgical series. One patient sustained a vascular injury to the right A1 vessel and required conversion to a craniotomy. Although it is a risk in any surgery, it is conceivable that iMRI might encourage surgeons to remove tumor from locations where it might have been prudent to leave residual tumor. Because of the added time, the surgeons reported that they tended to use the iMRI judiciously and concluded that iMRI will likely have limited use for purely sellar tumors and microadenomas.

In 2004, Nimsky et al. [52] reported on the use of the intraoperative high-field strength MRI in transsphenoidal surgery. Although operating within the high-magnetic field with MRI-compatible instruments is possible, the principal surgical position was at the 5-Gauss line, approximately 4 m from the center of the imager, where the microscope is positioned and standard microinstruments could be used. Intraoperative MRI was performed in 77 transsphenoidal operations, and resulted in a modification of surgical strategy through an extension of resection in 27 cases (35%). Among 48 patients with pituitary adenomas with distinct suprasellar extension that appeared to be respectable, findings at iMR led to repeated inspection in 29 cases (60%). Ten of these cases represented false-positive findings including fibrin glue, blood, and a suprasellar diaphragmatic fold. Of the remaining 19 patients, 15 were found to have residual tumor that was resected in its entirety, thereby increasing the rate of complete tumor removal in this subset of patients with pituitary adenomas from 56.2 (27/48) to 87.5% (42/48). No adverse events were reported because of the high-magnetic field strength. Additionally, early visualization of tumor remnants that are not removed via the transsphenoidal route make them amenable to immediate planning for postoperative treatment.

At this time, each available iMRI system is a prototype. The balancing of expense, signal-to-noise ratio and resolution, ease of access during surgery, and time efficiency have made the development of the ideal system difficult. Of course, it would be one that provides rapid high-quality multiplanar images with maximal access to the patient in a variety of surgical positions without requiring new surgical equipment or instruments. We are confident that the shortcomings are temporary and that iMRI will find its place in the resection of certain pituitary tumors. Unresectable tumors will remain so, and purely sellar lesions will likely not benefit from iMRI. To substantiate and solidify its presence as a necessary imaging technique in transsphenoidal surgery, long-term results will be needed to assess whether iMRI decreases recurrence in nonfunctioning adenomas or improves the biochemical remission rate in secreting adenomas. Although it may be that direct endoscopic inspection of possible tumor remnants will be adequate for most tumors, there is an obvious advantage of iMRI in assessing the adequacy of resection of the suprasellar portion of the tumor.

Conclusions

Major advances in radiology have played a key role in the decrease in morbidity and mortality once associated with pituitary surgery [23, 24, 53, 54]. As intraoperative image guidance techniques such as frameless stereotaxy and iMRI advance the concept of immediate feedback to the operating neurosurgeon, it is imperative that we maintain an understanding of economic restraints and global availability of such expensive neuronavigational modalities. The judicious use of appropriate resources based on the level of intraoperative guidance that will be required and an understanding of the relative utility and limitations of each modality will limit the superfluous use of advanced neuroimaging techniques (table 1). The use of intraoperative neuroimaging is not a replacement for surgical experience and a thorough knowledge of regional anatomy, but provides another tool by which the neurosurgeon can reduce the risk associated with surgical access and treatment of pituitary pathology.

Table 1. Utility and limitations of selected image-guidance technologies

Imaging modality		Indications	Utility	Limitations
Intraoperative video fluoroscopy	–	Exposure of intrasellar pathology in patients whose midline structures remain intact	Establishes target trajectory in the vertical axis Identifies superior and inferior borders of the sella turcica Real-time feedback regarding depth but not laterality within the operative field Simple and accurate	No information on midline approach to the sella in the horizontal axis No image based feedback regarding extent of tumor resection Intraoperative radiation exposure Cumbersome and bulky equipment
	In conjunction with air encephalography		Indirect information regarding extent of tumor resection	Lumbar intrathecal drain placement required

Table 1. (continued)

Imaging modality		Indications	Utility	Limitations
Frameless stereotaxy	–	Transsphenoidal surgery in which midline structures are disrupted/not dependable	Decrease intraoperative radiation exposure Multiplanar information aids in the midline approach to the sella	Requires fixation of array to skull Increases setup time (preoperative films required) Inescapable degree of inaccuracy
	Fluoroscopy-based		Images acquired preoperatively, at the time of surgery	
	CT-based		Bone thickness variation and sphenoid sinus asymmetry better appreciated	Poor soft tissue imaging Expense (additional cost of CT scan) Preoperative imaging required
	MRI-based		Direct trajectory to anterior skull base lesions and suprasellar lesions can be ascertained	Intraoperative shift of soft tissues structures Expense (additional cost of MRI scan) Preoperative imaging required
Ultrasonography	–	Large invasive tumors with significant suprasellar components	Direct, real-time imaging of tumor No radiation exposure Identification of major vascular structures with duplex color Doppler imaging Cost-effective	Poor image resolution Concurrent surgical procedure needed
iMRI	–	Large invasive tumors with significant suprasellar components	Improved resolution and differentiation of soft tissue structures Improve suprasellar and extratumoral imaging Early visualization of tumor remnants that are not removable allows immediate planning for postoperative treatment	Image acquisition lengthens surgical time Although intraoperative images are relatively up-to-date, not true real-time imaging Significant capital investment required

References

1 Caton R, Paul FT: Notes on a case of acromegaly treated by operation. Br Med J 1893;ii: 1421–1423.
2 Roentgen W: Ueber eine neue Art von Strahlen: vorläufige Mitteilung. Sitzungsber Physmed Ges Würzburg 1895;137:132–141.
3 Cushing H: Haematomyelia from gunshot wound of the cervical spine. Bull Johns Hopkins Hosp 1897;8:195–197.
4 Medvei VC: The birth of endocrinology – part II; in Medvei VC (ed): The History of Clinical Endocrinology, ed 2. New York, Parthenon, 1993, pp 159–194.
5 Schloffer H: Erfolgreiche Operationen eines Hypophentamors auf nasalem Wege. Wien Klin Wochenschr 1907;20:621–624.
6 Schuller A: Röntgendiagnostik der Erkrankungen des Kopfes. Vienna, Holder, 1912.
7 Dandy W: Ventriculography following the injection of air into the cerebral ventricles. Ann Surg 1918;68:5–11.
8 Dandy W: Roentgenography of the brain after the injection of air into the spinal canal. Ann Surg 1919;70:397–403.
9 Frazier C: An approach to the hypophysis through the anterior cranial fossa. Ann Surg 1913;57: 145–150.
10 Hardy J: L'exérèse des adénomes hypophysaires par voie transsphénoïdale. Union Med Can 1962;91:933–945.
11 Hardy J, Wigser SM: Trans-sphenoidal surgery of pituitary fossa tumors with televised radiofluoroscopic control. J Neurosurg 1965;23:612–619.
12 Moniz E: Arterial encephalography: importance in the localization of cerebral tumours. Rev Neurol (Paris) 1927;34:72–90.
13 Loman J, Myerson A: Visualization of the cerebral vessels by direct intracarotid injection of thorium dioxid (thorotrast). Am J Roentgenol 1936;35:188–193.
14 Littleton J, Runbaugh C, Winter F: Polydirectional body section tomography: a new diagnostic method. Am J Roentgenol 1963;89:1179–1193.
15 Kern EB, Pearson BW, McDonald TJ, Laws ER Jr: The transseptal approach to lesions of the pituitary and parasellar regions. Laryngoscope 1979;89(suppl 15):1–34.
16 Riskaer N, Fog CV, Hommelgaard T: Transsphenoidal hypophysectomy in metastatic cancer of the breast. Arch Otolaryngol 1961;74:483–493.
17 Bateman GH: Trans-sphenoidal hypohysectomy. A review of 70 cases treated in the past two years. Trans Am Acad Ophthalmol Otolaryngol 1962;66:103–110.
18 Gisselsson L: Transsphenoidale Hypophysenektomie. Photogr Forsch Zeiss Ikon Dienst Wiss 1959;8:77–80.
19 Hardy J: Surgery of the pituitary gland, using the trans-sphenoidal approach. Comparative study of 2 technical methods (in French). Union Med Can 1967;96:702–712.
20 Hardy J, Ciric IS: Selective anterior hypophysectomy in the treatment of diabetic retinopathy. A transsphenoidal microsurgical technique. JAMA 1968;203:73–78.
21 Hardy J: Transphenoidal microsurgery of the normal and pathological pituitary. Clin Neurosurg 1969;16:185–217.
22 Macbeth RG: An approach to the pituitary via a nasal osteoplastic flap. J Laryngol Otol 1961;75:70–77.
23 Ciric I, Ragin A, Baumgartner C, Pierce D: Complications of transsphenoidal surgery: results of a national survey, review of the literature, and personal experience. Neurosurgery 1997;40:225–237.
24 Laws ER Jr, Kern EB: Complications of trans-sphenoidal surgery. Clin Neurosurg 1976;23: 401–416.
25 Kennedy DW, Cohn ES, Papel ID, Holliday MJ: Transsphenoidal approach to the sella: the Johns Hopkins experience. Laryngoscope 1984;94:1066–1074.
26 Jane JA Jr, Thapar K, Alden TD, Laws ER Jr: Fluoroscopic frameless stereotaxy for transsphenoidal surgery. Neurosurgery 2001;48:1302–1308.
27 Elias WJ, Chadduck JB, Alden TD, Laws ER Jr: Frameless stereotaxy for transsphenoidal surgery. Neurosurgery 1999;45:271–277.

28 McCutcheon IE, Kitagawa RS, Demasi PF, Law BK, Friend KE: Frameless stereotactic navigation in transsphenoidal surgery: comparison with fluoroscopy. Stereotact Funct Neurosurg 2004;82: 43–48.
29 Lee JY, Lunsford LD, Subach BR, Jho HD, Bissonette DJ, Kondziolka D: Brain surgery with image guidance: current recommendations based on a 20-year assessment. Stereotact Funct Neurosurg 2000;75:35–48.
30 Sandeman D, Moufid A: Interactive image-guided pituitary surgery. An experience of 101 procedures. Neurochirurgie 1998;44:331–338.
31 Jane JA Jr, Thapar K, Kaptain GJ, Maartens N, Laws ER Jr: Pituitary surgery: transsphenoidal approach. Neurosurgery 2002;51:435–444.
32 Metson R, Gliklich RE, Cosenza M: A comparison of image guidance systems for sinus surgery. Laryngoscope 1998;108:1164–1170.
33 Walker DG, Ohaegbulam C, Black PM: Frameless stereotaxy as an alternative to fluoroscopy for transsphenoidal surgery: use of the InstaTrak-3000 and a novel headset. J Clin Neurosci 2002;9:294–297.
34 Suzuki R, Asai J, Nagashima G, Itokawa H, Chang CW, Noda M, Fujimoto M, Fujimoto T: Transcranial echo-guided transsphenoidal surgical approach for the removal of large macroadenomas. J Neurosurg 2004;100:68–72.
35 Atkinson JL, Kasperbauer JL, James EM, Lane JI, Nippoldt TB: Transcranial-transdural real-time ultrasonography during transsphenoidal resection of a large pituitary tumor. Case report. J Neurosurg 2000;93:129–131.
36 Jane JA Jr, Dumont AS, Sheehan JP, Laws ER Jr: Surgical techniques in transsphenoidal surgery: what is the standard of care in pituitary adenoma surgery? Curr Opin Endocrinol Diabetes 2004;11:264–270.
37 Wen P, Teoh S, Black PM: Clinical, imaging, and laboratory diagnosis of brain tumors; in Kaye A, Laws ER Jr (eds): Brain Tumors. London, Churchill Livingstone, 2001, pp 217–248.
38 Bronen RA: Epilepsy: the role of MR imaging. AJR Am J Roentgenol 1992;159:1165–1174.
39 Jolesz FA: Blumenfeld SM: Interventional use of magnetic resonance imaging. Magn Reson Q 1994;10:85–96.
40 Black PM, Moriarty T, Alexander E 3rd, Stieg P, Woodard EJ, Gleason PL, Martin CH, Kikinis R, Schwartz RB, Jolesz FA: Development and implementation of intraoperative magnetic resonance imaging and its neurosurgical applications. Neurosurgery 1997;41:831–845.
41 Albayrak B, Samdani AF, Black PM: Intra-operative magnetic resonance imaging in neurosurgery. Acta Neurochir (Wien) 2004;146:543–557.
42 Fahlbusch R, Ganslandt O, Buchfelder M, Schott W, Nimsky C: Intraoperative magnetic resonance imaging during transsphenoidal surgery. J Neurosurg 2001;95:381–390.
43 Lipson AC, Gargollo PC, Black PM: Intraoperative magnetic resonance imaging: considerations for the operating room of the future. J Clin Neurosci 2001;8:305–310.
44 Martin CH, Schwartz R, Jolesz F, Black PM: Transsphenoidal resection of pituitary adenomas in an intraoperative MRI unit. Pituitary 1999;2:155–162.
45 Kanner AA, Vogelbaum MA, Mayberg MR, Weisenberger JP, Barnett GH: Intracranial navigation by using low-field intraoperative magnetic resonance imaging: preliminary experience. J Neurosurg 2002;97:1115–1124.
46 McPherson CM, Bohinski RJ, Dagnew E, Warnick RE, Tew JM: Tumor resection in a shared-resource magnetic resonance operating room: experience at the University of Cincinnati. Acta Neurochir Suppl 2003;85:39–44.
47 Bohinski RJ, Warnick RE, Gaskill-Shipley MF, Zuccarello M, van Loveren HR, Kormos DW, Tew JM Jr: Intraoperative magnetic resonance imaging to determine the extent of resection of pituitary macroadenomas during transsphenoidal microsurgery. Neurosurgery 2001;49:1133–1144.
48 Levivier M, Wikler D, De Witte O, Van de Steene A, Baleriaux D, Brotchi J: PoleStar N-10 low-field compact intraoperative magnetic resonance imaging system with mobile radiofrequency shielding. Neurosurgery 2003;53:1001–1007.
49 Tummala RP, Chu RM, Liu H, Truwit CL, Hall WA: Optimizing brain tumor resection: high-field interventional MR imaging. Neuroimaging Clin N Am 2001;11:673–683.

50 Lewin JS, Metzger A, Selman WR: Intraoperative magnetic resonance image guidance in neurosurgery. J Magn Reson Imaging 2000;12:512–524.
51 Sutherland GR, Kaibara T, Louw D, Hoult DI, Tomanek B, Saunders J: A mobile high-field magnetic resonance system for neurosurgery. J Neurosurg 1999;91:804–813.
52 Nimsky C, Ganslandt O, Von Keller B, Romstock J, Fahlbusch R: Intraoperative high-field-strength MR imaging: implementation and experience in 200 patients. Radiology 2004;233: 67–78.
53 Henderson W: The pituitary adenomata: A follow-up study of the surgical results in 338 cases (Dr. Harvey Cushing's series). Br J Surg 1939;26:809–921.
54 Bakay L: The results of 300 pituitary adenoma operations (Prof. Herbert Olivecrona's series). J Neurosurg 1950;7:240–255.

Ashok R. Asthagiri, MD
Department of Neurological Surgery, Health Sciences Center
University of Virginia, PO Box 800212
Charlottesville, VA 22908 (USA)
Tel. +1 434 982 3244, Fax +1 434 924 9656, E-Mail ara5x@virginia.edu

Laws ER Jr, Sheehan JP (eds): Pituitary Surgery – A Modern Approach.
Front Horm Res. Basel, Karger, 2006, vol 34, pp 64–82

Endoscopic Endonasal Cavernous Sinus Surgery, with Special Reference to Pituitary Adenomas

Giorgio Frank, Ernesto Pasquini

Centre of Surgery for Pituitary Tumours, Department of Neuroscience, Bellaria Hospital, Bologna, Italy

Abstract

Cavernous sinus surgery has always been a surgical challenge because of the high functional importance of this region and the associated high morbidity. The augmented peripheral vision of the endoscope has led to the development of surgical approaches that allow adequate exposure of the cavernous sinus, with a reduction in surgical morbidity. Since 1998, 65 patients with pituitary adenomas and intraoperative evidence of cavernous sinus invasion were treated with a purely endoscopic approach. Follow-up was of at least 6 (mean 51.2) months. There was no perioperative mortality and extremely low morbidity. Radical tumor removal was obtained in 21/35 cases with nonfunctioning adenomas. Hormonal remission was obtained in 13/30 functioning adenomas. One patient with partial hypopituitarism and 1 patient with persistent diabetes insipidus were seen. Three patients with delayed CSF leaks required endoscopic repair. In 1 patient with hemorrhagic infarction in a residual tumor, reintervention with craniotomy was necessary. We advocate the central role of surgery in the treatment of cavernous sinus tumors, since it allows definition of true cavernous sinus involvement, histopathological diagnosis and, when cure is not feasible, tumor volume reduction, which might be an important factor in the response to adjuvant therapy.

Copyright © 2006 S. Karger AG, Basel

Introduction

Cavernous sinus surgery has always been a surgical challenge due to the anatomical complexity and the high functional value of the structures contained in this 'jewelry box'.

Winslow [1] gave the cavernous sinus its name in 1734, probably relating it to the cavernous body of the penis. For centuries this anatomical structure was dismissed or misunderstood by anatomists, and for surgeons it was a 'no man's land'. Although its original denomination remains in current use, it is criticized by those who have underlined that it is not a dural sinus, but a venous plexus [2].

Since the 1960s when Parkinson [3] deliberately entered the cavernous sinus to treat a long-standing arteriovenous fistula, surgical interest in this region has increased together with anatomical knowledge. Parkinson [2] also proposed a more appropriate name for this region: the 'lateral sellar compartment', containing the 'parasellar plexus'.

Transcranial surgery was initially used for the treatment of cavernous sinus tumors, mainly due to the safety given by the proximal and distal control of the internal carotid artery (ICA). This type of surgery has increasingly decreased, partly due to the appearance of alternative non-surgical therapies, such as radiosurgery, and partly due to its high morbidity. One of the most famous skull base neurosurgeons indeed wrote about cavernous sinus surgery that 'very early enthusiasm will undoubtedly be tempered in time by the poor results and complications that will be encountered in some patients' [4].

Currently cavernous sinus surgery is criticized by some authors [5]. However, the aim is to achieve clinical improvement and avoiding damaging the cavernous sinus. The therapy of cavernous sinus tumors is mainly multidisciplinary, involving primarily the endocrinologist, oncologist, radiotherapist and surgeon. Surgery still remains a cornerstone in the treatment of cavernous sinus neoplasms because it allows a true definition of cavernous sinus invasion, histopathological diagnosis, tumor debulking and, in some cases, a cure of the patient. A single golden standard in cavernous sinus surgery does not exist, since the technique has to be adapted to the biological and anatomical features of the tumor. The transcranial approach remains the main procedure for meningiomas and vascular malformation, or for tumors with a major intradural component. Interest has increased though for the use of anterior extracranial approaches in the treatment of non-meningeal tumors.

Pituitary surgeons have always adventured in the lateral sellar compartment to remove intracavernous extensions of sellar tumors. In these circumstances a gentle, though mostly blind, use of the curettes was performed.

The first anterior extracranial approach to the cavernous sinus was described by Laws et al. [6] in 1979 for the treatment of a carotid-cavernous fistula through a contralateral ethmoid-sphenoidal approach. Later several microscopic anterior approaches were proposed for the treatment of cavernous sinus pathologies: transphenoethmoidal [7], transmaxillosphenoidal [8], transmaxillary [9] transmaxillary-transnasal [10], and recently an extended transphenoidal approach with submucosal posterior ethmoidectomy [11]. These approaches

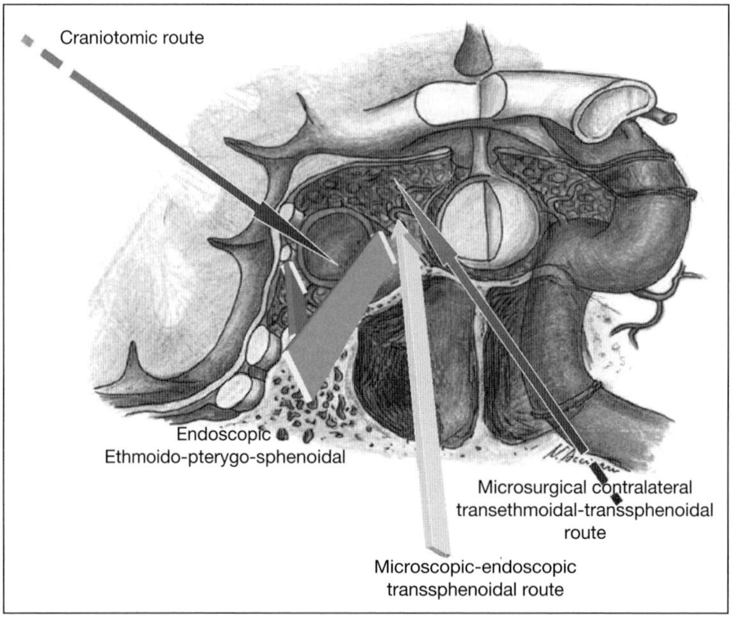

Fig. 1. Different surgical route to the cavernous sinus. The EPSea creates a frontal exposure of the cavernous sinus giving access to the medial and lateral compartments. The surgeon is able to work coaxially to the cavernous sinus (CS), avoiding blind and/or crossing maneuvers.

were suggested to overcome the limit of every microscopic technique: a reduced peripheral vision. These techniques impose the creation of a wide surgical channel to allow adequate exposure of the surgical field. Still, as these channels are relatively narrow in anterior approaches, conical and converging, they do not allow wide and direct view of cavernous sinus especially on its lateral compartment [12, 13].

The introduction of the endoscope in the armamentarium of pituitary surgeons [14] has permitted the possibility of a wide peripheral and endocavitary vision through a limited surgical channel and, above all, an adequate lateral control of the cavernous sinus regions by means of different angled endoscopes. The results attained in the treatment of pituitary adenomas, the development of the specific technology and instrumentation pushed us to apply endoscopic endonasal surgery to the treatment of cavernous sinus tumors. Detailed anatomical studies [15, 16] have recently shown the feasibility and efficacy of the endoscope in exploring the lateral sellar compartment (fig. 1).

Since 1998, at the Bellaria Hospital of Bologna, we have used the endoscopic endonasal technique in the surgical treatment of more than 500 lesions

Table 1. Histopathological diagnosis of the 84 lesions invading the cavernous sinus which were treated from 1998 to December 2004

Histopathology	Patients	
	n	%
Pituitary adenomas	65	77.3
Chordomas	10	14.2
Neurinoma V c.n.	2	2.3
Inflammatory disease (Toulosa-Hunt)	2	2.3
Hemangiomas	2	2.3
Chondrosarcomas	2	2.3
Meningiomas	1	1.1

involving the sellar region. Patients operated from May 1998 to February 2005 and clinically evaluated until July 2005 for lesions with cavernous sinus invasion were selected (table 1). Here only patients affected by pituitary adenomas are evaluated because they are the most representative and homogeneous group of patients.

Patients, Material and Methods

Between May 1998 and February 2005, 84 patients affected by tumors involving the cavernous sinus were treated at the Bellaria Hospital of Bologna (table 1). Pituitary adenomas are the most representative and homogenous group of patients in this series; they represent 15.5% (n = 65: 36 males and 29 females) of all the pituitary adenomas (n = 435) treated in this period. Pituitary adenomas compressing and not invading the cavernous sinus were excluded.

Ages ranged from 18 to 70 (mean 51.2) years. Follow-up was at least 6 (mean 36; maximum 67) months.

The classification of Knosp et al. [17] was used to describe cavernous sinus involvement as evidenced by MRI.

We performed an intraoperative evaluation of cavernous sinus invasion in each case, which was classified according to 5 grades: 0 = no involvement; 1 = compression/invagination of the medial wall with no invasion (fig. 2); 2 = focal extension through one or more little pit holes of the medial wall (fig. 3, 4); 3 = multifocal invasion without encasement of ICA (fig. 5), and 4 = total encasement of the ICA. Therefore patients included in this work had an Intraoperative Cavernous Sinus Invasion index (ICSI) of 2 or more.

Pituitary adenomas were histologically and immunohistochemically investigated. They are classified as functioning (GH-, PRL- and ACTH-secreting adenomas) or nonfunctioning adenomas in relation to the clinical activity. The proliferative index (Ki-67) was measured in all cases; p53 was measured only in some patients and therefore was not included in the overall evaluation.

Endocrinological cure was defined as follows. In GH adenomas, remission was defined by basal serum GH level of <2.5 ng/ml, normal sex- and age-adjusted IGF-1 level, GH nadir <1 ng/ml after OGTT [18]. In PRL-secreting adenomas, remission is defined as having normal serum PRL levels (<30 ng/ml in females, <15 ng/ml in males) at the latest check-up, without

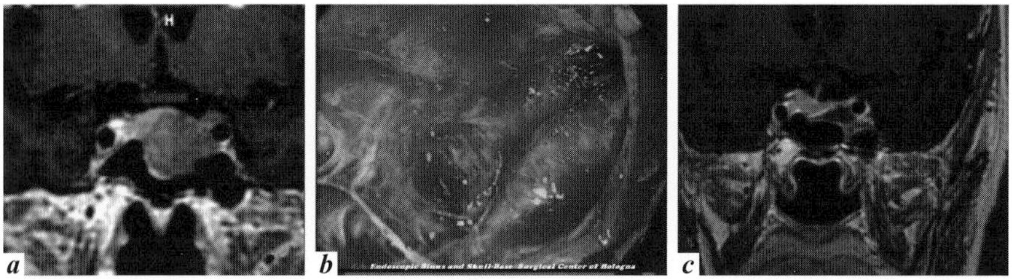

Fig. 2. RM, a 73-year-old female affected by nonfunctioning adenoma stage 2 of the Knosp classification complaining of mild visual disturbances. ***a*** Presurgical MRI. ***b*** Intraoperative view with 30° endoscope after tumor removal using the FEPS procedure. The medial wall of the left cavernous sinus is clearly visible without interruption. ICSI grade 1. ***c*** Five months after surgery, MRI confirms the gross total removal of the tumor.

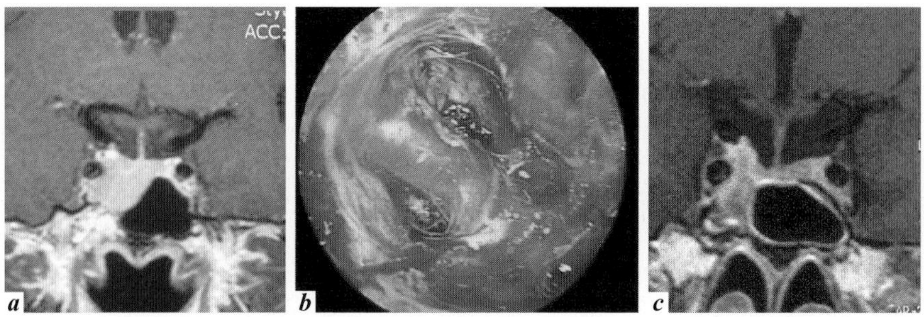

Fig. 3. SL, a 53-year-old male affected by acromegaly due to a GH adenoma, stage 2 of the Knosp classification. ***a*** Presurgical MRI. ***b*** Intraoperative view with 30° endoscope after tumor removal using the FEPS procedure. Two focal dehiscences of the right cavernous sinus medial wall are clearly visible superior and inferior to the ICA. ICSI grade 2. ***c*** The postoperative MRI control documenting the total tumor removal (postoperative MRI evaluation grade 1). The endocrinological remission was obtained (clinical evaluation grade 1) and the patient was classified as being in grade 1 of the comprehensive classification.

previously having had dopaminergic therapy for at least 2 months [19]. In ACTH adenomas, remission is defined by an early morning cortisol level of <50 nmol/l, requiring substitutive therapy and then by the normalization of 24-hour urinary free cortisol levels [20].

All patients were classified at follow-up in relation to three parameters (table 2): the entity of tumor removal at the 3- to 6-month follow-up MRI; evaluation of clinical symptoms and/or endocrinological status, and a comprehensive evaluation crossing the MRI and clinical data at the 6-month follow-up.

Tumor removal was judged on the basis of MRI control: 1 = radical, no evidence of residual tumor; 2 = subtotal, residual tumor of <20%; 3 = partial, residual tumor of <50%, and 4 = insufficient, residual tumor of >50%.

We defined the clinical parameter as follows: 1 = cure, complete symptom resolution in nonfunctioning adenomas and endocrinological cure in functioning adenomas; 2 = improvement,

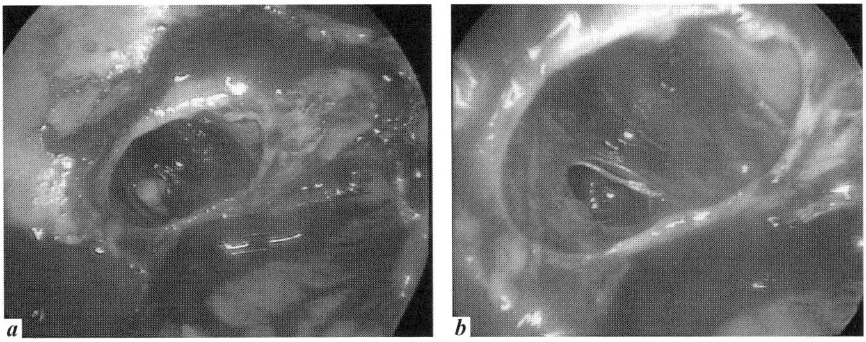

Fig. 4. OG, a 56-year-old man affected by acromegaly due to a GH microadenoma. Intraoperative view during the FEPS procedure with a 0° endoscope. ***a*** After removal of the intrasellar portion of the adenoma a residual was visible infiltrating the right cavernous sinus medial wall. ***b*** After removal of the focal invasion of the cavernous sinus (ICSI grade 2), the pit hole in the medial wall is visible.

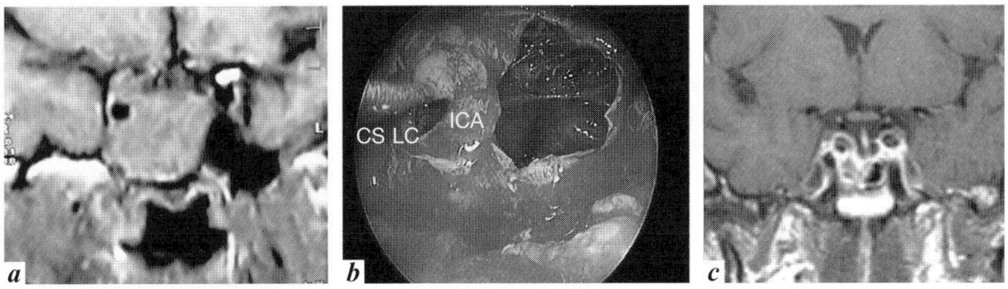

Fig. 5. GA, a 70-year-old male affected by acromegaly due to a GH- and PRL-secreting adenoma in MEN-1 syndrome. The preoperative Knosp classification was grade 2. ***a*** Presurgical MRI. ***b*** Intraoperative view with 0° endoscope during tumor removal by EPSea. Tumor invasion in the medial as well as lateral right cavernous sinus (CS) compartment. ***c*** Postoperative MRI documenting total tumor removal (postoperative MRI evaluation grade 1). Endocrinological remission was obtained (clinical evaluation grade 1) and the patient was classified as being in grade 1 of the comprehensive classification.

partial resolution of symptoms (i.e. sensible improvement of hemianopia or clinical improvement without hormonal remission), and 3 = no cure, no symptom resolution.

Finally, the comprehensive evaluation was defined as: 1 = cured, radical removal and clinical cure; 2 = controlled, subtotal removal with symptoms resolution; 3 = improved, radical removal with amelioration of symptoms and/or biohumoral parameters, without resolution, and 4 = not cured, residual tumor with persistent symptoms.

Fisher's exact test was used for statistical analysis.

Preoperative and Postoperative Evaluation

All patients underwent preoperative endocrinological, neuroradiological and neuro-ophthalmological evaluation. After an overnight fast, plasma samples were collected for the

Table 2. Parameters used for surgical outcome analysis

MRI evaluation	Clinical evaluation	Comprehensive evaluation
Radical removal No residue	Symptoms resolution and/or endocrinological cure	Cured (no residual; no symptoms; endocrinological remission)
Remnant <20%	Partial resolution	Controlled (residual without symptoms)
Remnant <50%	Unchanged	Improved (no residual tumor; mild symptoms)
Remnant >50%	–	Not cured (residual tumor with symptoms)

measurement of cortisol, free thyroxine, thyrotropin, corticotropin (ACTH), prolactin (PRL), growth hormone (GH), luteinizing hormone, follicle-stimulating hormone, insulin-like grown factor-I, testosterone (in males) and estradiol (in females). A 24-hour urine collection was obtained for the measurement of urinary free cortisol.

All patients underwent radiological assessments by means of MRI and CT scans. All patients received short-term prophylaxis with 1 g cefazolin intravenously during the induction and 1 g intravenously after 6 h. Patients with secondary hypoadrenalism received a loading dose of a 50- to 100-mg infusion of hydrocortisone.

Our postoperative protocol consists of an endocrinological evaluation on the 3rd day and again at 1, 3 and 6 months. MRI follow-up is performed routinely at 3 and 6 months postoperatively and then yearly. Early neuroradiological examinations by MRI or CT are carried out for specific indications. An endoscopic rhinologic evaluation is carried out 1 month postoperatively to evaluate the normalization of the nasal and sphenoid cavities. A neuro-ophthalmological control is performed 3 months after surgery only in case of preoperative dysfunction or postoperatively referred visual disturbances.

Instrumentation

The instrumentation used in the endoscopic technique is a Xenon 300-watt cold light fountain source, an endoscopic video camera and a video recorder. The endoscopes are 0°, 30° and 45° Hopkins® telescopes, 4 mm in diameter, and 18 mm long. A cleansing system with pedal control is used to reduce the necessity of extracting the telescope from the nose every time the vision becomes unclear. During the tumor removal phase, we use a mechanical holder for the endoscope to allow the surgeon to work with both hands. The camera zoom allows a better definition of anatomical features and the positioning of the endoscope further away from the surgical field, reducing the possibility of contamination of the tip of the telescope by blood.

Technical Adjuncts

Computer-assisted navigation and microdoppler are often used in the cavernous sinus to localize the ICA before incision of the cavernous sinus wall and during tumor debulking.

Surgical Technique

Surgery is carried out under general anesthesia using orotracheal intubation; the patient is placed in a half-sitting position with his head turned towards the surgeon and resting freely in the horseshoe head holder. When the neuronavigator is required the head is fixed in a three-pin holder (Mayfield). The oropharynx is packed with moist gauze to prevent blood and secretions from reaching the stomach from the operative site. The nose and face are cleaned with soap and aqueous solutions. The nasal mucous membranes are decongested with Xilocaine® 5%. The periumbilical abdomen is routinely prepared for the eventual harvest of a free fat graft.

Two different surgical approaches can be used for pituitary adenomas involving the cavernous sinus: the classic functional endoscopic pituitary surgery (FEPS) or the ethmoid-pterygoid-sphenoidal endoscopic approach (EPSea). The choice of the approach is based on the grade and type of cavernous sinus invasion. When the invasion is confined to the medial and postero-superior compartment, FEPS may be sufficient. When the tumor invades the antero-inferior and lateral compartments of the cavernous sinus, EPSea is required (fig. 1).

The operation is usually performed through one nostril, which is the one with the larger cavity in FEPS and homolateral to the involved cavernous sinus in EPSea.

Functional Endoscopic Pituitary Surgery (FEPS)

The surgical procedure can be schematically divided into 3 stages.

Stage I: Localization of Sellar Wall

The lateral dislocation of the middle and upper turbinate allows the localization of the sphenoethmoidal recess and the natural ostium of the sphenoid sinus.

The opening of the sphenoid sinus starts with the enlargement of the natural ostium, with a Kerrison or a Stammberger punch. A semilunar incision is made in the vomer to separate the mucoperiostium from the bone of the vomer and the natural ostium of the sphenoid sinuses. In cases of difficult exposition of the sphenoid ostium, the entry point to the sphenoid sinus may be obtained through a direct perforation of the anterior wall at the junction of the keel of the sphenoid bone and the posterior nasal septum, approximately 1 cm above the rim of the choana and close to the septum.

The access to the sphenoid sinus should be widened, extending from the roof to the floor of the sphenoid vertically and exceeding the sphenoid ostia laterally. All the intersinusal septa, which reduce the vision and limit the maneuverability in front of the sella, have to be removed. It is not necessary to remove the sphenoid mucosa because with the opening of the natural ostium the risk of postoperative mucocele is very low; preserving the mucosa indeed permits faster postoperative stabilization of the sphenoid cavity with a decreased incidence of sphenoid flogosis or disventilation.

The opening of the sellar floor should be extended to the bone overlying the invaded cavernous sinus.

Stage II: Adenomectomy

After dural opening the pituitary adenoma is removed with the combined use of curettes and aspirator. Subsequently either the opening of the medial wall created by the tumor is used to enter the medial compartment of the cavernous sinus or an incision of the medial wall is performed in a safe area. Recognition of this area is possible either through the identification of the bulging created by the tumor itself or through the accurate location of the ICA, by means of microdoppler and neuronavigation. The removal of the tumor inside the cavernous sinus is relatively safe due to the absence of cranial nerves and is always performed under direct view, avoiding any blind procedure.

Stage III: Final Exploration and Closure of the Surgical Field

After hemostasis is obtained using cotton packing, free hand exploration into the surgical field with angled 30° and 45° optic scopes is recommended to localize and remove any remnant tumor.

In the absence of CSF leaks, the surgical cavity is packed with Gelfoam®; if a CSF leak is detected or suspected, autologous fat is applied in the sellar cavity and the dural gap may also be closed with a middle turbinate mucoperiostial graft.

The sphenoid sinus is gently packed with Gelfoam® and, finally, the middle turbinate is medially displaced from its normal position. Nasal packing is not routinely required if the middle turbinate has not been resected. Lumbar drainage is not usually used.

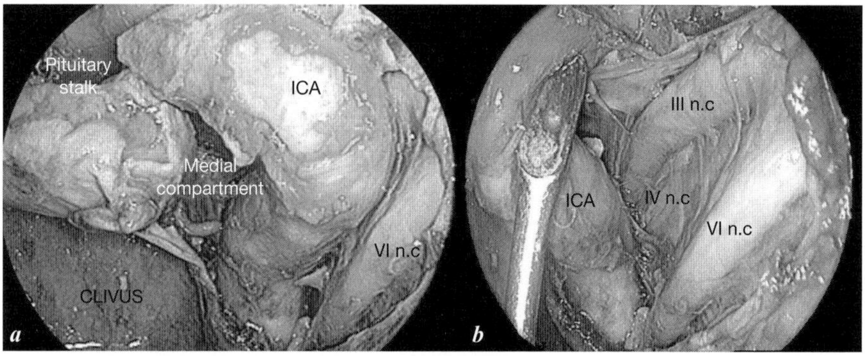

Fig. 6. Anatomical dissection of the left cavernous sinus. ***a*** The medial compartment lies between the ICA and the medial wall of the cavernous sinus. No nerves cross over this area. The meningo-hypophysial artery is clearly visible running in the inferior portion. ***b*** The antero-inferior and lateral compartments are exposed. The 6th n.c. runs free inferior and lateral to the ICA. The 3rd, 4th and 5th are embedded and protected between the endosteal and meningeal layers of the lateral wall.

Ethmoid-Pterygoid-Sphenoidal Endoscopic Approach

EPSea is used for tumors whose major component is in the cavernous sinus. This type of procedure permits the total exposure of the cavernous sinus with the possibility of a direct control of the lateral as well as the medial compartment of the cavernous sinus (fig. 6). The procedure can be schematically divided into 3 stages.

Stage I: Approach to the Parasellar Area

The procedure is performed in a freehand fashion by means of a 0° endoscope or more rarely a 30° endoscope.

An ethmoidal route is used and a complete sphenoethmoidectomy with a wide meatotomy is required. The medial portion of the posterior wall of the maxillary sinus is resected to expose the posterior wall of maxillary antrum and the vertical process of palatine bone. Resection of the middle and superior turbinate allows a peripheral view of all the sellar and parasellar region and improves the maneuverability of surgical instruments in the region. The vertical portion of insertion at the skull base of the middle turbinate is usually kept in place. The sphenoid sinus and its septa are removed as in the FEPS. After ligation of the sphenopalatine artery, the medial pterygoid process is drilled out. Resection of the medial pterygoid process enables exposure of the inferolateral portion of cavernous sinus. Partial resection of the pterygoid process is carried out taking into account the degree of pneumatization of the lateral recess of the sphenoid and the need for visualization of the lateral and inferior walls of the sphenoid sinus.

Stage II: Opening of the Cavernous Sinus and Removal of the Tumor

This stage is performed after the endoscope has been fixed on its holder. With the exception of a tumor exclusively located in the lateral portion of the cavernous sinus, the dural opening is made in the sellar region and progressively enlarged following the tumor from its medial to its lateral portion.

The tumor may displace the ICA medially or laterally when involving the lateral or medial compartments of cavernous sinus, respectively. Moreover, besides the displacement in a coronal plane of the ICA, it is also important to remember changes in position in the axial and sagittal

Table 3. Referral symptoms

Symptoms	Patients	
	n	%
Endocrine symptoms	23	35
Regrowth/residual	14	21.5
Visual deficits	12	18.5
Pituitary apoplexy	5	8
Neurological deficits	6	9
Incidentaloma	5	8

planes. In cases of lesions involving the antero-inferior compartment of cavernous sinus, the ICA is generally displaced posteriorly. In this case, the lesion covers the vessel and thereby renders the opening of the dura less dangerous. On the other hand, in cases of lesions arising postero-superiorly, the ICA is displaced anteriorly and behind the dura. In this latter case, it is mandatory to exactly locate the position of the ICA before any dura incision is performed; this is accomplished with the combined use of neuronavigation and microdoppler.

After dural incision, by means curettes it is possible to mobilize the tumor fragments before their suction and/or removal.

Stage III: Final Exploration and Closure of the Surgical Defect

Venous bleeding is usually not noteworthy and is generally well controlled with Gelfoam® and cotton packing. After tumor removal venous bleeding is possible and is well controlled with the usual hemostatic agents.

At the end of the tumor resection, inspection of the surgical field through angled endoscopes, such as the 30° and the 45°, permits the detection and removal of neoplastic residues.

Nasal packing with a single Merocel® is usually kept in place for 2 days.

Results

All patients harbored macroadenomas, invading the cavernous sinus. Referral symptoms are shown in table 3.

FEPS was used in 32 patients, while in the remaining 33 the EPSea was performed. The median surgical time was 45 (35–90) min for the FEPS and 90 (60–180) min for the EPSea. There was no perioperative mortality. Patients' hospital stay was between 2 and 91 (median 4) days.

Neuroradiological Classification and Intraoperative Cavernous Sinus Invasion

Table 4 shows the comparison of the preoperative Knosp classification and ICSI. For this work, only pituitary adenomas that had evidence of ICSI were included (i.e. all adenomas with an ICSI of 2 or more).

Table 4. Comparison of the preoperative Knosp classification and the intraoperative classification of cavernous sinus invasion

MRI Knosp	Intraoperative cavernous sinus invasion		
	2	3	4
0	2	0	0
1	0	0	0
2	11	5	0
3	9	12	3
4	0	15	8
Total	22 (34%)	32 (49%)	11 (17%)

Table 5. Comprehensive evaluation of this series

Type of tumor	Comprehensive evaluation				
	n	1	2	3	4
GH	16	7 (44%)	0	3 (18.5%)	6 (37.5%)
PRL	11	4 (36.5%)	0	0	7 (63.5%)
ACTH	3	2 (66.5%)	0	0	1 (33.5%)
Nonfunctioning	35	21 (60%)	9 (25.5%)	0	5 (14.5%)
Total	65	34 (52%)	9 (14%)	3 (5%)	19 (29%)

Endocrinological Results

Thirty patients presented functioning adenomas: of these 13 patients had complete remission of the endocrinological picture (table 5). Four of 11 PRL-secreting adenomas, which were operated due to resistance to medical therapy, obtained endocrinological cure. Two of 3 ACTH-secreting adenomas were cured. Seven of 16 acromegalics were in remission after surgery.

Visual and Neurological Outcome

Visual function improved in the majority of patients (25/28) and was unchanged in 2 cases. In 1 case visual worsening was due to overpacking of the surgical cavity.

Table 6. Postoperative outcome of neurological symptoms

Neurological symptoms	Preoperative	Postoperative
Oculomotor nerve	3	0
Abducens nerve	5	1
Trigeminal pain	5	0

Table 7. Complications seen in the series

	Patients	
	n	%
Surgical complications		
Postoperative CSF leak	3	4.5
Hematoma	1	1.5
Overpacking	1	1.5
Medical complications		
Adrenocortical insufficiency	1	1.5
Transient DI	1	1.5
Permanent DI	1	1.5

All preoperative neurological symptoms (table 6) resolved after surgery except an abducens nerve palsy. There was no additional cranial nerve palsy after surgery.

Complications

Surgical and medical complications are summarized in table 7.

In 10 cases there was intraoperative evidence of a CSF leak making a reconstruction procedure necessary with the use of abdominal fat or fascia lata, together with mucoperiostium of the middle turbinate. Three patients experienced delayed postoperative CSF leak, which required reintervention.

In 1 case worsening of a visual deficit was observed. It was related to overpacking of the sella and was only partially corrected by early surgical revision. One patient who underwent partial removal of the tumor was re-operated using a transcranial approach due to residual tumor hemorrhagic infarction in the temporal lobe.

Among the medical complications, we experienced 1 patient with ACTH insufficiency which required substitutive therapy, 1 patient with transient and 1 patient with permanent diabetes insipidus.

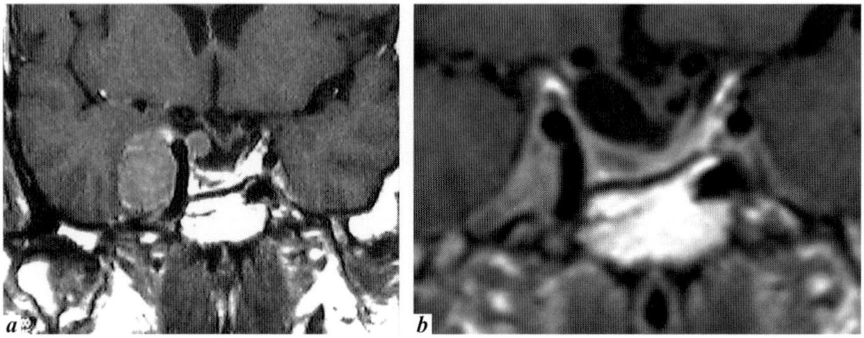

Fig. 7. NE, a 65-year-old man affected by a recurring PRL pituitary adenoma unresponsive to medical treatment. ***a*** Presurgical MRI documenting invasion of the lateral right cavernous sinus compartment; a proliferative index (Ki-67) of more than 10% was evident after the tumor removal. ***b*** MRI control 3 years after surgery and radiosurgical treatment.

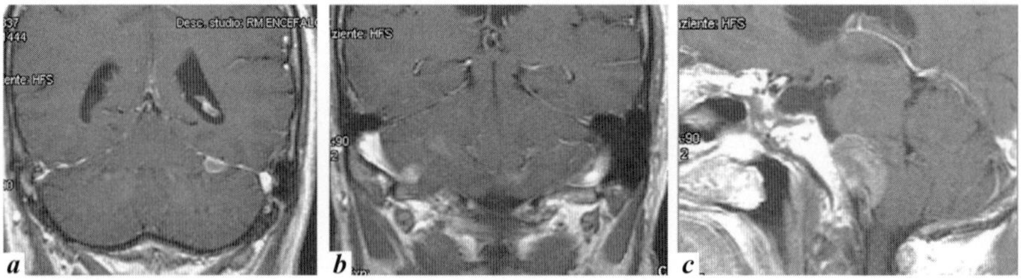

Fig. 8. NE, follow-up after 6 years. The MRI control shows 3 different metastases: tentorial (***a***), right cerebellar (***b***) and retroclival (***c***) clival metastases. The last one required a retrosigmoid approach.

One patient died 3 months after surgery due to tumor progression; multiple brain metastases were discovered at autopsy. One patient died after 2 years due to unrelated myocardial ischemia. Six years after surgery, 1 patient developed multiple brain metastases; he underwent a retrosigmoid approach for removal of symptomatic clival lesions and is still alive (fig. 7, 8).

No recurrences have yet been observed in the patients who underwent total resection.

Histopathological Findings

Table 8 shows the immunohistochemical diagnosis in the present series. In every surgical specimen the Ki-67 proliferative index was measured: in the majority of cases it was less than 3% (<1%, n =23; 1–3%, n = 27); in 13 cases it was between 3 and 10%.

Table 8. Proliferative index and comprehensive evaluation

Ki-67	Comprehensive evaluation		
	n	cure (1)	no cure (2, 3, 4)
<3%	50	31	19
>3%	15	3	12
Total		34 (52%)	31 (48%)

Table 9. Results of MRI control 3–6 months after surgery

Type of tumor	Follow-up MRI				
	n	1	2	3	4
GH	16	11	4	1	0
PRL	11	4	6	1	0
ACTH	3	2	1	0	0
Nonfunctioning	35	21	8	5	1
Total		38 (58.5%)	19 (29%)	7 (11%)	1 (1.5%)

In 2 cases the proliferative index was higher than 10%. These 2 cases were both positive for p53 and developed metastases (fig. 7, 8).

The proliferative index of the tumors was not statistically associated with the ICSI (Fisher's exact test, $p = 0.7565$).

When the Ki-67 proliferative index was matched with the final clinical outcome, the two-sided p value was very significant ($p = 0.0065$; table 8): patients harboring pituitary adenomas with a proliferative index of <3% had a better chance of remission at the 6-month follow-up.

MRI Results

The first follow-up MRI documented (table 9): no residual tumor in 58.5% of the cases; 29% with subtotal removal; 11% with partial, and 1.5% with insufficient removal.

Overall Evaluation of Surgical Results

Finally, we judged the patients as: cured in 52%; improved in 6%; controlled in 17%, and not cured in 29% of the cases (table 5).

Discussion

The choice of surgical procedure (i.e. transcranial or extracranial) for cavernous sinus tumors is planned on the basis of morphology, direction of growth and biological behavior of the tumor. Intradural tumors that tend to infiltrate surrounding vessels, such as meningiomas, are better approached through a transcranial approach. Extradural neoplasia growing antero-inferiorly are better approached through an anterior extracranial approach, which follows the direction of growth: from the sella in case of pituitary adenomas, and from the clivus in chordomas or chondrosarcomas.

The transsphenoidal approach is the most used among the anterior extracranial approaches [21], and although neurosurgeons were reluctant to extend surgery laterally in the cavernous sinus, parasellar tumors have been operated on via this route for a long time [13]. Its main limit in cavernous sinus surgery is the strictly median access, which carries the risk during the blind use of curettes when the lateral sellar compartment is not adequately exposured.

This limit is witnessed by the search for variations in the classic microscopic transsphenoidal approach with the aim of improving surgical exposure of the cavernous sinus. In 1979, Laws et al. [6] proposed a cross-court approach using a contralateral transethmoidal-transsphenoidal approach providing an improved exposure of the contralateral medial compartment of the cavernous sinus. Lalwani et al. [7] resorted to this route using a Lynch incision and combined this with a medial maxillectomy when necessary. Arita et al. [22], using a slightly modified speculum, proposed another 'cross-court' approach. Fraioli et al. [8], developing on the anatomic study by Inoue et al. [23], suggested an infero-medial exposure of the cavernous sinus adding a maxillary osteotomy or fracturing the medial wall of the maxillary sinus in the standard transsphenoidal approach, and the use of a modified speculum. A distant lateral infero-medial route combined with a transmaxillary transsphenoidal approach was proposed by Sabit et al. [9] to allow a safe extradural lateral to medial passage in the parasellar region. Recently, Kitano and Taneda [11] suggested an extended microscopic transsphenoidal approach with a submucosal posterior ethmoidectomy.

In spite of the wider exposure allowed by these different approaches, the surgical route to the cavernous sinus remains narrow, rigid, with limited lateral visualization due to the use of the speculum and the optical features of the microscope.

At the same time the improvements in radiotherapeutic techniques lead to the increasing application of radiation therapy, especially radiosurgery, in the treatment of cavernous sinus tumors [24]. The efficacy and extremely low morbidity of these alternative techniques has led to the growing philosophy of refraining from surgery in the cavernous sinus [5].

Recently, the endoscope has been introduced in the armamentarium of the pituitary surgeon and has lead to the introduction of new approaches to the cavernous sinus, encouraged by the peripheral view given by the endoscope. Detailed anatomical studies [15, 16] have recently shown the feasibility and efficacy of the endoscope in exploring the lateral sellar compartment. Alfieri and Jho [15] described three different endoscopic routes to the cavernous sinus in their cadaveric dissection: the paraseptal as a median one; the middle turbinectomy as a lateral approach, and the middle meatal as a far lateral approach.

We have used two different endoscopic endonasal approaches to deal with tumors invading the cavernous sinus: FEPS, a median one, and EPSea, a lateral one. The choice of the approach is based on the grade and type of cavernous sinus invasion. When the invasion is confined to the medial and postero-superior compartment FEPS may be sufficient. When the tumor also invades the antero-inferior and lateral compartments of the cavernous sinus, EPSea is required.

The complication rate in our series of pituitary adenomas invading the cavernous sinus appears to be extremely low. Our data favorably compare with the recently published experience with the microscopic transsphenoidal extended approach [5].

We therefore believe that the central role of surgery in cavernous sinus tumors should be reevaluated, considering that it remains the only technique that allows an inspective diagnosis of the cavernous sinus invasion, a histopathological diagnosis, and early tumoral volume decompression.

Definition of True Cavernous Sinus Involvement

Numerous studies have dealt with the predictive value of preoperative neuroimaging of cavernous sinus invasion. Knosp et al. [17] suggested a specific classification of cavernous sinus invasion based on the position of the lateral portion of the tumor in relation to the ICA. We classified all our pituitary adenomas according to the Knosp classification and compared them to intraoperative findings: statistical analysis showed a good predictive value for low and high grades but a low predictive value was evident for grade-2 adenomas [Frank and Pasquini, unpublished data].

This finding confirms other authors' reports [17, 25] of a low predictive value for grade-2 cavernous sinus invasion in the Knosp classification. Our data could also be explained by the increased visualization allowed by the endoscope which permitted the visualization of minor tumoral extensions through small focal dehiscences of the medial wall of the cavernous sinus; we found these minor cavernous sinus invasions in pituitary adenomas independent of their size. This might explain the higher percentage of pituitary adenomas in this series in comparison to others [13, 26].

The specificity of the remaining Knosp classification grades is high but not absolute. We have indeed experienced cavernous sinus invasion when none was expected from the neuroradiological study and found no invasion when the MRI was highly suggestive of cavernous sinus invasion. The limits of neuroradiological studies are due to the present inability of clearly demonstrating the medial wall of the cavernous sinus, especially in the presence of a lesion in the sellar area. Surgery remains the only way to ascertain the presence or absence of cavernous sinus invasion.

Histopathological Evaluation

The aim of histopathological diagnosis is equally important. Tissue analysis is extremely important in the specific therapeutic management of each patient. Statistical analysis of the results of our series indicated that the proliferative index Ki-67 was the most significant factor for patient's outcome (table 5). These data suggest the high significance of the proliferative index, which should therefore be included among the factors that influence the postoperative treatment of the patient (for example, radiosurgery of a small asymptomatic residue with a high proliferative index or clinical follow-up if there is a low Ki-67).

The proliferative index was not statistically associated with the ICSI grading; this was not related to the overall evaluation grading. However, the biological features of the tumor are the most important factor for the patient's prognosis.

Tumor Debulking

From a therapeutic point of view the ideal goal is the cure of the patient, which can be obtained only in a few cases. In our series in functional adenoma remission was obtained in 13/30 cases. In nonfunctioning adenomas radical removal of the adenoma without any new deficit was obtained in 21/35 cases.

Improvement of symptoms can be obtained by surgical decompression, even with long-lasting pre-surgical deficits, as reported by other authors [13]. In our experience 34/38 cranial nerve deficits improved after surgery.

As well as having a rapid effect on neurological deficits, tumoral volume reduction might play an important role in the response of the tumor to adjuvant therapies.

Tumor debulking is important to achieve safety and efficacy of radiation therapy because it reduces the tumor residual volume and increases the distance from radiosensitive structures, such as optic nerves and chiasm [27].

Petrossians et al. [28] recently reported that tumor debulking increases the likelihood of achieving biochemical disease control with somatostatin analogs in acromegalic patients with adenomas that were not amenable to complete surgical resection and in whom primary somatostatin analog therapy was unable to achieve good biochemical control.

Conclusions

In our experience the endoscopic endonasal approach allows safe and effective management of the tumors with cavernous sinus extension, probably due to the increased visualization with avoidance of blind curettage. FEPS can be adequate for minor extension limited to the medial or postero-superior compartments. We have used the extended approach (EPSea) for major lateral or antero-inferior involvement of the cavernous sinus.

The aim of surgery is to confirm the cavernous sinus invasion, to reach a histological diagnosis, which should include the measurement of the proliferative index, and to remove the tumor as radically and safely as possible.

The actual lower complication rates and the important benefits that can be obtained with endoscopic endonasal cavernous sinus surgery should lead to a reevaluation of the role of surgery in the challenging multidisciplinary pathology of pituitary adenomas invading the cavernous sinus.

Acknowledgement

The authors thank Dr. Francesco Doglietto for his invaluable support in the manuscript preparation and Prof. Manfred Tschabitscher for his anatomic assistance.

References

1 Winslow JB: Exposition anatomique de la structure du corps humain, vol II. London, Prevast, 1734, p 29.
2 Parkinson D: Lateral sellar compartment O.T. (cavernous sinus): history, anatomy, terminology. Anat Rec 1998;251:486–490.
3 Parkinson D: A surgical approach to the cavernous portion of the carotid artery. Anatomical studies and case report. J Neurosurg 1965;23:474–483.
4 Sekhar LN, Goel A, Sen CN: Cavernous sinus tumours; in Apuzzo MLJ (ed): Brain Surgery: Complication Avoidance and Management. New York, Churchill Livingstone, 1993, pp 2197–2218.
5 Couldwell WT, Weiss MH, Rabb C, Liu JK, Apfelbaum RI, Fukushima T: Variations on the standard transsphenoidal approach to the sellar region, with emphasis on the extended approaches and parasellar approaches: surgical experience in 105 cases. Neurosurgery 2004;55:539–547.
6 Laws ER Jr, Onofrio BM, Pearson BW, McDonald TJ, Dirrenberger RA: Successful management of bilateral carotid-cavernous fistulae with a trans-sphenoidal approach. Neurosurgery 1979;4:162–167.
7 Lalwani AK, Kaplan MJ, Gutin PH: The transsphenoethmoid approach to the sphenoid sinus and clivus. Neurosurgery 1992;31:1008–1014.
8 Fraioli B, Esposito V, Santoro A, Iannetti G, Giuffre R, Cantore G: Transmaxillosphenoidal approach to tumors invading the medial compartment of the cavernous sinus. J Neurosurg 1995;82:63–69.

9 Sabit I, Schaefer SD, Couldwell WT: Extradural extranasal combined transmaxillary transsphenoidal approach to the cavernous sinus: a minimally invasive microsurgical model. Laryngoscope 2000;110:286–291.
10 Rabadan A, Conesa H: Transmaxillary-transnasal approach to the anterior clivus: a microsurgical anatomical model. Neurosurgery 1992;30:473–482.
11 Kitano M, Taneda M: Extended transsphenoidal approach with submucosal posterior ethmoidectomy for parasellar tumors. Technical note. J Neurosurg 2001;94:999–1004.
12 Hashimoto N, Kikuchi H: Transsphenoidal approach to infrasellar tumors involving the cavernous sinus. J Neurosurg 1990;73:513–517.
13 Fahlbusch R, Buchfelder M: Transsphenoidal surgery of parasellar pituitary adenomas. Acta Neurochir 1988;92:93–99.
14 Jho HD, Carrau RL: Endoscopic endonasal transsphenoidal surgery: experience with 50 patients. J Neurosurg 1997;87:44–51.
15 Alfieri A, Jho HD: Endoscopic endonasal approaches to the cavernous sinus: surgical approaches. Neurosurgery 2001;49:354–360.
16 Cavallo LM, Cappabianca P, Galzio R, Iaconetta G, de Divitiis E, Tschabitscher M: Endoscopic transnasal approach to the cavernous sinus versus transcranial route: anatomic study. Neurosurgery 2005;56(suppl):379–389.
17 Knosp E, Steiner E, Kitz K, Matula C: Pituitary adenomas with invasion of the cavernous sinus space: a magnetic resonance imaging classification compared with surgical findings. Neurosurgery 1993;33:610–617.
18 Giustina A, Barkan A, Casanueva FF, Cavagnini F, Frohman L, Ho K, Veldhuis J, Wass J, Von Werder K, Melmed S: Criteria for cure of acromegaly: a consensus statement. J Clin Endocrinol Metab 2000;85:526–529.
19 Losa M, Mortini P, Barzaghi R, Gioia L, Giovanelli M: Surgical treatment of prolactin-secreting pituitary adenomas: early results and long-term outcome. J Clin Endocrinol Metab 2002;87: 3180–3186.
20 Nishizawa S, Oki Y, Ohta S, Yokota N, Yokoyama T, Uemura K: What can predict postoperative 'endocrinological cure' in Cushing's disease? Neurosurgery 1999;45:239–244.
21 Jane JA Jr, Thapar K, Kaptain GJ, Maartens N, Laws ER Jr: Pituitary surgery: transsphenoidal approach. Neurosurgery 2002;51:435–444.
22 Arita K, Kurisu K, Tominaga A, Ohba S, Ikawa F, Iida K, Yoshioka H: Transsphenoidal 'cross court' approach using a slightly modified speculum to reach pituitary adenomas with lateral growth. Acta Neurochir 2000;142:1055–1058.
23 Inoue T, Rhoton AL Jr, Theele D, Barry ME: Surgical approaches to the cavernous sinus: a microsurgical study. Neurosurgery 1990;26:903–932.
24 Shin M, Kurita H, Sasaki T, Tago M, Morita A, Ueki K, Kirino T: Stereotactic radiosurgery for pituitary adenoma invading the cavernous sinus. J Neurosurg 2000;93(suppl 3):2–5.
25 Pinker K, Ba-Ssalamah A, Wolfsberger S, Mlynarik V, Knosp E, Trattnig S: The value of high-field MRI (3T) in the assessment of sellar lesions. Eur J Radiol 2005;54:327–334.
26 Ahmadi J, North CM, Segall HD, Zee CS, Weiss MH: Cavernous sinus invasion by pituitary adenomas. AJR Am J Roentgenol 1986;146:257–262.
27 Liu JK, Schmidt MH, MacDonald JD, Jensen RL, Couldwell WT: Hypophysial transposition (hypophysopexy) for radiosurgical treatment of pituitary tumors involving the cavernous sinus. Technical note. Neurosurg Focus 2003;14:e11.
28 Petrossians P, Borges-Martins L, Espinoza C, Daly A, Betea D, Valdes-Socin H, Stevenaert A, Chanson P, Beckers A: Gross total resection or debulking of pituitary adenomas improves hormonal control of acromegaly by somatostatin analogs. Eur J Endocrinol 2005;152:61–66.

Giorgio Frank, MD
Centre of Surgery for Pituitary Tumours, Department of Neuroscience, Bellaria Hospital
Via Altura 3
IT–40100 Bologna (Italy)
Tel. +39 051 6225111, Fax +39 051 6225347, E-Mail giorgio.frank@ausl.bo.it

Laws ER Jr, Sheehan JP (eds): Pituitary Surgery – A Modern Approach.
Front Horm Res. Basel, Karger, 2006, vol 34, pp 83–104

Diagnosis and Management of Pediatric Sellar Lesions

Jay Jagannathan, Aaron S. Dumont, John A. Jane, Jr.

Department of Neurological Surgery, Health Sciences Center, University of Virginia, Charlottesville, Va., USA

Abstract

Pituitary region tumors in pediatric patients are largely comprised of craniopharyngiomas and pituitary adenomas, each with their unique considerations. Craniopharyngiomas account for the majority of pediatric sellar masses. Pituitary adenomas are relatively uncommon during childhood, although the incidence increases during adolescence. The diagnosis of sellar lesions involves a multidisciplinary effort, and detailed endocrinologic, ophthamologic and neurologic testing are critical. The management of pituitary tumors varies depending on the entity. For most tumors, other than prolactinomas, transsphenoidal resection remains the mainstay of treatment. Less invasive modalities such as endoscopic transsphenoidal surgery, and stereotactic radiosurgery have shown promise as primary and adjuvant treatment modalities, respectively.

Copyright © 2006 S. Karger AG, Basel

Introduction

Pediatric sellar and parasellar lesions represent a diverse group of tumors, the majority of which are benign. Craniopharyngiomas comprise 80–90% of tumors arising in the pituitary region with pituitary adenomas being the next most common lesion. Germinomas, dermoid/epidermoid cysts, lipomas, teratomas and hamartomas also can occur in the sellar region, but are much less common. Other sellar tumors such as meningiomas or gliomas are uncommonly symptomatic during childhood and adolescence. Over the last 30 years, advances in microneurosurgery, neuroimaging and molecular biology have significantly altered the diagnosis and management of sellar lesions. This review focuses on current concepts in understanding these diverse pathological entities.

Classification

Given the variety of tumor types and clinical presentations, an assortment of systems have been proposed to classify pituitary tumors. The most commonly used approaches classify them according to size and functional status. Pituitary adenomas that are $\leq$10 mm are termed microadenomas; those $>$10 mm are identified as macroadenomas.

In addition to classifying tumors based on size, adenomas are also classified based on their functional status. This allows a broad classification into clinically non-secreting adenomas, and those that secrete active hormone(s). These hormonally active tumors include prolactinomas, growth hormone (GH) adenomas, corticotroph adenomas (ACTH) and thyrotroph (TSH) adenomas. Each is associated with specific clinical syndromes. Prolactinomas are associated with galactorrhea, GH excess, causes acromegaly or gigantism, ACTH adenomas cause Cushing's disease, and TSH adenomas are associated with hyperthyroidism.

Confusing the picture somewhat are those tumors that secrete more than one clinically significant hormone. The most common plurihormonal tumors secrete both GH and prolactin (PRL) either in a mixed population of cells or by a single cell population secreting both hormones [1–3]. Further, although the clinical and biochemical functional status generally correlates with the immunohistochemical findings, exceptions do exist. Not all tumors that immunoreact for ACTH, GH or TSH are associated with elevated serum hormone levels. These tumors are considered clinically 'silent'. For example, the silent corticotroph adenoma does not produce hypercortisolemia and the stigmata of Cushing's disease, but stains positively for ACTH. The most comprehensive classification schema that accounts for these exceptions is that of the World Health Organization which codifies tumors based upon: (1) clinical presentation and biochemical secretory activity; (2) size and invasiveness (i.e. micro- versus macroadenoma); (3) histologic features (adenoma versus carcinoma); (4) immunohistochemical profile, and (5) ultrastructural features on electron microscopy [4].

Overview and Epidemiology

Pituitary Adenomas

Pituitary adenomas are the most common cause of pituitary disease in adults but rarely present during childhood (although the incidence increases during adolescence) [5]. Pituitary adenomas constitute less than 3% of supratentorial tumors in children [5], with an average annual incidence of about 0.1/million children [6]. Pituitary carcinomas are rare in adults and even more uncommon in children.

An increased prevalence of pituitary adenomas in females has been reported, most likely reflecting the relative predominance of the two main types of adenomas, PRL- and ACTH-secreting adenomas which are more common in women [5, 6]. Prolactinomas are the most frequent adenoma subtype in children [6, 7]. Between 11 and 15 years of age, ACTH-secreting adenomas are the most frequent cause of adrenal hyperfunction [8]. Most commonly these tumors are small – macroadenomas rarely cause Cushing's disease (CD) in children [8, 9].

GH-secreting adenomas have a prevalence of 50–80 cases/million people [10] in adulthood. Gigantism is extremely rare with approximately 100 reported cases to date. In childhood, GH-secreting adenomas account for 5–15% of all pituitary adenomas. In less than 2% of the cases excessive GH secretion is caused by hypothalamic or ectopic GH-releasing hormone (GHRH)-producing tumor (i.e. bronchial or pancreatic carcinoid) [10].

TSH-secreting adenomas are rare in adulthood and extremely uncommon in childhood and adolescence with only a few case reports in the literature [11]. These tumors frequently occur as macroadenomas, presenting with mass effect symptoms such as headache, visual disturbance, together with variable symptoms and signs of hyperthyroidism. TSH-secreting adenomas must be differentiated from thyroid hormone resistance [4, 11]. In most cases, the classical criteria of a lack of TSH response to thyrotropin-releasing hormone stimulation, elevation of serum α-subunit levels, and a high α-subunit/TSH ratio along with a pituitary mass on magnetic resonance imaging (MRI), are diagnostic of a TSH-secreting adenoma [11, 12].

Craniopharyngiomas

Craniopharyngiomas are a group of slowly growing, benign epithelial neoplasms of the sellar and suprasellar region. Craniopharyngiomas account for the overwhelming majority (~90%) of neoplasms, arising in the pituitary region in the pediatric population [12]. Craniopharyngiomas constitute between 3 and 5% of all intracranial masses [12, 13] and account for 6% of all expanding brain tumors during the pediatric years [14]. These tumors show a bimodal age distribution during the first and second decade of life and then in the fifth, without apparent gender predilection [12–17]. Craniopharyngiomas are generally sporadic, and the molecular pathogenesis remains poorly defined [18].

Embryologically, craniopharyngiomas arise from squamous epithelial remnants along the involuted craniopharyngeal duct [19, 20]. During the 4th week of gestation, a diverticulum of embryonic stomodeum (oral cavity roof) gives rise to Rathke's pouch which subsequently migrates cranially to meet with the infundibulum (derived from diencephalic neuroectoderm). The path along which Rathke's pouch migrates gives rise to the craniopharyngeal duct. Rathke's pouch will eventually separate to form Rathke's vesicle (surrounding the infundibulum) which gives rise to the constituents of the adenohypophysis, namely, the pars distalis, pars tuberalis and the pars intermedia [21]. Craniopharyngiomas are postulated to originate from squamous cell rests deposited along the path of the primitive craniopharyngeal duct and adenohypophysis (either from remnants of the craniopharyngeal duct or from metaplasia of adenohypophyseal cells of the pituitary stalk) [21].

Grossly, craniopharyngiomas can be cystic, solid or both. Histologically, there are 2 variants of craniopharyngioma, adamantinomatous and papillary, that have correspondingly unique clinical and radiological features. Adamantinomatous craniopharyngiomas are epithelial neoplasms that arise in the suprasellar region and bear resemblance to odontogenic tumors [21]. These tumors typically affect a juvenile population (first 2 decades of life) [20]. Internally, these tumors may contain a conglomeration of cysts, necrotic debris, fibrous tissue, calcification and fluid filled with cholesterol particles [21]. This fluid, likened to machinery oil, may incite an intense sterile inflammatory reaction if spilled into the cerebrospinal fluid (CSF) space during surgery or through spontaneous rupture [22–25]. Histologically, adamantinomatous craniopharyngiomas may be arranged in patterns of sheets, nodular whorls, trabeculae and 'clover leaves' and cysts lined by attenuated epithelium [21]. The epithelial cells (all squamous in origin and immunoreactive for epithelial membrane antigen) are arranged in a peripheral palisaded layer of columnar cells (stellate reticulum) and an intervening layer of polygonal cells [21]. Another characteristic feature of this variant is the so-called 'wet keratin', formed by congregations of desquamated cells often undergoing calcification (accounting for the calcification observed grossly and on imaging) [21]. These lesions are also known to adhere to neurovascular structures and this can be observed histologically where intensive gliosis and Rosenthal formation is observed at the tissue-tumor interface [26].

Papillary craniopharyngiomas are well-differentiated pseudopapillary tumors of squamous origin arising in the suprasellar region or third ventricle. The papillary craniopharyngioma variant, in contrast, occurs almost exclusively in adults [27]. Papillary craniopharyngiomas are mostly solid on gross inspection with papillations, but may exhibit a smaller cystic component and lack the cholesterol-rich machinery oil contents, calcification and adherence to neurovascular structures as with adamantinomatous variants [21].

Most craniopharyngiomas originate in the intrasellar and suprasellar region (70%) with suprasellar localizations (20%) or solely intrasellar lesions (10%) occurring less frequently [28].

Table 1. Presenting signs and symptoms

	Presenting signs/symptoms
Mass effect	diminished growth velocity, short stature, delayed puberty, hypogonadism; visual changes; headache, nausea vomiting, papilledema (increased ICP); memory problems, behavioral changes, decline in school performance
Hypersecretion	
i PRL	Galactorrhea, delayed growth, delayed or arrested puberty, hypogonadism, menstrual irregularity
ii ACTH	Obesity, striae, hypertension, thin skin, glucose intolerance, growth arrest, pubertal arrest, virilization
iii GH	Pre-pubertal children – tall stature, enlarged hands/feet, thickened skin, prognathism
	Post-pubertal children – enlargement of hands/feet, overgrowth of skull/facial bones, macroglossia, sleep apnea, hypertension, glucose intolerance, arthritis, carpal tunnel syndrome, hyperhydrosis

Clinical Presentation and Diagnostics

Symptoms and clinical signs of pituitary tumors in the pediatric patient depend upon the type and size of the tumor and age of the patient (table 1). The patient may be asymptomatic and the lesion discovered during imaging for an unrelated condition.

Mass effect from a sellar tumor may produce variable endocrinological and neurological manifestations. Diminished growth velocity or short stature is a common feature in many children harboring pituitary adenomas; this may be accompanied by delayed puberty or hypogonadism. Mass effect can also produce galactorrhea (from hyperprolactinemia resulting from disturbance of the pituitary stalk and loss of tonic inhibition of PRL, the 'stalk effect'). Visual changes, including diminished acuity or visual field deficits, may result from tumor compression of the optic apparatus. Mass effect producing increased intracranial pressure may evoke headache, nausea, vomiting and papilledema. Memory problems, behavioral changes and a decline in school performance may also be seen.

All pediatric patients suspected of harboring a pituitary adenoma should undergo a complete neurological, ophthalmological, endocrinological, and radiological work-up. A neurological examination is performed noting any focal neurological deficits including cranial neuropathies. All patients old enough to cooperate should undergo formal visual field testing, acuity testing and dilated fundoscopic examination. Each facet of the hypothalamic-pituitary-end organ axis is assessed. Diabetes insipidus is assessed with careful questioning of the

Table 2. Patient evaluation

Neurological	Complete neurological examination including assessment of cranial nerve function
Ophthalmological	Formal visual field testing, acuity testing, dilated fundoscopic examination
Endocrinological	– Clinical history supplemented by serum electrolytes and urinalysis (for DI) – Radiograph to assess bone age in comparison to chronological age – Serum PRL, free thyroxine, TSH, morning cortisol, GH, IGF-1, serum gonadotropins – Suspected Cushing's disease – 24-hour urine free cortisol, +/– dexamethasone suppression test, inferior petrosal sinus sampling – Suspected GH hypersecretion – oral glucose tolerance test
Radiological	– Dedicated MRI of the sellar region (with and without contrast – CT scan in younger patients to assess aeration of sphenoid sinus

Table 3. Tumor classification

Size	
Microadenoma	Diameter ≤10 mm
Macroadenoma	Diameter >10 mm
Functional status	
Non-functioning adenoma	Null cell; gonadotroph immunoreactivity
Functioning adenoma	
Cushing's disease	ACTH immunoreactivity
Prolactinoma	PRL immunoreactivity
Gigantism or acromegaly	GH immunoreactivity
TSH-secreting	TSH immunoreactivity

parents and child where a classical history of polydipsia, polyuria and nocturia may be ascertained. Serum electrolytes and urinalysis may also provide confirmatory evidence; however, the sodium may be normal despite voluminous, dilute urine in the setting of intact thirst mechanisms and the ability to drink (table 2).

Serum PRL levels should be evaluated in all patients with pituitary tumors. Mild elevation may be due to a 'stalk effect' (loss of tonic inhibition) while levels of >200 ng/ml support the presence of a PRL-secreting adenoma. Thyroid function is evaluated by measuring free thyroxine, thyroxine and thyroid-stimulating hormone. Adrenal function is assessed by a morning serum cortisol measurement. In case of suspected CD, 24-hour urine free cortisol is evaluated (age permitting) and a dexamethasone suppression test can be performed. Rarely, inferior petrosal sinus sampling is performed in pediatric patients with suspected CD. To evaluate for GH status, serum GH and insulin-like growth factor (IGF)-1 levels are measured. A radiograph can be obtained to assess bone age in comparison with chronological age. An oral glucose tolerance test can be performed when possible in cases of suspected GH-secreting tumors. Serum gonadotropins should also be measured in older children and in those with signs of pubertal development (table 3).

Radiological evaluation is achieved with dedicated MRI of the sellar region. At times, a computed tomographic (CT) scan may be useful to assess the degree of aeration of the sella, particularly in younger patients where the sella has not yet become fully pneumatized.

PRL-Secreting Adenomas

PRL-secreting adenomas are usually diagnosed at the time of puberty or in the post-pubertal period [5, 28], and clinical manifestations vary depending on the age and sex of the child. Pre-pubertal children generally present with a combination of headache, visual disturbances, growth failure, and primary amenorrhea. Post-pubertal children present with amenorrhea and galactorrhea. Although males may experience galactorrhea, they more often come to clinical attention secondary to mass effect and often report headache, visual disturbance, diminished libido and loss of vitality.

The biochemical diagnosis of prolactinoma is typically straightforward. Some pitfalls in the diagnosis must be avoided. Certain drugs (dopamine antagonists, estrogens), renal and liver failure, hypothyroidism, and 'stalk effect' can produce moderate elevations in basal PRL levels. Nevertheless, serum PRL levels of >200 ng/ml are consistent with the diagnosis of a PRL-secreting adenoma.

Another pitfall is the serum PRL 'hook effect' that may misdiagnose a macroprolactinoma as a non-secreting adenoma [28] in the absence of serial dilutions. In fact, this may apply in any situation in which extremely high PRL levels are encountered (micro- and macroadenomas, although most common with macroadenomas). Patients with macroadenomas and moderate elevations in PRL levels (or in any situation in which extremely high PRL levels are suspected but not initially confirmed biochemically) should have repeated serum PRL testing with serial dilutions.

Cushing's Disease

The clinical manifestations of CD are mostly the consequence of excessive cortisol production. The clinical presentation is highly variable, with signs and symptoms that can range from subtle to obvious. The diagnosis is generally delayed since a decrease in growth rate may be the only symptom for a some time. Growth failure in CD may be due to a decrease in free IGF-1 levels and/or a direct negative effect of cortisol on the growth plate [29].

Other physical manifestations of CD include facial plethora; atrophic striae in the abdomen, legs and arms, muscular weakness, hypertension, and osteoporosis. Results of bone mineral density or bone metabolism in children with CD have been reported only in some patients, and marked osteopenia was also found in affected children [29]. Recent reports indicate that a long period of time (often more than 2 years) is necessary to restore bone mass after the cure of CD, so other therapeutic approaches may be indicated to limit bone loss and/or accelerate bone recovery in these patients [30].

Children with CD may also have impaired carbohydrate tolerance (although diabetes mellitus is uncommon). Excessive adrenal androgens may cause acne and excessive hair growth, or premature sexual development in the first decade of life. On the other hand, hypercortisolism may cause pubertal delay in adolescent patients. Peculiarly, young patients with CD may with present neuropsychiatric symptoms which differ from those of adult patients. Frequently, they tend to be obsessive and are high performers at school [29].

The differential diagnosis of CD includes adrenal tumors, ectopic ACTH production (rare in the pediatric population), and ectopic corticotrophin-releasing hormone (CRH)-producing tumors. In a child/adolescent with suspected CD the diagnosis can be problematic not only because these tumors are often not evident on MRI, but because pseudo-Cushing's states can be difficult to distinguish definitively from true CD. Pseudo-Cushing's syndrome results in a hypercortisolemic state and may also include physical features indistinguishable from those of CD. It results from an underlying disease process, such as depression or obesity, although the precise mechanism remains unclear. It appears to be centrally mediated and may involve excessive hypothalamic secretion of CRH [31–36]. However, this condition resolves with treatment of the underlying disease. Hence, the initial examination of a patient suspected of having CD should screen for disorders that may lead to pseudo-Cushing's syndrome.

Nonetheless, hypercortisolemia can be screened using a 24-hour urinary free cortisol (UFC) or a low-dose dexamethasone suppression test. UFC values of >220–330 nmol/24 h (80–120 μg/24 hours) are sensitive, but relatively nonspecific, for the diagnosis Cushing's syndrome [34, 35]. Failure to suppress morning (08:00 h) serum cortisol levels to 100–200 nmol/l (3.6–7.2 μg/dl) the morning following a midnight dose of 0.5–2.0 mg dexamethasone is also indicative of Cushing's syndrome [37, 38]. Suppression to <50 nmol/l or 1.8 μg/dl is highly specific for the exclusion of Cushing's syndrome. When doubt remains as to the possibility of pseudo-Cushing's, a combined CRH-low-dose dexamethasone suppression test may be used [39]. As described, patients are administered 0.5 mg dexamethasone every 6 h for 24 h and then are given a 1-μg/kg intravenous dose of CRH. In patients with Cushing's syndrome, CRH should overcome the suppressive effects of dexamethasone, and serum cortisol level at 15 min should be >1.4 μg/dl.

Once the presence of Cushing's syndrome has been established, the source of cortisol excess must be determined. Although low ACTH levels (<5 pg/ml) exclude CD, higher levels require further testing to distinguish a pituitary from an ectopic source of ACTH secretion [40]. No single test provides an absolute distinction, but the combined results of several tests generally provide a preponderance of evidence. These tests include the high-dose dexamethasone suppression test, metyrapone (750 mg every 4 h for 6 doses), CRH (1 μg/kg intravenously), and inferior petrosal sinus sampling.

The high-dose dexamethasone test compares steroid levels (either serum cortisol, 24-hour urinary 17-hydroxycorticosteriods, or 24-hour UFC) prior to and the morning after either 2 mg dexamethasone every 6 h for 48 h or a single evening (23:00 h) 8-mg dexamethasone dose. Patients with pituitary-dependent ACTH secretion should suppress serum cortisol >50%, UFC >90%, and 17-hydroxycorticosteroids >64–69% [41, 42].

GH-Secreting Adenomas

In post-pubertal young adults, chronic GH hypersecretion causes acromegaly which is characterized by hyperostosis and hypertrophy of soft tissue. In children and adolescents whose epiphyseal plates are open, GH hypersecretion leads to gigantism (because of associated secondary hypogonadism). The two disorders may be considered along a spectrum of GH excess, with principal manifestations determined by the developmental stage during which such excess originates. Supporting this model has been the observation of clinical overlap between the two entities, with approximately 10% of acromegalics exhibiting tall stature [43], and the majority of giants eventually demonstrating features of acromegaly [43].

The diagnosis of acromegaly is clinical, and often apparent on physical examination. However, biochemical confirmation is imperative and easily obtained. Because GH secretion is pulsatile, random serum GH levels are of limited diagnostic value. Nevertheless, serum IGF-1 levels and GH levels following a standard glucose load (oral glucose tolerance test) may be used to diagnose acromegaly and to monitor for remission and recurrence [44]. Serum GH levels are drawn in the fasting patient at –30, 0, 30, 60, 90, and 120 min around the time of an oral glucose load of 75–100 g. Failure to suppress GH levels to <1 μg/l (<2 mU/l) confirms the diagnosis.

Occasionally, the presence of different GH isoforms in patients with gigantism/acromegaly may represent a diagnostic problem [44]. A greater sensitivity of the GH assay may facilitate the distinction between symptomatic and normal subjects, as shown by the use of a chemiluminescence GH assay [44, 45]. It may also help in demonstrating the persistence of GH hypersecretion after surgery or during medical therapy. In case of clinical and laboratory findings suggestive of a GH-producing adenoma, a pituitary MRI must be performed to localize and characterize the tumor.

Craniopharyngiomas

Neurological disturbances, such as headache and visual field defects along with manifestations of endocrine deficiency such as growth retardation and delayed puberty are the common presenting symptoms of craniopharyngiomas. Craniopharyngiomas can stretch the diaphragm sellae and cause headaches. Obstruction of the cerebral aqueduct and the foramen of Monro may also occur, making a CSF-diversion procedures necessary [45]. At diagnosis, endocrine dysfunction is found in up to 80% of patients [45, 46]. Reduced GH secretion is the most frequent endocrinopathy and can be present in up to 75% of patients. This is followed by FSH/LH deficiency, which can be seen in 40% of patients, and then ACTH and TSH deficiency in 25% [47–48].

Despite the fact that craniopharyngiomas are frequently large at presentation, the pituitary stalk is usually not disrupted, and hyperprolactinemia secondary to pituitary stalk compression is found in only 20% of patients. Diabetes insipidus is relatively uncommon, occurring in 9–17% of patients [48]. The recent availability of high resolution MRI has greatly improved the visualization and radiological diagnosis of craniopharyngiomas.

The neuroradiological diagnosis of craniopharyngiomas is based on the features of the lesion itself and on its relations with the surrounding structures. The diagnosis is mainly based on the three characteristic components of the tumor: cystic, solid and calcified [44–49]. The cystic component constitutes the most important part of the tumor, and shows variable signals depending on the chemical-physical properties of its content [47]. A fluid content will appear hypointense in T1 and hyperintense in T2 while a lipid (due to cholesterol) methemoglobin or protein content will appear as hyperintense in T1 and T2 sequences. The solid portion shows an isointense signal in T1 and a hyperintense signal in T2 with an enhancement after gadolinium, at variance with the cystic component. However, contrast enhancement is not a consistent feature [47]. Calcifications can appear as areas of low signal in all sequences, but are generally visualized better with CT scans [47].

Treatment

PRL-Secreting Adenomas

In the absence of complications necessitating immediate surgery, such as rapidly progressing visual loss, hydrocephalus, or CSF leak, pharmacotherapy with dopamine agonists should be considered the first-line treatment approach. Dopamine agonists, including bromocriptine, pergolide, and cabergoline, effectively normalize PRL levels in as many as 89% of patients [48–51]. These medications are not only effective biochemically, tumor volume decreases by at least 50% in more than two thirds of patients within the first few months of therapy, and, more importantly, visual field deficits improve in all but 10% of patients [52]. Quinagolide and cabergoline, both selective dopamine receptor subtype-2 agonists, have also been reported to be effective in reducing PRL secretion and tumor size in adult patients with prolactinoma, even in those previously shown to be poorly responsive or intolerant to bromocriptine [52]. Cabergoline in particular has received attention for its tolerability and high compliance rates [51, 52]. Cabergoline has a longer half-life than bromocriptine and normalizes serum PRL levels and restores gonadal function in the majority of patients with microprolactinomas [52]. Its convenient weekly administration also makes it an excellent therapeutic alternative in children with prolactinomas.

Bromocriptine has been used in several thousand women who became pregnant while taking the medication [53]. There appeared to be no increased risk of birth defects in more than 2,000 babies born to women taking bromocriptine [54]. More limited experience exists with cabergoline in women taking this medication during pregnancy, but the body of data at present suggests no increased risk above baseline in terms of birth defects in babies exposed to this medication during gestation [55].

Although medical therapy can be highly effective, some patients are intolerant of the medications, and some tumors are resistant to pharmacotherapy. Tumor resistance is characterized by either failure to normalize PRL levels or inadequate tumor volume reduction. In these situations, we have advocated transsphenoidal surgery.

Transsphenoidal surgery is most successful in obtaining remission in the setting of microprolactinomas. In this population, PRL levels can be normalized in 50–90%, with experienced centers reporting results around 85% [56–59]. Not unexpectedly, results with macroprolactinomas are less successful. Surgical remission may be expected in 28–56%, with most experienced centers reporting remission in about half the patients [56–59].

Cushing's Disease

Transsphenoidal resection is the treatment of choice for ACTH-secreting adenomas. Surgical excision is successful in the majority of children, with initial remission rates of 70–98% and long-term cure of 50–98% in most studies [60–63]. The success rate decreases when the patients are followed up for more than 5 years [64], and the outcome cannot be predicted either by preoperative or postoperative tests [65]. The morbidity is low when the procedure is carried out by an experienced team [66]. Transsphenoidal microsurgery is considered successful when it is followed by remission of signs and symptoms of hypercortisolism and by normalization of laboratory values. Surgery is usually followed by adrenal insufficiency and patients require hydrocortisone replacement for 6–12 months. After normalization of cortisol levels, resumption of normal growth or even catch-up growth can be observed. Generally, final height is compromised compared to target height [32, 33]. However, some children do achieve a normal final stature [32].

The treatment modality in patients who have relapses after transsphenoidal adenomectomy is still controversial. Some authors recommend repeated surgery [66–71], while others favor radiation therapy [72, 73]. Radiotherapy with or without concomitant mitotane treatment may be indicated in patients with macroadenoma [71–73], although caution must be used as the long-term risks of side effects, such as new neoplasms and radiation necrosis, are unknown. Although surgery can induce panhypopituitarism, or permanent diabetes insipidus, hypothalamic-pituitary dysfunction is an early and frequent complication of radiation [73]. Bilateral adrenalectomy may be the last therapeutic option in case of failure of both surgery and radiotherapy. Stereotactic radiosurgery with either the gamma knife or a linear accelerator is a promising modality that minimizes the toxic effects of radiation on the brain, while still controlling tumor growth and ACTH secretion [73] (fig. 1). However, the long-term effects in the pediatric population are not well known.

GH-Secreting Adenomas

The objectives of treatment of GH excess are tumor removal with resolution of its mass effect, restoration of normal basal and stimulated GH secretion, relief of symptoms caused by GH excess and prevention of the disease sequelae (i.e. hypertension, insulin resistance, diabetes mellitus and lipid abnormalities) [74]. The currently available treatment options for acromegaly include surgery, radiotherapy, and pharmacological suppression of GH levels by means of dopamine agonists or somatostatin analogs [74–81]. Although medical therapy is increasingly improving, transsphenoidal surgery remains the first-line therapy for GH adenomas. Surgery can achieve biochemical remission (normal IGF-1 levels, nadir GH <1 μg/l during oral glucose tolerance test) in about 85% of patients with microadenomas and 50% of those with macroadenomas [81–86], and in pediatric patients with gigantism, transsphenoidal surgery was found to be as safe as in adults [87]. The success rate of surgery is further improved when

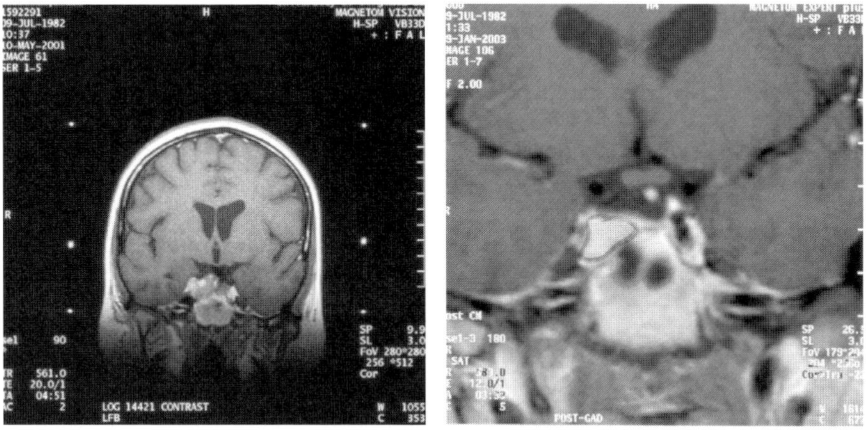

a b

Fig. 1. ***a*** 18-year-old female with Cushing's disease treated with gamma knife and for a residual pituitary macroadenoma involving the cavernous sinus. ***b*** 2-years post-gamma knife follow-up revealed 60% decrease in tumor size, and endocrinologic remission from Cushing's disease.

performed by a surgeon who specializes in transsphenoidal surgery [83–87]. Once in remission, about 8% of patients recur at 10 years [87]. Of these patients, 48% can achieve remission with repeated transsphenoidal surgery [85–87].

Somatostatin is a native factor that inhibits GH secretion. Somatostatin analogs (such as octreotide) may be more suppressive of GH than native somatostatin and more suppressive of GH secretion than insulin [88]. Debate lingers as to the possible beneficial effects of preoperative octreotide therapy. Although some investigators report reduced morbidity and improved biochemical results, consensus is lacking [88, 89]. Preoperative GH levels of >50 μg/l predict failure of remission [83, 84]. Early postoperative GH levels of <2 μg/l are predictive of remission. Patients with known cavernous sinus invasion and large incompletely removed tumors require adjuvant therapy [80–83, 90].

Impressive advances have occurred with regard to the medical therapy of GH adenomas. Until recently, the two options for medical therapy were dopamine agonists and somatostatin analogs. Dopamine agonists provide symptomatic relief in the majority of patients, but normalize IGF-1 levels in only about 20–40% of patients [90–92]. Somatostatin analogs (octreotide, sandostatin-LAR, lanreotide, lanreotide-SR) can normalize IGF-1 levels in up to 60% of patients and have a more favorable side-effect profile compared to dopamine agonists [91–95]. However, the recently introduced GH receptor antagonist, pegvisomant, has normalized IGF-1 levels in 90–100% of patients with refractory disease, although reported experience with administration for more than 2 years is limited [96].

Clinically Non-Functioning Adenomas

The first approach to these adenomas is transsphenoidal resection to debulk the tumor and decompress parasellar/suprasellar structures. As in the other adenoma histotypes, surgery has a low morbidity and leads to an improvement in visual symptoms in the majority of cases [97]. New endocrine deficits, seen more frequently in macroadenomas, have been reported in up to 40% [97–99]. However, recent results indicate that only 3% of patients with microadenomas and 5% of patients with macroadenomas with preoperative normal pituitary function experience new hormonal deficits following surgery [100]. Immediate postoperative polyuria occurs in about 30% of patients, but in only 3–10% does this polyuria persist beyond the first week of surgery [100]. Delayed hyponatremia, occurring most often 7–10 days after surgery, is evident in 1–2.4% [100, 101]. Worsening in preoperative vision can be seen in 1–4% [100–102]. Anatomic complications include nasal septal perforations in 7% and fat graft hematomas in 4% [102]. Postoperative CSF leaks and meningitis are reported in 0.5–3.9% [100–103].

Recurrences do develop over time and as many as 16% of patients may experience recurrent disease at 10 years [96]. However, recurrence requiring repeat surgery occurs in only 6% of patients. Completeness of resection as judged on postoperative MRI can predict recurrence. Although one third of patients with residual tumor have recurrent tumor growth, fewer than 3% with complete resection experience recurrent disease (mean follow-up of 3.3 years) [103]. For tumors with incomplete resection, radiosurgery, medical and radiation therapy can be considered. Neither medical therapy nor radiation therapy is recommended as primary treatment, as the long-term effects are unknown.

The recent development of the endoscopic transsphenoidal approach to the pituitary region [94, 95], which has the similar indications to conventional transsphenoidal microsurgery, offers some potential advantages over traditional surgical approaches due to its minimal invasiveness and panoramic visualization. This procedure involves no fractures of the facial bones, or sublabial incisions. Furthermore, a wider surgical vision of the operating field is obtained, which potentially improves the likelihood of a better and safer tumor removal. Endoscopic treatments can result in shorter hospitalization, and a rapid recovery for the child [94, 95, 104].

Craniopharyngiomas

In small intrasellar or enclosed tumors, total resection is often achievable, and adjunctive radiotherapy is unnecessary [106]. Radiotherapy or radiosurgery is often implemented in cases of incomplete tumor removal as occurs frequently with extrasellar craniopharyngiomas (the majority of cases) [17, 48, 106]. Surgical morbidity depends on tumor size and invasiveness, the experience of the

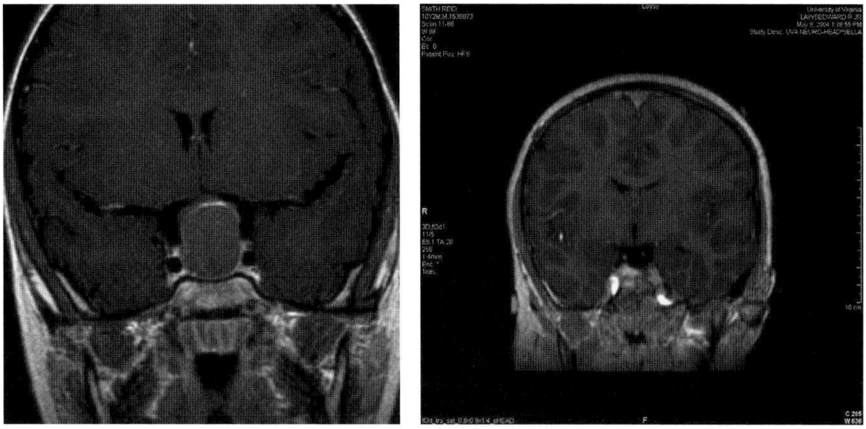

a b

Fig. 2. Pre- (*a*) and 36-month postoperative (*b*) MRIs of a 16-year-old male with cystic craniopharyngioma, who presented with visual loss and failure to achieve secondary sex characteristics. Patient was treated using a sublabial transsphenoidal approach and a fat graft.

surgeon, and the route of surgical approach. The risk of hypothalamic damage is significantly greater in large invasive tumors treated by a transcranial approach. Near total excision of the tumor by an experienced pituitary surgeon sparing the hypothalamus, carotids, and visual apparatus, followed by radiosurgery or fractionated radiotherapy provides the best hope of low long-term morbidity and longer survival [48, 106–110] (fig. 2). Regardless of the approach, the incidence of endocrine dysfunction is high following surgical treatment [106–113], although it is lower after the transsphenoidal approach [107].

Localized intracavity Yttrium, P^{32}, and other radioactive implants, given as additional treatment, have proven useful for recurrent tumors with a predominant cystic component [113, 114]. Hyperfractionated multiportal stereotactic radiotherapy and gamma knife radiosurgery are promising therapeutic adjuvants to standard radiotherapy, due to their potential ability to reduce treatment-associated morbidity in this condition. In children, however, the benefit of any additional radiation treatment should be balanced against the relatively high risk of inducing hypopituitarism later in life [113, 114].

Prognosis

Prognosis for pediatric pituitary adenomas is dependent upon patient status, comorbid conditions, tumor size and extension, and functional status of the tumor.

For prolactinomas, medical therapy can be effective in achieving normalization of PRL levels. In those patients that eventually require surgery, the size of the tumor, invasive characteristics and pretreatment PRL levels appear to influence success [5]. Males often present with macroadenomas in the pubertal years and normalization of PRL levels are achieved in less than 30% of patients [5]. In contrast, female patients often present with secondary amenorrhea and galactorrhea secondary to microadenomas and over 75% will achieve biochemical remission [5]. With combinations of therapy, tumor control can be achieved in the majority of patients.

As mentioned, patients with CD can achieve remission with transsphenoidal surgery in the majority of instances (70–98%). However, late recurrences are known to occur and patients must be followed carefully. Re-treatment, however, can result in long-term remission [80].

The reported experience with pediatric GH-secreting tumors is limited, however, a cure with surgery alone appears less likely in this population. Combinatorial therapy with transsphenoidal surgery, medical therapy (somatostatin analogs) and possibly radiation therapy appears to result in remission in the majority of patients.

The largest division in the treatment of craniopharyngiomas is in whether to perform a gross total resection, versus a subtotal resection followed by adjuvant therapy (i.e. radiation). Recurrences are more likely to occur with subtotal resection. In the majority of cases, if a recurrence does occur, it happens within 3 years of treatment. Recurrences are associated with higher degrees of morbidity and mortality, although fluoroscopic navigation can help reduce the risk of damage to eloquent structures (fig. 3).

Follow-Up

Pediatric patients being treated for pituitary adenomas must be followed long-term, generally with serial clinical, ophthalmological, endocrinological and radiological evaluations. In particular, height, weight and pubertal status must be carefully monitored in relevant age groups. Serial visual field examinations and screening should be performed. Questioning directed at assessing hormonal status (screening for hypothyroidism, adrenal insufficiency, diabetes insipidus, etc.) should be directed to the patient and family. Serial testing of thyroid function and GH status (with IGF-1 levels and provocative testing when applicable) should be undertaken. Tanner staging, skeletal maturation, LH, FSH and sex hormone levels should be performed serially. Patients with functioning tumors should be investigated as appropriate (for example, 24-hour UFC testing in patients with CD). Patients already on hormonal replacement should have

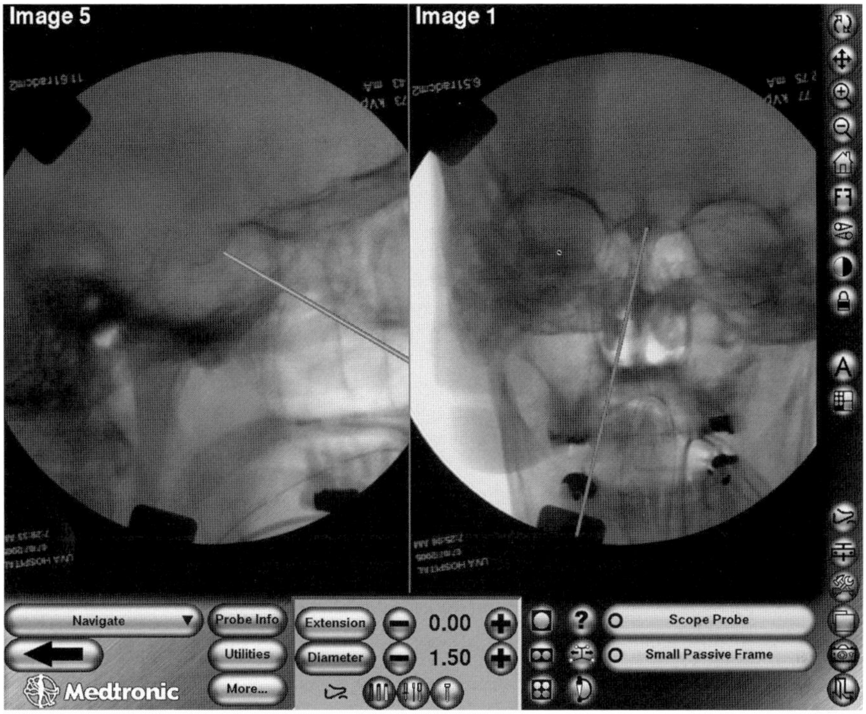

Fig. 3. Fluoroscopic neuronavigation allows realtime visualization of the bony anatomy around the sellar, and is useful when the normal sellar anatomy is disrupted.

their replacement therapy adjusted as necessary. Finally, serial MRI should be performed to assess for tumor recurrence. Generally, an initial postoperative study is performed 6 weeks to 3 months following treatment and repeated yearly thereafter (or more frequently as indicated).

Conclusions

The management of pituitary adenomas and other sellar lesions must account for both the endocrine and neurological sequelae of these tumors. Patients require thorough pre- and post-treatment evaluation by neuroendocrinologists, neurosurgeons, neuroophthalmologists, and neuroradiologists. Medical therapy is the primary therapy for prolactinomas and recent advances have brought forward the expectation of effective pharmacotherapy for GH adenomas as well. Transsphenoidal surgery offers effective relief of mass effect and not only restoration but the preservation of normal endocrine function in the majority of patients. Radiosurgery or radiation therapy can offer remission for some patients with medically and surgically refractory tumors, but patients must be observed closely for evidence of radiation necrosis and the presence of new endocrinopathies. With improved understanding of the molecular pathogenesis, future therapy will treat these tumors more effectively.

References

1 Guyda H, Robert F, Colle E, Hardy J: Histologic, ultrastructural and hormonal characterization of a pituitary tumor secreting both HGH and prolactin. J Clin Endocrinol Metab 1973;36:531–547.

2 Horvath E, Kovacs K, Scheithauer BW, et al: Pituitary adenomas producing growth hormone, prolactin, and one or more glycoprotein hormones: a histologic, immunohistochemical, and ultrastructural study of four surgically removed tumors. Ultrastruct Pathol 1983;5:171–183.

3 Landolt AM, Rothenbuhler V: Extracellular growth hormone deposits in pituitary adenoma. Virchows Arch A Pathol Anat Histol 1978;378:55–65.

4 Kovacs K, Scheithauer BW, Horvath E, Lloyd RV: The World Health Organization classification of adenohypophysial neoplasms. A proposed five-tier scheme. Cancer 1996;78:502–510.

5 Mindermann T, Wilson CB: Pediatric pituitary adenomas. Neurosurgery 1995;36:259–269.

6 Blackwell RE, Younger BJ: Long-term medical therapy and follow up of pediatric adolescent patients with prolactin-secreting macroadenomas. Fertil Steril 1986;45;713–716.

7 Boop FA, Teo C, Pihoker K: Pediatric pituitary tumors; in Krisht AF, Tindall GT (eds): Comprehensive Management of Pituitary Disorders. Philadelphia, Lippincott Williams & Wilkins, 1999, pp 315–326.

8 Lafferty AR, Chrousos GP: Pituitary tumors in children and adolescents. J Clin Endocrinol Metab 1999;84:4317–4323.

9 Leinung MC, Kane LA, Scheithauer BW, et al: Long term follow-up of transsphenoidal surgery or the treatment of Cushing's disease in childhood. J Clin Endocrinol Metab 1985;80:2475–2479.

10 Abe T, Tara LA, Lüdecke DK: Growth hormone-secreting pituitary adenomas in childhood and adolescence: features and results of transnasal surgery. Neurosurgery 1999;45:1–10.

11 Beck-Peccoz P, Bruckner-Davis F, Persani L, Smallridge RC, Weintraub BD: Thyrotropin-secreting pituitary tumors. Endocr Rev 1996;17:610–638.

12 Abe T, Lüdecke DK, Saeger W: Clinically nonsecreting pituitary adenomas in childhood and adolescence. Neurosurgery 1998;42:744–751.

13 Bunin GR, Surawicz TS, Witman PA, et al: The descriptive epidemiology of craniopharyngioma. J Neurosurg 1998;89:547–551.

14 Hayward R: The present and future management of childhood craniopharyngioma. Childs Nerv Syst 1999;15:764–776.

15 Hetelekidis S, Barnes PD, Tao ML, et al: 20-year experience in childhood craniopharyngioma. Int J Radiat Oncol Biol Phys 1993;27:189–195.

16 Thomsett MJ, Conte FA, Kaplan SL, Grumbach MM: Endocrine and neurologic outcome in childhood craniopharyngioma: review of effect of treatment in 42 patients. J Pediatr 1980;97: 728–735.

17 Weiner HL, Wisoff JH, Rosenberg ME, et al: Craniopharyngiomas: a clinicopathological analysis of factors predictive of recurrence and functional outcome. Neurosurgery 1994;35:1001–1011.

18 Rickert CH, Paulus W: Lack of chromosomal imbalances in adamantinomatous and papillary craniopharyngiomas. J Neurol Neurosurg Psychiatry 2003;74:260–261.

19 Harrison MJ, Morgello S, Post KD: Epithelial cystic lesions of the sellar and parasellar region: a continuum of ectodermal derivatives? J Neurosurg 1994;80:1018–1025.

20 FitzPatrick M, Tartaglino LM, Hollander MD, Zimmerman RA, Flanders AE: Imaging of sellar and parasellar pathology. Radiol Clin North Am 1999;37:101–121.

21 Moore KD, Couldwell WT: Craniopharyngiomas; in Bernstein M, Berger MS (eds): Neuro-Oncology. The Essentials. New York, Thieme Medical, 2000, pp 409–418.
22 Burger PC, Scheithauer BW, Vogel FS: Region of the Sella Turcica. Surgical Pathology of the Nervous System and its Coverings, ed 4. New York, Churchill Livingstone, 2002, pp 437–497.
23 Maeda T, Kazumi T, Hotta K, et al: Aseptic localized peritonitis in a patient with chemical meningitis associated with craniopharyngioma cysts. Intern Med 1993;32:340–342.
24 Satoh H, Uozumi T, Arita K, et al: Spontaneous rupture of craniopharyngioma cysts. A report of five cases and review of the literature. Surg Neurol 1993;40:414–419.
25 Shida N, Nakasato N, Mizoi K, Kanaki M, Yoshimoto T: Symptomatic vessel narrowing caused by spontaneous rupture of craniopharyngioma cyst – case report. Neurol Med Chir (Tokyo) 1998;38: 666–668.
26 Kulkarni V, Daniel RT, Pranatartiharan R: Spontaneous intraventricular rupture of craniopharyngioma cyst. Surg Neurol 2000;54:249–253.
27 Kahn EA, Gosch HH, Seeger JF, Hicks SP: Forty-five years experience with the craniopharyngiomas. Surg Neurol 1973;1:5–12.
28 Akimura T, Kamleda H: Infrasellar craniopharyngioma. Neuroradiology 1989;31:180–183.
29 Blackwell RE, Younger BJ: Long-term medical therapy and follow up of pediatric adolescent patients with prolactin-secreting macroadenomas. Fertil Steril 1986;45;713–716.
30 Colao A, Annunziato L, Lombardi G: Treatment of prolactinomas. Ann Med 1998;30:452–459.
31 St-Jean E, Blain F, Comtois R: High prolactin levels maybe missed by immunoradiometric assay in patients with macroprolactinomas. Clin Endocrinol (Oxf) 1996;44:305–309.
32 Di Somma C, Pivonello R, Loche S: Effect of 2 years of cortisol normalization on the impaired bone mass and turnover in adolescent and adult patients with Cushing's disease. Clin Endocrinol (Oxf) 2003;58:302–308.
33 Johnston LB, Grossmann AB, Plowman PN, et al: Normal final height and apparent cure after pituitary irradiation for Cushing's disease in childhood: long-term follow-up of anterior pituitary function. Clin Endocrinol (Oxf) 1998;48:663–667.
34 Kirkman S, Nelson DH: Alcohol-induced pseudo-Cushing's disease: a study of prevalence with review of the literature. Metabolism 1988;37:390–394.
35 Newell-Price J, Trainer P, Besser M, Grossman A: The diagnosis and differential diagnosis of Cushing's syndrome and pseudo-Cushing's states. Endocr Rev 1998;19:647–672.
36 Tsigos C, Chrousos GP: Differential diagnosis and management of Cushing's syndrome. Annu Rev Med 1996;47:443–461.
37 Cizza G, Nieman LK, Doppman JL, et al: Factitious Cushing syndrome. J Clin Endocrinol Metab 1996;81:3573–3577.
38 Mengden T, Hubmann P, Muller J, Greminger P, Vetter W: Urinary free cortisol versus 17-hydroxycorticosteroids: a comparative study of their diagnostic value in Cushing's syndrome. Clin Investig 1992;70:545–548.
39 Yanovski JA, Cutler GB Jr, Chrousos GP, Nieman LK: Corticotropin-releasing hormone stimulation following low-dose dexamethasone administration. A new test to distinguish Cushing's syndrome from pseudo-Cushing's states. JAMA 1993;269:2232–2238.
40 Raff H, Findling JW: A new immunoradiometric assay for corticotropin evaluated in normal subjects and patients with Cushing's syndrome. Clin Chem 1989;35:596–600.
41 Dichek HL, Nieman LK, Oldfield EH, Pass HI, Malley JD, Cutler GB Jr: A comparison of the standard high dose dexamethasone suppression test and the overnight 8-mg dexamethasone suppression test for the differential diagnosis of adrenocorticotropin-dependent Cushing's syndrome. J Clin Endocrinol Metab 1994;78:418–422.
42 Flack MR, Oldfield EH, Cutler GB Jr, et al: Urine free cortisol in the high-dose dexamethasone suppression test for the differential diagnosis of the Cushing syndrome. Ann Intern Med 1992;116: 211–217.
43 Eugster EA, Pescovitz OH: Gigantism. J Clin Endocrinol Metab 1999;84:4379–4384.
44 Giustina A, Barkan A, Casanueva FF, et al: Criteria for cure of acromegaly: a consensus statement. J Clin Endocrinol Metab 2000;85:526–529.

45 Chapman IM, Hartman ML, Straume M, et al: Enhanced sensitivity growth hormone (GH) chemiluminescence assay reveals lower postglucose nadir GH concentrations in men than in women. J Clin Endocrinol Metab 1994;78:1312–1319.
46 Fahlbusch R, Honegger J, Paulus W, et al: Surgical treatment of craniopharyngiomas: experience with 168 patients. J Neurosurg 1999;90:237–250.
47 Freeman M, Kessler R, Allen JH, Price AC: Craniopharyngioma: CT and MR imaging in nine cases. J Comput Assist Tomogr 1987;5:810–814.
48 Adamson TE, Wiestler OD, Kleihues P, Yasargil MG: Correlation of clinical and pathological features in surgically treated craniopharyngiomas. J Neurosurg 1990;73:12–17.
49 Acquati S, Pizzocaro A, Tomei G, et al: A comparative evaluation of effectiveness of medical and surgical therapy in patients with macroprolactinoma. J Neurosurg Sci 2001;45:65–69.
50 Molitch ME, Elton RL, Blackwell RE, et al: Bromocriptine as primary therapy for prolactin-secreting macroadenomas: results of a prospective multicenter study. J Clin Endocrinol Metab 1985;60:698–705.
51 Liuzzi A, Dallabonzana D, Oppizzi G, et al: Low doses of dopamine agonists in the long-term treatment of macroprolactinomas. N Engl J Med 1985;313:656–659.
52 Webster J, Piscitelli G, Polli A, Ferrari CI, Ismail I, Scanlon MF: A comparison of cabergoline and bromocriptine in the treatment of hyperprolactinemic amenorrhea. Cabergoline Comparative Study Group. N Engl J Med 1994;331:904–909.
53 Vance ML: Medical treatment of functional pituitary tumors. Neurosurg Clin North Am 2003;14: 81–87.
54 Turkalj I, Braun P, Krupp P: Surveillance of bromocriptine in pregnancy. JAMA 1982;247: 1589–1591.
55 Robert E, Musatti L, Piscitelli G, Ferrari CI: Pregnancy outcome after treatment with the ergot derivative, cabergoline. Reprod Toxicol 1996;10:333–337.
56 Gokalp HZ, Deda H, Attar A, Ugur HC, Arasil E, Egemen N: The neurosurgical management of prolactinomas. J Neurosurg Sci 2000;44:128–132.
57 Randall RV, Laws ER Jr, Abboud CF, Ebersold MJ, Kao PC, Scheithauer BW: Transsphenoidal microsurgical treatment of prolactin-producing pituitary adenomas. Results in 100 patients. Mayo Clin Proc 1983;58:108–121.
58 Molitch ME: Pathologic hyperprolactinemia. Endocrinol Metab Clin North Am 1992;21:877–901.
59 Feigenbaum SL, Downey DE, Wilson CB, Jaffe RB: Transsphenoidal pituitary resection for preoperative diagnosis of prolactin-secreting pituitary adenoma in women: long term follow-up. J Clin Endocrinol Metab 1996;81:1711–1719.
60 Semple PL, Vance ML, Findling J, Laws ER: Transsphenoidal surgery for Cushing's disease: outcome in patients with a normal magnetic resonance imaging scan. Neurosurgery 2000;46:553–559.
61 Lopez J, Barcelo B, Lucas T, et al: Petrosal sinus sampling for diagnosis of Cushing's disease: evidence of false negative results. Clin Endocrinol (Oxf) 1996;45:147–156.
62 Blevins LS, Christy JH, Khajavi M, Tindall GT: Outcomes of therapy for Cushing's disease due to adrenocorticotropin-secreting pituitary macroadenomas. J Clin Endocrinol Metab 1998;83:63–67.
63 Yap LB, Turner HE, Adams CB, Wass JA: Undetectable postoperative cortisol does not always predict long-term remission in Cushing's disease: a single centre audit. Clin Endocrinol (Oxf) 2002;56:25–31.
64 Chee GH, Mathias DB, James RA, Kendall-Taylor P: Transsphenoidal pituitary surgery in Cushing's disease: can we predict outcome? Clin Endocrinol (Oxf) 2001;54:617–626.
65 Simmons NE, Alden TD, Thorner MO, Laws ER Jr: Serum cortisol response to transsphenoidal surgery for Cushing disease. J Neurosurg 2001;95:1–8.
66 Sheehan JM, Lopes MB, Sheehan JP, Ellegala D, Webb KM, Laws ER Jr: Results of transsphenoidal surgery for Cushing's disease in patients with no histologically confirmed tumor. Neurosurgery 2000;47:33–39.
67 Invitti C, Giraldi FP, de Martin M, Cavagnini F: Diagnosis and management of Cushing's syndrome: results of an Italian multicentre study. Study Group of the Italian Society of Endocrinology on the Pathophysiology of the Hypothalamic-Pituitary-Adrenal Axis. J Clin Endocrinol Metab 1999;84:440–448.
68 Chou SC, Lin JD: Long-term effects of ketoconazole in the treatment of residual or recurrent Cushing's disease. Endocr J 2000;47:401–406.

69 Sonino N, Boscaro M: Medical therapy for Cushing's disease. Endocrinol Metab Clin North Am 1999;28:211–222.
70 Sonino N, Boscaro M, Paoletta A, Mantero F, Ziliotto D: Ketoconazole treatment in Cushing's syndrome: experience in 34 patients. Clin Endocrinol (Oxf) 1991;35:347–352.
71 Savage MO, Lienhardt A, Lebrethon MC, et al: Cushing's disease in childhood: presentation, investigation, treatment and long-term outcome. Horm Res 2001;55(suppl 1):24–30.
72 Estrada J, Boronat M, Mielgo M, et al: The long-term outcome of pituitary irradiation after unsuccessful transsphenoidal surgery in Cushing's disease. N Engl J Med 1997;336:172–177.
73 Sheehan JM, Vance ML, Sheehan JP, et al: Radiosurgery for Cushing's disease after failed transsphenoidal surgery. J Neurosurg 2000;93:738–747.
74 Trainer PJ, Drake WM, Katznelson L, et al: Treatment of acromegaly with the growth hormone-receptor antagonist pegvisomant. N Engl J Med 2000;342:1171–1177.
75 Parkinson C, Trainer PJ: Growth hormone receptor antagonists therapy for acromegaly. Baillieres Best Pract Res Clin Endocrinol Metab 1999;13:419–430.
76 Drake WM, Parkinson C, Akker SA, Monson JP, Besser GM, Trainer PJ: Successful treatment of resistant acromegaly with a growth hormone receptor antagonist. Eur J Endocrinol 2001;145: 451–456.
77 Herman-Bonert VS, Zib K, Scarlett JA, Melmed S: Growth hormone receptor antagonist therapy in acromegalic patients resistant to somatostatin analogs. J Clin Endocrinol Metab 2000;85:2958–2961.
78 Cozzi R, Barausse M, Asnaghi D, Dallabonzana D, Lodrini S, Attanasio R: Failure of radiotherapy in acromegaly. Eur J Endocrinol 2001;145:717–726.
79 Powell JS, Wardlaw SL, Post KD, Freda PU: Outcome of radiotherapy for acromegaly using normalization of insulin-like growth factor I to define cure. J Clin Endocrinol Metab 2000;85: 2068–2071.
80 Morange-Ramos I, Regis J, Dufour H, et al: Gamma-knife surgery for secreting pituitary adenomas. Acta Neurochir (Wien) 1998;140:437–443.
81 Landolt AM, Haller D, Lomax N, et al: Stereotactic radiosurgery for recurrent surgically treated acromegaly: comparison with fractionated radiotherapy. J Neurosurg 1998;88:1002–1008.
82 Laws ER, Vance ML, Thapar K: Pituitary surgery for the management of acromegaly. Horm Res 2000;53(suppl 3):71–75.
83 Shimon I, Cohen ZR, Ram Z, Hadani M: Transsphenoidal surgery for acromegaly: endocrinological follow-up of 98 patients. Neurosurgery 2001;48:1239–1245.
84 Kreutzer J, Vance ML, Lopes MB, Laws ER Jr: Surgical management of GH-secreting pituitary adenomas: an outcome study using modern remission criteria. J Clin Endocrinol Metab 2001;86: 4072–4077.
85 Gittoes NJ, Sheppard MC, Johnson AP, Stewart PM: Outcome of surgery for acromegaly – the experience of a dedicated pituitary surgeon. QJM 1999;92:741–745.
86 Swearingen B, Barker FG 2nd, Katznelson L, et al: Long-term mortality after transsphenoidal surgery and adjunctive therapy for acromegaly. J Clin Endocrinol Metab 1998;83:3419–3426.
87 Laws ER Jr: Acromegaly and gigantism; in Wilkins RA, Rengachary SS (eds): Neurosurgery, ed 2. New York, McGraw-Hill, 1996, vol 1, pp 1317–1320.
88 Plewe G, Beyer J, Krause U, Neufeld M, del Pozo E: Long-acting and selective suppression of growth hormone secretion by somatostatin analogue SMS 201–995 in acromegaly. Lancet 1984;ii:782–784.
89 Biermasz NR, van Dulken H, Roelfsema F: Direct postoperative and follow-up results of transsphenoidal surgery in 19 acromegalic patients pretreated with octreotide compared to those in untreated matched controls. J Clin Endocrinol Metab 1999;84:3551–3555.
90 Sheaves R, Jenkins P, Blackburn P, et al: Outcome of transsphenoidal surgery for acromegaly using strict criteria for surgical cure. Clin Endocrinol (Oxf) 1996;45:407–413.
91 Colao A, Ferone D, Marzullo P, et al: Effect of different dopaminergic agents in the treatment of acromegaly. J Clin Endocrinol Metab 1997;82:518–523.
92 Abs R, Verhelst J, Maiter D, et al: Cabergoline in the treatment of acromegaly: a study in 64 patients. J Clin Endocrinol Metab 1998;83:374–378.
93 Jaffe CA, Barkan AL: Treatment of acromegaly with dopamine agonists. Endocrinol Metab Clin North Am 1992;21:713–735.

94 Cozzi R, Attanasio R, Barausse M, et al: Cabergoline in acromegaly: a renewed role for dopamine agonist treatment? Eur J Endocrinol 1998;139:516–521.
95 Wass JA, Thorner MO, Morris DV, et al: Long-term treatment of acromegaly with bromocriptine. Br Med J 1977;i:875–878.
96 Trainer PJ, Drake WM, Katznelson L, et al: Treatment of acromegaly with the growth hormone-receptor antagonist pegvisomant. N Engl J Med 2000;342:1171–1177.
97 Colao A, Cerbone G, Cappabianca P, et al: Effect of surgery and radiotherapy on visual and endocrine function in nonfunctioning pituitary adenomas. J Endocrinol Invest 1998;21:284–290.
98 Kurosaki M, Ludecke DK, Flitsch J, Saeger W: Surgical treatment of clinically nonsecreting pituitary adenomas in elderly patients. Neurosurgery 2000;47:843–849.
99 Laws ER Jr: Pituitary tumors – long-term outcomes and expectations. Clin Neurosurg 2001;48: 306–319.
100 Laws ER Jr, Thapar K: Pituitary surgery. Endocrinol Metab Clin North Am 1999;28:119–131.
101 Hensen J, Henig A, Fahlbusch R, Meyer M, Boehnert M, Buchfelder M: Prevalence, predictors and patterns of postoperative polyuria and hyponatraemia in the immediate course after transsphenoidal surgery for pituitary adenomas. Clin Endocrinol (Oxf) 1999;50:431–439.
102 Woollons AC, Balakrishnan V, Hunn MK, Rajapaske YR: Complications of trans-sphenoidal surgery: the Wellington experience. Aust NZ J Surg 2000;70:405–408.
103 Losa M, Franzin A, Mangili F, et al: Proliferation index of nonfunctioning pituitary adenomas: correlations with clinical characteristics and long-term follow-up results. Neurosurgery 2000;47: 1313–1319.
104 Cappabianca P, Alfieri A, Colao A, et al: Endoscopic endonasal transsphenoidal approach: an additional reason in support of surgery in the management of pituitary lesions. Skull Base Surg 1999;9:109–117.
105 Jho HD, Carrau RL: Endoscopic endonasal transsphenoidal surgery: experience with 50 patients. J Neurosurg 1997;87:44–51.
106 Van Effenterre R, Boch AL: Craniopharyngioma in adults and children: a study of 122 surgical cases. J Neurosurg 2002;97:3–11.
107 Kahn EA, Gosch HH, Seeger JF, Hicks SP: Forty-five years experience with the craniopharyngiomas. Surg Neurol 1973;1:5–12.
108 Hoffman HJ: Surgical management of craniopharyngioma. Pediatr Neurosurg 1994;21(suppl 1): 44–49.
109 Hoffman HJ, De Silva M, Humphreys RP, Drake JM, Smith ML, Blaser SI: Aggressive surgical management of craniopharyngiomas in children. J Neurosurg 1992;76:47–52.
110 de Vries L, Lazar L, Phillip M: Craniopharyngioma: presentation and endocrine sequelae in 36 children. J Pediatr Endocrinol Metab 2003;16:703–710.
111 Sklar CA: Craniopharyngioma: endocrine abnormalities at presentation. Pediatr Neurosurg 1994;21(suppl 1):18–20.
112 Merchant TE, Kiehna EN, Sanford RA, et al: Craniopharyngioma: the St. Jude Children's Research Hospital experience 1984–2001. Int J Radiat Oncol Biol Phys 2002;53:533–542.
113 Hetelekidis S, Barnes PD, Tao ML, et al: 20-year experience in childhood craniopharyngioma. Int J Radiat Oncol Biol Phys 1993;27:189–195.
114 Jennings AS, Liddle GW, Orth DN: Results of treating childhood Cushing's disease with pituitary irradiation. N Engl J Med 1977;297:957–962.

Aaron S. Dumont, MD
Department of Neurological Surgery, Health Sciences Center
University of Virginia, PO Box 800212
Charlottesville, VA 22908 (USA)
Tel. +1 434 982 3244, Fax +1 434 243 2954, E-Mail asd2f@virginia.edu

Laws ER Jr, Sheehan JP (eds): Pituitary Surgery – A Modern Approach.
Front Horm Res. Basel, Karger, 2006, vol 34, pp 105–126

The Craniopharyngioma

Rod J. Oskouian[a], *Amir Samii*[b], *Edward R. Laws, Jr.*[a]

[a]Department of Neuorological Surgery, Health Sciences Center, University of Virginia, Charlottesville, Va., USA; [b]International Neuroscience Institute, Hannover, Germany

Abstract

The craniopharyngioma is one of the most common destructive lesions of the hypothalamus and pituitary gland. It still remains one of the most difficult tumors to treat effectively since complete resection is often impossible and is associated with frequent recurrence. Current therapy is multimodal and focuses on a combination of surgical decompression, medical treatment, as well as stereotactic radiosurgery. This chapter reviews the embryology, neuroanatomy, current treatment strategies, clinical features and the several surgical approaches to its treatment.

Copyright © 2006 S. Karger AG, Basel

Introduction

In 1909, A.E. Halstead of Chicago successfully operated on a craniopharyngioma through the transsphenoidal approach [1]. Nearly a century has passed since then, and despite advances in our basic science understanding, cell biology, genetics, biologic behavior and technological capabilities, there still remains controversy in the optimal management of craniopharyngiomas. The actual term 'craniopharyngioma' was coined by Charles Frazier in 1931 and was popularized by Harvey Cushing in 1932 [2]. In 1932, Cushing in his writings on 'The Craniopharyngiomas' astutely recognized the difficulty to cure or even effectively resect these lesions [2]. Craniopharyngiomas are congenital and benign tumors that are thought to result from disorders of embryogenesis of the normal pituitary. Although benign in their biological behavior they are often located adjacent to the hypothalamus, infundibulohypophyseal axis, sellar, suprasellar and parasellar regions which are difficult to access surgically [3]. The hypothalamus has vital connections to the pituitary, brainstem, cortex, and injury to these connections contribute to the high mortality and morbidity rates that have been reported following radical surgery.

Craniopharyngiomas remain among the most challenging neoplasms both to diagnose and treat. The lesion is often situated at the cranial base, affects visual functions, and is often intimately associated with the hypothalamus and the pituitary gland. The surgical removal is technically demanding, associated with significant risks, and often these lesions cannot be totally resected because of their location [4–7]. The neurosurgeon has the ability to individualize the ideal treatment modality on the basis of magnetic resonance imaging (MRI) studies and has the advantage of intraoperative neuronavigation, radiosurgery and stereotactic aspiration. With the aid of these tools and our understanding of the microsurgical anatomy, the goal of total tumor excision has been accomplished with increased long-term survival as well as improved quality of life for the patient with optimal endocrinologic management postoperatively.

Epidemiology

The incidence of craniopharyngiomas is surprisingly low and most papers have cited that they account for 1–4% of all brain tumors. Historically craniopharyngiomas have been classified as brain tumors of childhood but large series have shown that there is actually a lower prevalence in childhood. In fact, the age distribution seems to have a bimodal pattern with a peak at 5–10 years of age and a second peak between the ages of 50–60. Sex distribution is equal with, perhaps, a slight male preponderance (males 55%, females 45%) [8]. There also seem to be no racial or genetic relationships in the pathogenesis of craniopharyngiomas.

Embryological Origin

Craniopharyngiomas are thought to arise from a small number of ectodermal cells found in the transitional area of the developing adenohypophysis which is why they so often involve the hypothalamus. These tumors are believed to be developmental in origin, arising from epithelial cell rests deposited between the hypothalamus, tuber cinereum and the pituitary gland. Squamous metaplasia of normal cells is an alternate possibility for their etiology. At about the same time in embryological development, the infundibulum forms as a downward growth of the neuroepithelium from the diencephalons [9, 10]. By the 8th week of gestation, Rathke's pouch has lost its connection with the oral cavity and is in contact with the infundibulum. The pars anterior develops from the anterior wall of the pouch between the 3rd and 5th months of gestation, but the posterior wall does not form glandular tissue and remains as the pars intermedia [11].

The embryogenesis of craniopharyngiomas is still controversial and is based on two opposing hypotheses. According to the first hypothesis, craniopharyngiomas arise from ectopic embryonic remnants of the craniopharyngeal duct. These cells initially connect Rathke's pouch with the stomodeum. As Rathke's pouch comes in contact with the infundibulum the neck separates itself from the oral epithelium. These same cells replicate and form the pars distalis of the hypophysis. The craniopharyngeal duct contains ectoblastic cells, and these have been proposed to be the origin of craniopharyngiomas [12].

The second theory entails the idea that craniopharyngiomas arise from metaplastic squamous epithelial cells in the adenohypophysis. There are residual epithelial cells that are found in the infundibulum and adenohypophysis which undergo metaplasia. This is supported by the fact that the squamous cell subtype of craniopharyngioma is rarely found in children but is often found in adults. Thus, it was suggested that craniopharyngiomas actually originate from metaplasia of mature cells rather than embryonic remnants.

Pathology

Craniopharyngiomas have a broad spectrum of size, content, and histology [13]. At one extreme there are tumors that form within a normal pituitary gland. At the other end of the spectrum there are giant tumors that extend superiorly and into the third ventricle and are intimately associated with the hypothalamus. The tumors can be entirely cystic or completely solid, but most tumors really have components of both. They are frequently calcified. The tumor cells can be squamous or cuboidal. The actual contents of the cyst fluid can be clear to the more typical yellow, brown, or chocolate, and the contents can be purulent in appearance with keratinized debris and cholesterol crystals. Some of the tumors are well encapsulated and separate easily from surrounding anatomic structures, while others can actually invade the brain, particularly the hypothalamus and third ventricle.

The anatomical origin of the tumor tends to determine its behavior and clinical presentation. Intrasellar craniopharyngiomas enlarge the sella and stretch the diaphragm. Purely suprasellar tumors can effect the stalk, hypothalamus, and chiasm and can cause obstructive hydrocephalus with compression of the third ventricle and the foramen of Monro. The myriad ways in which craniopharyngiomas present make it impossible to generalize about biologic behavior or any single mode of therapy. It is clearly evident that the craniopharyngioma in each patient is unique and must be considered individually.

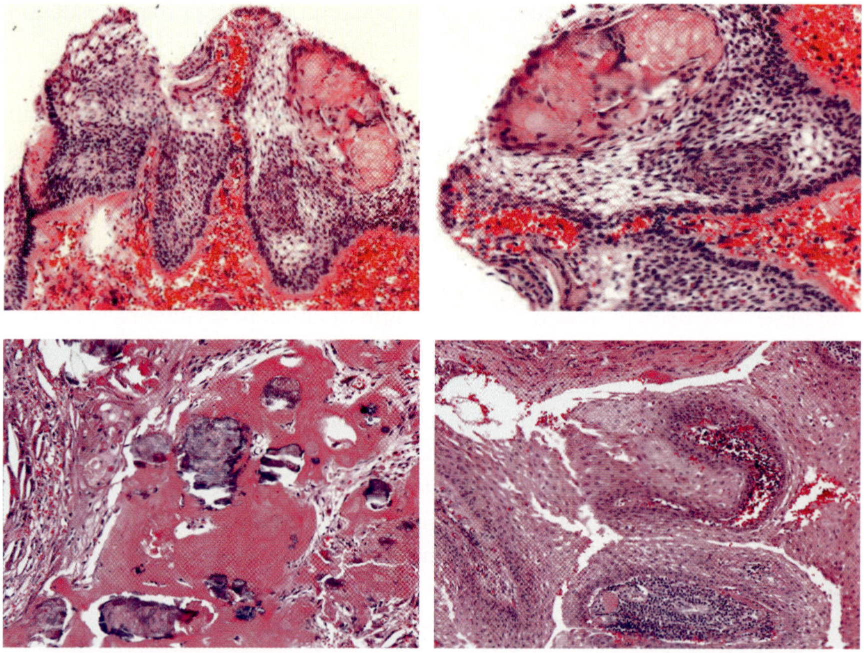

a b c d

Fig. 1. ***a*** Adamantinomatous craniopharyngioma. ×100. ***b*** Adamantinomatous craniopharyngioma. ×200. ***c*** Adamantinomatous craniopharyngioma exhibiting calcification and inflammatory reaction. ×200. ***d*** Papillary craniopharyngioma. ×100. All are HE stain and original magnifications.

There are two clinicopathologically separate types of craniopharyngiomas that have been categorized: the adamantinomatous and squamous papillary craniopharyngiomas (fig. 1). The adamantinomatous craniopharyngioma, found in children and in one quarter of adults, is usually cystic, with calcification, keratin nodules, cholesterol clefts, a suprasellar location, brain invasion and often has high recurrence rate. The squamous-papillary type, predominant in adults, is solid and characterized by a much lower incidence of calcification, keratin, recurrence, and brain invasion compared to the adamantinomatous type. We believe that craniopharyngiomas represent a continuum, and although there may be distinct histological and radiological differences, they often have no known prognostic or clinical significance. Pathologically, the epithelial elements comprising these tumors can range from cuboidal to columnar, or squamous in appearance. There has been an increasing tendency to distinguish craniopharyngiomas as being either classically adamantinomatous or papillary in nature. Although the latter has been proposed as a distinct clinicopathologically entity, featuring a predilection for adults, a less aggressive biology, and an overall favorable prognosis, so rigid a distinction may not be entirely justifiable, for papillary variants may simply reflect one component of the biological heterogeneity so characteristic of craniopharyngiomas in general. In fact, more recent studies indicate that no reliable prognostic differences exist between these two variants [14].

Rathke's Cleft Cysts and Craniopharyngiomas

Embryologically, the pituitary develops as the pars anterior, pars tuberalis, and pars intermedia which are all derived from the evagination of the stomodeal ectoderm. The residual lumen that is left between the anterior and intermediate lobes is what constitutes Rathke's cleft. Later in development, a small portion of the anterior wall of the pouch extends along the ventral aspect of the infundibulum and in the center of the infundibulum. This extension is termed the pars tuberalis. The pars tuberalis is above the diaphragma sellae and in humans has no functional relationship to the median eminence of the tuber cinereum. It can be found around the lower part of the hypophysial stalk where there are nests of squamous cells. Within the pars tuberalis, a combination of pituitary gland cells and squamous cells are frequently found. Both Rathke's cleft cysts and craniopharyngiomas are thought to arise from enlargement of this cleft. That is why both lesions are closely related and share a common cellular origin from Rathke's pouch. Thus, they constitute what many believe is really a spectrum from the simplest form, the Rathke's cleft cyst, through intermediate forms to the most complex form, the craniopharyngioma [15].

Neuroanatomical Considerations

A thorough understanding of the neuroanatomical relationships of the carotid artery, optic nerve, chiasm, third ventricle, subarachnoid cisterns and anterior clinoid process is fundamental to sellar, parasellar, suprasellar and suprachiasmatic lesions. The carotid artery and the optic nerve course medial to the anterior clinoid. The most common location for craniopharyngiomas is along the infundibulohypophyseal axis where they can be sellar or suprasellar extending up and into the suprasellar cisterns. The optic chiasm is often used as a critical reference point for suprasellar extension, but others consider the absolute vertical extension of the lesion as an important characteristic in classification (table 1) [16]. Our experience has shown that these tumors know no boundaries and may grow horizontally as well into the prechiasmatic and

Table 1. Classification of craniopharyngiomas according to Raybaud et al. [16]

Grade	Description
I	Intrasellar tumor
II	Intracisternal tumor with or without intrasellar component
III	Intracisternal tumor extending into the lower half of the third ventricle
IV	Intracisternal tumor extending into the upper half of the third ventricle
V	Intracisternal tumor extending into the septum pellucidum or into the lateral ventricle

subfrontal cisterns, laterally into the temporal area as well as posteriorly into the prepontine and interpeduncular cisterns and even on rare occasions to the cerebellopontine angle [17] (fig. 2).

It is unusual to have either a purely intrasellar or purely suprasellar craniopharyngioma. More often the tumor grows upward against the diaphragm and commonly breaks through allowing it to extend in any direction. Intrasellar craniopharyngiomas will often cause expansion of the sella and destruction of the pituitary gland with resultant panhypopituitarism. Prechiasmatic craniopharyngiomas will often extend anteriorly into the subfrontal space and can cause compression of the optic chiasm with visual deficits (fig. 3). The prechiasmatic craniopharyngiomas can achieve a very large size before they are diagnosed or cause any clinical symptoms. Retrochiasmatic craniopharyngiomas will grow posterior to the chiasm and can push the pituitary stalk as well as the chiasm forward as the tumor enlarges (fig. 4). There are also subchiasmatic craniopharyngiomas that can displace the chiasm upward and the stalk anteriorly or posteriorly.

Craniopharyngiomas can compress the hypothalamus and can result in obstruction of cerebrospinal fluid (CSF) flow through the foramen of Monro and impair drainage of CSF into the third ventricle with resultant obstructive hydrocephalus. There are also instances in which the lesions grow laterally with compression of the temporal lobe which can produce epilepsy.

Despite the variation in location of craniopharyngiomas, they are often adherent not only to the hypothalamus and chiasm but occasionally to vascular structures of the circle of Willis. The anterior as well as posterior circulation is at risk of injury during surgery, especially the small perforating vessels arising from the anterior communicating arteries, the anterior choroidal artery and the thalamoperforating vessels [18].

Tumors arising within the sella can often extend upward into the suprasellar cisterns to compress the floor of the third ventricle, the circle of Willis and hypothalamus [19] (fig. 5). The area involved by those tumors arising in the

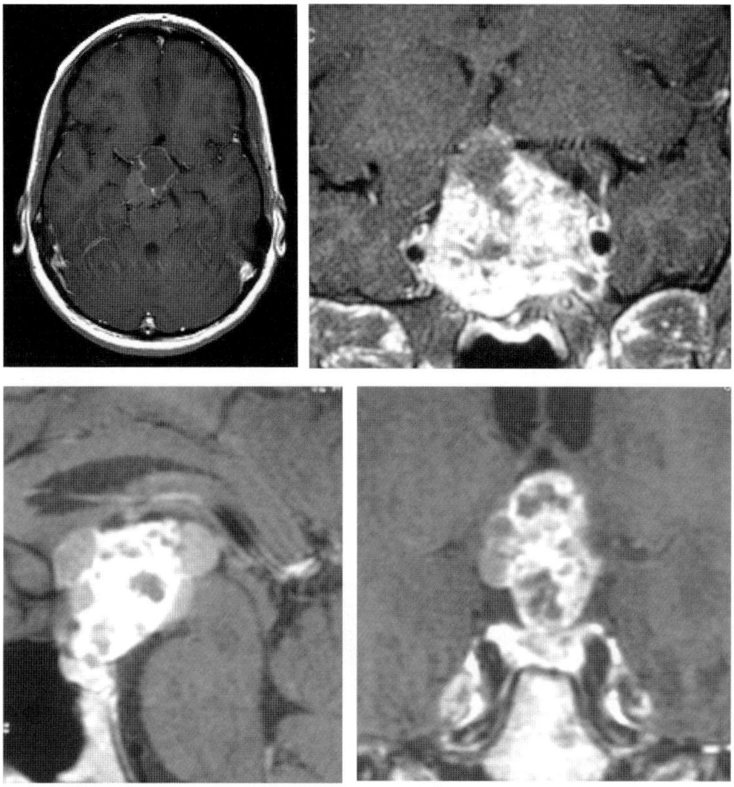

Fig. 2. Magnetic resonance imagings of craniopharyngiomas demonstrating the wide variety of anatomic locations of these lesions.

sella corresponds to the anterior incisural space located between the free edges of the tentorium and the anterior aspect of the midbrain. This space corresponds to the suprasellar area which from the anterior border of the midbrain extends anteriorly and around the optic chiasm. Below the optic chiasm, the suprasellar area has posterior walls that are formed by the cerebral peduncles. The anterior incisural space extends laterally to the sylvian fissure and is situated inferior to the anterior perforated substance.

When operating in the suprasellar cisterns and anterior incisural space it is important to note that there are several cranial nerves that traverse these cisterns. The optic and oculomotor nerves pass through the suprasellar region and are often compressed by or adherent to the wall of the tumor. The optic nerves travel medially to the anterior clinoid processes until they reach the chiasm.

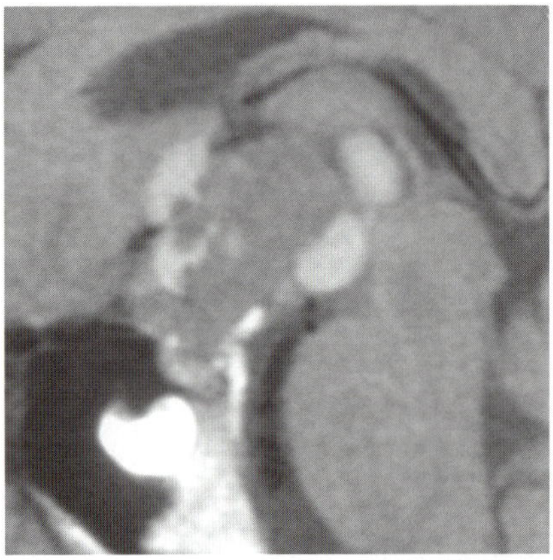

Fig. 3. MRI of a suprasellar craniopharyngioma with extension into the third ventricle and compression of the optic chiasm.

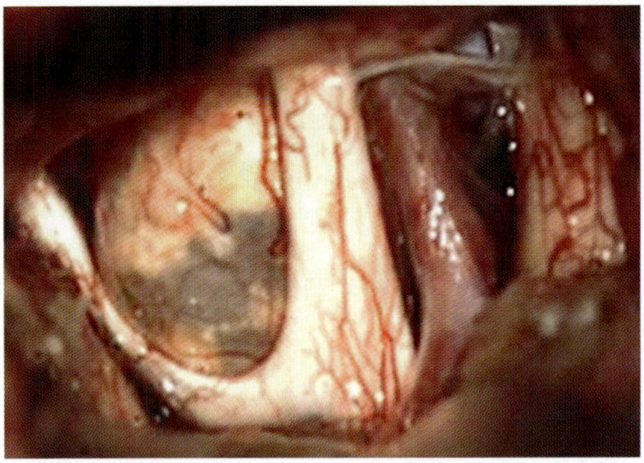

Fig. 4. Prechiasmatic craniopharyngiomas will often achieve a very large size before they are diagnosed or cause any clinical symptoms.

Posterior to the chiasm, the optic tracts continue in a posterolateral direction around the cerebral peduncles to enter the middle incisural spaces. Coagulation of the falciform ligament or dura above the optic nerve just proximal to the optic canal can lead to nerve injury. Compression of the optic nerve against the falciform ligament may result in a visual field deficit, as is seen with proximal carotid artery aneurysms. The optic nerve is usually separated from the sphenoid sinus by a very thin layer of bone, which can be absent in the case of a pneumatized sinus. The anterior cerebral and anterior communicating arteries,

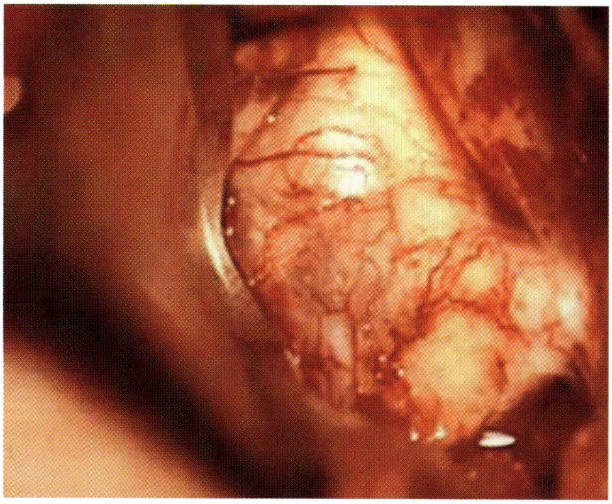

Fig. 5. Retrochiasmatic craniopharyngiomas will grow posterior to the chiasm and can push the pituitary stalk as well as the chiasm forward as the tumor enlarges. There are also subchiasmatic craniopharyngiomas that can displace the chiasm upward and the stalk anteriorly or even posteriorly as is shown here.

the lamina terminalis, and the third ventricle lie just above the chiasm. This anatomic relationship of the chiasm to the sella is important for determining surgical approaches. Normally the chiasm overlies the diaphragma sellae and the pituitary gland. The prefixed chiasm lies on the tuberculum sellae, and the postfixed chiasm is behind the dorsum sellae [20].

The oculomotor nerve arises in the interpeduncular cistern from the midbrain and forms the lateral border of Liliquist's membrane which separates the chiasmatic and interpeduncular cisterns. The oculomotor nerve enters the roof of the cavernous sinus and heads downward though the cavernous sinus. The trochlear nerve is the longest and smallest cranial nerve and enters the cavernous sinus just behind the tentorial attachment. The abducens nerve passes upward in the prepontine cistern to enter the posterior part of the cavernous sinus. The trigeminal nerve arises in the posterior fossa from the pons to enter Meckel's cave lateral to the cavernous sinus. The first division of the trigeminal nerve, the ophthalmic division, then courses to enter the lower part of the cavernous sinus.

Presenting Symptoms

The signs and symptoms of craniopharyngiomas are determined by the age of the patient, the size, and location of the tumor. Visual dysfunction referable to chiasmatic or optic nerve compression occurs in patients of all ages, though children are more tolerant of, and more difficult to test for, visual field deficits. The symptoms can include endocrine dysfunction, visual deficits, cognitive disturbances and even hydrocephalus. The most common presenting symptoms of any sellar mass are visual loss, pituitary dysfunction and headaches. Although headache is a common occurrence, more lesions are being diagnosed earlier since imaging technology has become more accessible and is less expensive.

All patients with suspected craniopharyngioma should have a comprehensive endocrine evaluation [21]. Visual performance should be documented with fundoscopic examination, tangent screen, and perimetry. With computed tomography (CT) or MRI, craniopharyngiomas typically appear as inhomogeneous lesions – ones in which cystic components can often be discerned from solid elements.

Endocrine symptoms are most prominent in children. Retardation of growth and sexual development are commonly seen. The sella is small and any size of lesion may produce headaches. The common historical features of a pituitary lesion in adolescents and adults include decreased libido and/or erectile dysfunction in men, irregular menses or amenorrhea in premenopausal women, and fatigue (thyroid hormone, cortisol, growth hormone (GH) deficiencies), weight gain, fatigue, difficulty with sleeping, irritability, depression, memory loss, difficulty with concentrating, and a general decline in executive functions. Development of diabetes insipidus is a relatively common occurrence in patients with a craniopharyngioma, a Rathke cleft cyst, or an infiltrative disease (lymphocytic hypophysitis, sarcoidosis and lymphoma) because these disorders often involve the pituitary stalk and the hypothalamic nuclei. The clinical history is that of frequent urination, particularly frequent nocturia. Men with hypogonadism will have testicular atrophy and diminished body hair which is indicative of testosterone deficiency. Fine wrinkling of the facial skin is characteristic and is likely to be a result of both a testosterone and GH deficiency.

Imaging

Craniopharyngiomas have a typical radiological appearance on CT and MRI often allowing one to infer correct preoperative differential diagnosis from other lesions: tuberculum sellae meningioma, optic or hypothalamic glioma, epidermoid tumor, Rathke's cleft cyst, suprasellar germinoma, or pituitary adenoma [22]. High-resolution CT scanning provides identification of the cystic calcified contents and details of the bony anatomy of the skull base (fig. 6).

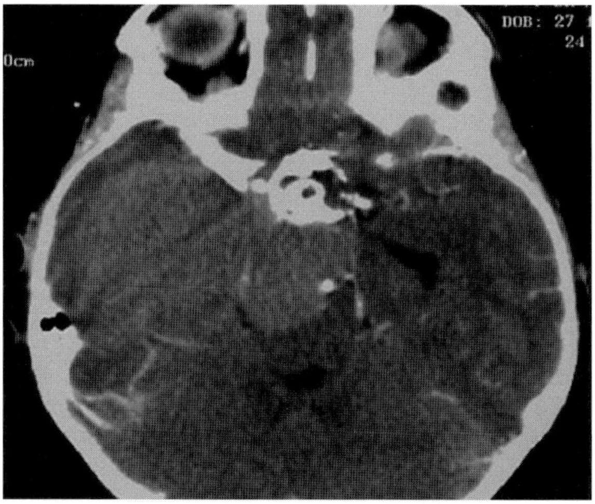

Fig. 6. Axial CT scan demonstrating calcification in the craniopharyngioma preoperatively.

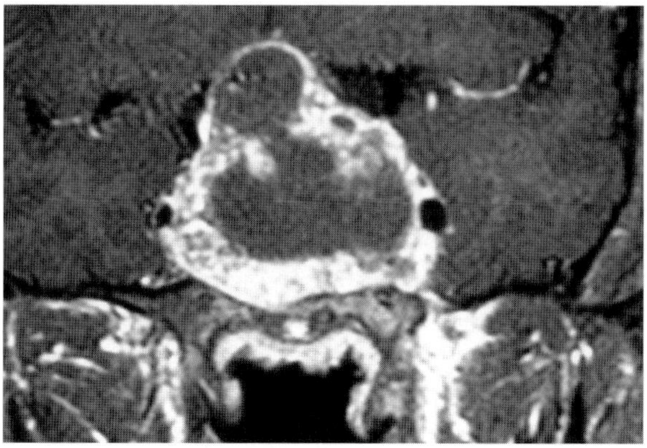

Fig. 7. MRI of a large craniopharyngioma demonstrating the cystic and solid portions of the lesion as well as the carotid arteries.

MRI is much better at identifying the soft tissue architecture such as the chiasm, hypothalamus, third ventricle and pituitary gland (fig. 7).

There are atypical imaging features that are sometimes present that can lead to misdiagnosis. Craniopharyngiomas often have a rather large suprasellar extension. Tuberculum sellae meningiomas show the typical homogeneous enhancement with a broad-based attachment frequently associated with a meningeal tail. Hypothalamic glioma, optic glioma and germinomas often invade brain tissue. Both epidermoids and Rathke's cleft cysts do not usually show significant contrast enhancement. However, Rathke's cleft cysts can also appear very similar to cystic craniopharyngiomas, with depiction of only a minimal contrast-enhanced, solid portion. We often obtain a CT scan in addition to MRI to demonstrate calcification which often has a curvilinear pattern along the periphery of the tumor. MRI is superior to CT in determining tumor extent, and provides valuable neuroanatomical information regarding the relationship of the tumor to the chiasm and intracranial arteries due to its multiplanar capabilities. We also recommend obtaining noncontrast, sagittal, coronal and axial T1-weighted images, which may enable identification of the normal pituitary, possibly leading to the diagnosis of craniopharyngioma. More recently, we have been obtaining three-dimensional CT angiography of the cranial base of large lesions that have significant suprasellar extension to better visualize the intracranial arteries and their relationship to the lesion.

Endocrinologic Evaluation

Craniopharyngiomas often cause loss of pituitary function, it is crucial to identify the need for hormone replacement in these patients. Since there is such a broad degree of pituitary dysfunction there may be a need for replacement of glucocorticoids, thyroid hormone, and vasopressin before surgery to minimize the risk of intraoperative and postoperative complications [21]. Diabetes insipidus should be anticipated postoperatively if there is involvement of the pituitary stalk or the hypothalamic nuclei and is often present preoperatively. The need for gonadal steroids and GH replacement therapy should be evaluated after surgery. Adrenal insufficiency, hypothyroidism, and diabetes insipidus must be identified and treated before surgery to reduce the risk of intraoperative and postoperative complications. Glucocorticoid (intravenous hydrocortisone or dexamethasone) administration at the time of surgery is a usual and appropriate neurosurgical practice. The general principle is to give a stress dose of a glucocorticoid at the time of surgery and for at least 24 h afterward intravenously. Because hospitalization for transsphenoidal surgery is short-term (2–3 days), at discharge many patients are given oral steroid replacement therapy with plans for reevaluation after surgical recovery (usually 6–8 weeks postoperatively) [23]. In this situation the patient should be given a short-acting glucocorticoid, hydrocortisone, to minimize the suppression of endogenous adrenocorticotropic hormone (ACTH). Typically, the hydrocortisone therapy is discontinued 2 days before the postoperative visit and the serum levels of cortisol and

ACTH are measured. Many patients have a GH deficiency both before and after surgery, and the definitive test of GH deficiency is the GH response to insulin-induced hypoglycemia. This test serves to diagnose both an impaired ACTH reserve and a GH deficiency, and should be reserved for the postoperative evaluation. GH replacement is beneficial in improving body composition with an increase in muscle mass, decrease in adipose mass, and improvement in muscle strength, and serum lipid levels.

Surgical Treatment

If a craniopharyngioma does arise within the confines of the sella below the diaphragm, then it will often enlarge the pituitary fossa and stretch the diaphragm above its dorsal aspect. This is the reason why an intrasellar craniopharyngioma can have the diaphragm of the sella continue to act as a barrier between the suprasellar portion of the craniopharyngioma and the intracranial structures such as the chiasm and hypothalamus. Enlargement of the sella therefore implies an origin of the craniopharyngioma below the diaphragm and the existence of an anatomic barrier that tends to prevent adherence or invasion of the tumor to vital structures [24].

The goals of surgery are to remove the tumor, relieve the mass effect, improve visual abnormalities and to preserve normal pituitary function. Surgery is very effective in relieving the mass effect; however, most patients harboring a large lesion will require additional treatment(s) to prevent re-growth of residual tumor, and most will require hormone replacement therapy to reestablish a normal hormonal balance.

Transsphenoidal Surgery

The transsphenoidal route may be ideally suited for craniopharyngiomas that begin within the sella turcica and extend in a direct suprasellar pathway [23–33]. The major indication for surgery in such lesions is, first and foremost, enlargement of the sella with compression of vital structures. The characteristics of the tumor also play a significant role in the decision of the surgical approach. For instance, it could be that an entirely cystic craniopharyngioma that has expanded the sella is best removed transsphenoidally. The ability to deflate the cyst and at the same time mobilize its capsule are important features in securing a satisfactory removal of the lesion. When a craniopharyngioma does arise within the sella turcica, it usually compresses the pituitary gland, which is the reason most patients present with hypopituitarism. If they do not

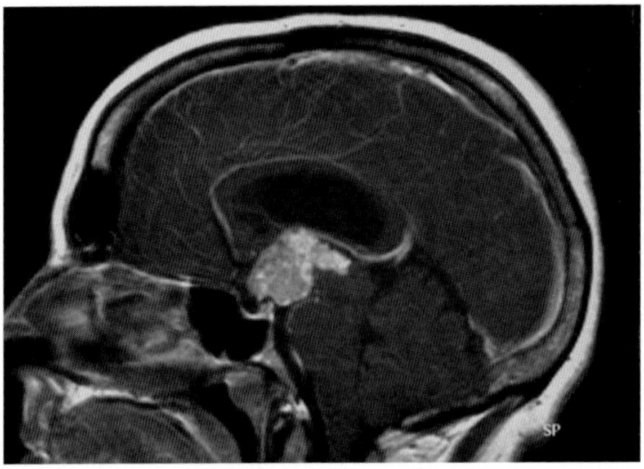

Fig. 8. A transsellar-transdiaphragmatic approach to reach the suprasellar cisterns was used to excise this lesion.

have pituitary dysfunction prior to surgery, many will have hypopituitarism after removal of an entirely intrasellar lesion since the gland is often compressed and densely adherent to the tumor. For this reason we tend to reserve transsphenoidal surgery as the primary approach for patients who have clinical evidence of pituitary dysfunction.

When pituitary function is intact, it is often easier to preserve function with a craniotomy, although preservation of the pituitary gland and its function is by no means certain. In recent years we have also become more aggressive with the transsphenoidal approach for tumors that have a significant suprasellar extension. We have found that patients tolerate the minimally invasive procedure of the transsphenoidal approach and often can go home in 2–3 days. Transsphenoidal surgery has been reserved for the removal of tumors involving the sella turcica and to the suprasellar extension of such tumors if the sella appears enlarged. Craniopharyngiomas located entirely within the suprasellar area with a normal sella have traditionally been managed through a craniotomy. The subfrontal, pterional or frontotemporal craniotomies have been used for the approach.

As minimally invasive techniques continue to be popularized there are two modified transsphenoidal approaches that can be used for midline lesions in the presence of a normal sella. A transsellar-transdiaphragmatic method of approaching the suprasellar cisterns has been reported in the excision of both craniopharyngiomas and pituitary adenomas [34]. We have used this approach in 35 cases of primarily suprasellar retrochiasmatic lesions (fig. 8). Alternatively, we have also used a presellar-transtuberculum extended skull base approach, through a widening of the surgical field obtainable with the standard procedure [35]. In this technique, bone is removed from the floor of the sella, tuberculum, and posterior portion of the planum sphenoidale, allowing a prediaphragmatic view of the basal cisterns. This is particularly helpful when the lesion is entirely cystic or has a major cystic component that can be drained from below either at surgery or, occasionally, with a permanent drain. We sometimes leave a Silastic shunt or tube to allow drainage of a cystic craniopharyngioma into the sphenoid sinus [24]. This can only be done when there is no evidence of a CSF leak during the operation. We have used this approach in a number of cases and the tubing eventually extrudes into the posterior nasal space. As with primary transsphenoidal operations, a large sella is desirable simply because it gives the surgeon room to manipulate instruments safely and at the same time visualize the sellar and suprasellar structures.

There are a number of situations in which transsphenoidal surgery is both difficult and inadvisable [23, 24]. The most challenging of these situations is the presence of a normal sella in a patient without evidence of pituitary dysfunction. Patients who have normal pituitary function do have significant risk of losing function following surgery. This may result from direct damage to anterior pituitary tissue or disconnection from the hypothalamic nuclei. If there is extensive involvement of the intracranial structures such as the chiasm or hypothalamus then it can be extremely hazardous to perform the operation from below. This is especially true when the capsule is adherent to the branches of the circle of Willis. Obviously, hemorrhage from suprasellar arteries is extremely difficult to control with the limited exposure of the transsphenoidal approach.

We generally avoid doing transsphenoidal surgery in growing children as the risk of pituitary damage and dysfunction postoperatively is significant and can alter normal growth [23]. In these circumstances it is reasonable to follow the child with serial imaging as well as close endocrinologic and ophthalmologic examinations. These same principles also apply to women of childbearing age who do not wish to have pituitary-hypothalamic dysfunction prior to conceiving.

Craniotomy

Several surgical approaches for the craniopharyngioma have been developed. Historically, the unilateral subfrontal approach has been the most popular. The craniotomy is usually performed on the side of the patient in which vision is worse. The bifrontal craniotomy with a subfrontal or interhemispheric approach has also been advocated. Heuer and Dandy in 1919 proposed a unilateral approach along the sphenoid wing for tumors in the hypophysis. Their

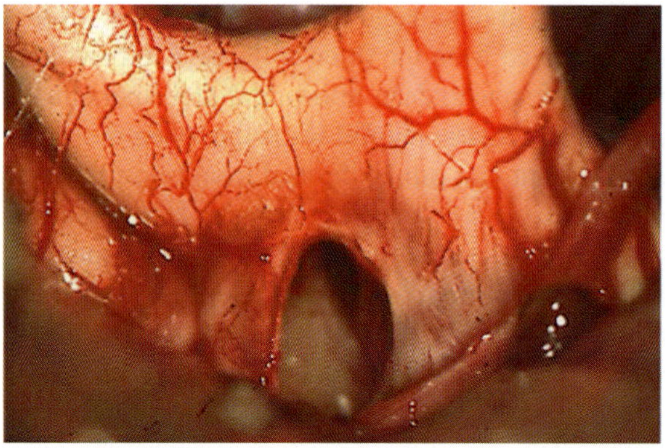

Fig. 9. An approach through the lamina terminalis has the advantage of excellent midline exposure, but limits visualization of the lateral extent of tumor.

approach has matured into the 'pterional' craniotomy that is now most favored [36, 37]. There are also transcallosal and transventricular approaches that have been advocated for tumors lying within the third ventricle or lateral ventricle. The choice of the approach depends on the anatomy of the tumor and its location [38–40].

Once the brain is exposed, access to the tumor can be achieved by several routes. Some lesions can be removed entirely between the optic nerves anteriorly. In many patients, especially children, the optic chiasm can be prefixed therefore limiting this approach. An approach through the lamina terminalis has the advantage of excellent midline exposure, but limits visualization of the lateral and posterior extent of the tumor [39] (fig. 9). An approach between the optic nerve and carotid artery allows great exposure of the lateral aspect of the tumor. However, this can be limited by the optic tract posteriorly, supraclinoid carotid and optic chiasm (fig. 10).

The pterional approach allows excellent access to the suprasellar region along the sphenoid wing [40]. We are able to immediately decompress the suprasellar compartment with drainage of CSF by way of the basal cistern which also aids in brain relaxation to minimize brain retraction. We carefully dissect the arachnoid around the basal cisterns and depending on our exposure will sometimes open the sylvian fissure. The fissure when opened will enable a wider window to view the carotid, chiasm and anterior cerebral artery. If the tumor is cystic then we often drain the cyst to further decompress the area and remove pressure from the optic nerves. While operating in the opticocarotid recess it is important not to damage the small perforators coming off the medial wall of the carotid artery that supply the chiasm and hypothalamus. The

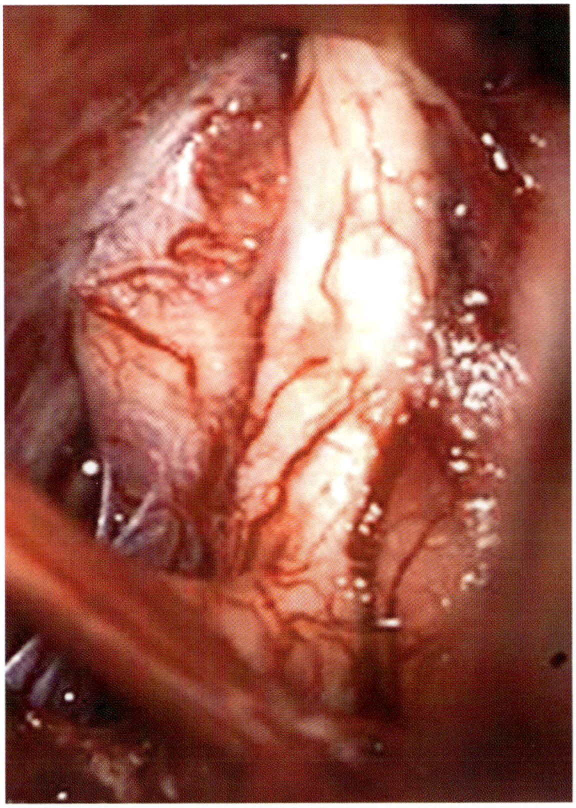

Fig. 10. An approach between the optic nerve and carotid artery allows great exposure of the lateral aspect of the tumor, however, this can be limited by the optic tract posteriorly, supraclinoid carotid and optic chiasm.

superior hypophyseal artery complex supplies the blood flow to the optic nerve, the optic chiasm and the pituitary stalk. We often open the lamina terminalis as well. Purely third ventricular tumors can be taken out through a transcallosal-transforaminal approach.

Other Treatments

The management of the recurrent craniopharyngioma is a complex subject and therapeutic goals must be well defined for each individual patient. In some cases, and despite the technical demands of reoperation, total resection can still

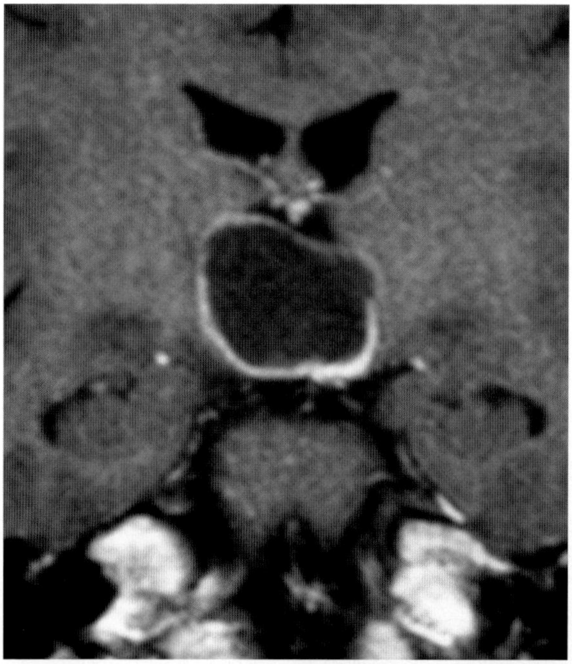

Fig. 11. Recurrent cystic lesions have been treated with stereotactic intracavitary instillation of radioactive solutions containing colloidal phosphorus, yttrium or gold.

be achieved. However, for many recurrent tumors palliative surgery is often the most realistic goal. Recurrent lesions with a significant cystic component can often be treated by repeat aspiration. This can be achieved by inserting a silastic tube attached to an Ommaya reservoir into the cyst cavity. Alternatively, the transsphenoidal insertion of a silastic tube from the tumor cavity into the posterior nasal space can provide prolonged drainage. In addition to conventional irradiation, there are several other radiotherapeutic options applicable for recurrent tumors. For cystic lesions, stereotactic intracavitary instillation of radioactive solutions containing colloidal phosphorus, yttrium, or gold has been of benefit (fig. 11). Solid recurrences have been treated with interstitial brachytherapy (the irradiation of lesions by insertion of an isotope within the tumor) and stereotactic radiosurgery.

Craniopharyngiomas have a tendency to recur, even after apparent total removal. The rate of recurrence ranges from 0 to 50% in cases of total removal and from 30 to 100% in cases of subtotal or partial removal [41]. Most recurrences develop in the first 3 years following surgery. The optimal treatment of recurrent craniopharyngioma remains elusive. We believe that surgery should be considered as the first choice of treatment among therapeutic modalities for recurrent craniopharyngiomas. Repeated surgery is more difficult than the primary one and has an increased risk of morbidity and mortality [42, 43]. Radiation is said to play an important role in reducing the rate of recurrence. Gamma knife surgery has been shown to be effective for achieving long-term control of tumors without compromising the quality of patient survival [44, 45]. However, there were few reports which analyzed the treatment outcomes of recurrent craniopharyngiomas for each modality.

Craniopharyngiomas are considered to be radiosensitive tumors. Radiation therapy whether it be conventional or stereotactic is most commonly used as adjuvant treatment after incomplete tumor resection or tumor recurrence. In patients with a large tumor in whom the resection is incomplete, radiotherapy or radiosurgery can reduce the risk of residual tumor enlargement and offer a chance of tumor control without further surgery. We feel that radiosurgery should be considered in cases where it is thought that the tumor cannot be removed safely and completely by surgery. Current radiosurgical technology minimizes radiation damage to adjacent neural structures as long as there is a safe distance between the tumor and the optic chiasm and hypothalamus. Gamma knife surgery is effective for achieving long-term control of tumors without compromising the quality of patient survival and can be delivered in one treatment session [46–49]. These patients need careful endocrine follow-up since pituitary dysfunction can present in a delayed fashion. While conventional radiotherapy carries the risk of damaging the hypothalamus and the optic pathway, it would appear that stereotactic, i.e. gamma knife, proton beam, cyberknife radiosurgery, may be superior in this respect if this treatment modality is applicable.

Conclusion

The management of the craniopharyngioma must be individualized to the patient and to the anatomy and biology of the specific tumor. Total removal is a reasonable goal in many patients, especially in those that have an enlarged sella and can be managed entirely through transsphenoidal surgery. In infants and children who are growing normally and neurologically stable, it can be prudent to delay surgery until growth is complete. For many patients, satisfactory results can follow subtotal removal and subsequent radiation therapy. The effects of radiation, particularly on the immature brain, optic apparatus and the neuroendocrine system, must be carefully considered.

In patients who have persistent or recurrent craniopharyngioma, the goals of therapy must also be thoroughly analyzed. Although in some cases total removal can be accomplished, in most cases subtotal resection is reasonable in light of hypothalamic or visual dysfunction. The immediate goals of surgery should include decompression of the optic apparatus, aspiration of a cystic portion of the tumor, and decreasing intracranial pressure in the setting of obstructive hydrocephalus.

Therefore the goal of treatment, a neurologically intact patient living a normal life, is accomplished with a judicious combination of surgery, meticulous medical and endocrine management, and appropriate radiosurgery or fractionated radiation therapy when indicated. Improvements in our ability to diagnose as well as treat the craniopharyngioma, with medical, surgical and radiosurgical techniques, should lead to continuing improvement in the management of this formidable tumor.

References

1 Halstead AE: Remarks on an operative treatment of tumors of the hypophysis. Surg Gynecol Obstet 1910;10:494–502.

2 Cushing HW: The Craniopharyngiomas. Intracranial Tumors: Notes upon a Series of Two Thousand Verified Cases with Surgical Mortality Percentage Pertaining Thereto. Springfield, Thomas, 1932, pp 93–98.

3 Bergland RM, Ray BS, Torack RM: Anatomical variations in the pituitary gland and adjacent structures in 225 human autopsy cases. J Neurosurg 1968;28:93–99.

4 Baskin DS, Wilson CB: Surgical management of craniopharyngiomas: a review of 74 cases. J Neurosurg 1986;65:22–27.

5 Carmel PW: Craniopharyngiomas; in Wilkins RH, Rengachary SS (eds): Neurosurgery. New York, McGraw-Hill, 1985, vol 1, pp 905–916.

6 Effenterre RV, Boch AL: Craniopharyngioma in adults and children: a study of 122 surgical cases. J Neurosurg 2002;97:3–11.

7 Fahlbusch R, Honegger J, Paulus W, Huk W, Buchfelder M: Surgical treatment of craniopharyngiomas: experience with 168 patients. J Neurosurg 1999;90:237–250.

8 Nomura K: Report of Brain Tumor Registry of Japan (1969–1993), ed 10. Neurol Med Chir 2000;40(suppl):47–48.

9 Rougerie J: Intrasellar and suprasellar tumors of the infant and adolescent; in Bushe KA, Spoerri O, Shaw J (eds): Progress in Pediatric Neurosurgery. Proceedings of the 3rd European Congress of Paediatric Neurosurgery, Göttingen 1972. Stuttgart, Hippokrates, 1974, pp 34–45.

10 Choux M, Lena G, Genitori L: Le craniopharyngiome de l'enfant. Neurochirurgie 1991;37.

11 Hayward R: The present and future management of childhood craniopharyngioma. Childs Nerv Syst 1999;15:764–769.

12 Erdheim J: Über Hypophysenganggeschwülste und Hirncholesteatome. Sitzungsber Kaiserliche Akad Wiss (Wien) 1904;113(sect 3):537–726.

13 Petito CK, DeGirolami U, Earle KM: Craniopharyngiomas: a clinical and pathological review. Cancer 1976;37:1944–1952.

14 Adamson TE, Wiestler OD, Kleihues P, Yasargil MG: Correlation of clinical and pathological features in surgically treated craniopharyngiomas. J Neurosurg 1990;73:12–17.

15 Harrison MJ, Morgello S, Post KD: Epithelial cystic lesions of the sellar and parasellar region: a continuum of ectodermal derivatives? J Neurosurg 1994;80:1018–1025.

16 Raybaud C, Rabehanta P, Girard N: Aspects radiologiques des craniopharyngiomes. Neurochirurgie 1991;37:44–58.
17 Laws ER Jr: Transsphenoidal approach to lesions in and about the sella turcica; in Schmidek HH, Sweet WH (eds): Operative Neurosurgical Technique. Indications, Methods, and Results. New York, Grune & Stratton, 1982, pp 327–341.
18 Samii M, Tatagiba M: Surgical management of craniopharyngiomas: a review. Neurol Med Chir (Tokyo) 1997;37:141–149.
19 Yasargil MG, Curcic M, Kis M, Siegenthaler G, Teddy PJ, Roth P: Total removal of craniopharyngiomas. Approaches and long-term results in 144 patients. J Neurosurg 1990;73:3–11.
20 Samii M, Bini W: Surgical treatment of craniopharyngiomas. Zentralbl Neurochir 1991;52:17–23.
21 Vance ML: Treatment of patients with a pituitary adenoma: one clinician's experience. Neurosurg Focus 2004;16:E1.
22 Lindgren E, Di Chiro G: Suprasellar tumours with calcification. Acta Radiol 1951;36:173–195.
23 Laws ER Jr: Transsphenoidal surgery; in Apuzzo MLJ (ed): Brain Surgery. Complication Avoidance and Management. New York, Churchill Livingstone, 1993, pp 357–361.
24 Laws ER Jr: Transsphenoidal removal of craniopharyngioma. Pediatr Neurosurg 1994;21: 57–63.
25 Ciric IS, Cozzens JW: Craniopharyngiomas: transsphenoidal method of approach – for the virtuoso only? Clin Neurosurg 1980;27:169–187.
26 Laws ER Jr: Transsphenoidal microsurgery in the management of craniopharyngioma. J Neurosurg 1980;52:661–666.
27 Fahlbusch R, Honegger J, Paulus W, Huk W, Buchfelder M: Surgical treatment of craniopharyngiomas: experience with 168 patients. J Neurosurg 1999;90:237–250.
28 Hardy J: Transsphenoidal approach to the pituitary gland; in Wilkins RH, Rengachary SS (eds): Neurosurgery, ed 2. New York, McGraw-Hill, 1996, vol 2, pp 1375–1384.
29 Hardy J: Transsphenoidal hypophysectomy. J Neurosurg 1971;34:582–594.
30 Hardy J: Transsphenoidal microsurgery of the normal and pathological pituitary. Clin Neurosurg 1969;16:185–217.
31 Hardy J, Lalonde JL: Exérèse par voie trans-sphénoïdale d'un craniopharyngiome géant. Union Med Can 1963;92:1124–1129.
32 Hardy J, Maira G: Microsurgical anatomy in trans-sphenoidal hypophysectomy. J Neurosurg Sci 1977;21:151–157.
33 Hardy J, Vezina JL: Transsphenoidal neurosurgery of intracranial neoplasm. Adv Neurol 1976;15:261–274.
34 Kaptain GJ, Vincent DA, Sheehan JP: Transsphenoidal approaches for the extracapsular resection of midline suprasellar and anterior cranial base lesions. Neurosurgery 2001;49:94–101.
35 Kato T, Sawamura Y, Abe H: Transsphenoidal-transtuberculum sellae approach for supradiaphragmatic tumours: technical note. Acta Neurochir 1998;140:715–719.
36 Al-Mefty O, Hassounah M, Weaver P, Sakati N, Jinkins JR, Fox JL: Microsurgery for giant craniopharyngiomas in children. Neurosurgery 1985;17:585–595.
37 Maira G, Anile C, Rossi GF, Colosimo C: Surgical treatment of craniopharyngiomas: an evaluation of the transsphenoidal and pterional approaches. Neurosurgery 1995;36:715–724.
38 Pang D: Surgical management of craniopharyngioma; in Sekhar LN, Janeka IP (eds): Surgery of Cranial Base Tumors. New York, Raven Press, 1993, pp 787–807.
39 Maira G, Anile C, Colosimo C: Craniopharyngiomas of the third ventricle: trans-lamina terminalis approach. Neurosurgery 2000;47:857–865.
40 Maira G, Anile C, Rossi GF: Surgical treatment of craniopharyngiomas: an evaluation of the transsphenoidal and pterional approaches. Neurosurgery 1995;36:715–724.
41 Weiner HL, Wisoff JH, Rosenberg ME, Kupersmith MJ, Cohen H, Zagzag D, Maher TS, Flamm ES, Epstein FJ, Miller DC: Craniopharyngiomas: a clinicopathological analysis of factors predictive of recurrence and functional outcome. Neurosurgery 1994;35:1001–1011.
42 Hoffman HJ, Silva MD, Humphreys RP, Drake JM, Smith ML, Blaser SI: Aggressive surgical management of craniopharyngiomas in children. J Neurosurg 1992;76:47–52.
43 Wisoff JH: Surgical management of recurrent craniopharyngiomas. Pediatr Neurosurg 1994;21 (suppl 1):108–113.

44 Amacher AL: Craniopharyngioma: the controversy regarding radiotherapy. Childs Brain 1980;6: 57–64.
45 Wara MW, Sneed PK, Larson DA: The role of radiation therapy in the treatment of craniopharyngioma. Pediatr Neurosurg 1994;21(suppl 1):98–100.
46 Chung WY, Pan DH, Shiau CY, Guo WY, Wang LW: Gamma knife radiosurgery for craniopharyngiomas. J Neurosurg 2000;93(suppl 3):47–56.
47 Kobayashi T, Tanaka T, Kida Y: Stereotactic gamma radiosurgery of craniopharyngiomas. Pediatr Neurosurg 1994;21(suppl 1):69–74.
48 Manaka S, Teramoto A, Takakura K: The efficacy of radiotherapy for craniopharyngioma. J Neurosurg 1985;62:648–656.
49 Mokry M: Craniopharyngiomas: a six year experience with gamma knife radiosurgery. Stereotact Funct Neursurg 1999;72(suppl 1):140–149.

Edward R. Laws, Jr., MD, FACS
Department of Neurological Surgery, Health Sciences Center
University of Virginia, PO Box 800212
Charlottesville, VA 22908 (USA)
Tel. +1 434 924 2650, Fax +1 434 924 5894, E-Mail el5g@virginia.edu

Laws ER Jr, Sheehan JP (eds): Pituitary Surgery – A Modern Approach.
Front Horm Res. Basel, Karger, 2006, vol 34, pp 127–157

Rathke's Cleft Cysts

Adam S. Kanter, Charles A. Sansur, John A. Jane, Jr., Edward R. Laws, Jr.

Department of Neurological Surgery, Health Sciences Center, University of Virginia, Charlottesville, Va., USA

Abstract

Rathke's cleft cysts are typically regarded as benign cystic lesions of the sella that may affect the pituitary gland and on occasion the visual apparatus. They are most commonly incidental and rarely of clinical significance. As medical neuroimaging and surgical technologies have rapidly advanced, so too has the discovery, experience, knowledge, and intrigue concerning this relatively rare disease entity. Nevertheless, numerous controversies still exist regarding its natural history, recurrence rate, predictive variables, and optimal surgical management. This chapter aims to review the pathogenesis, symptomatologic manifestations, radiographic, morphologic and histopathological characteristics, treatment strategies and outcomes in the cysts of Rathke's cleft.

Copyright © 2006 S. Karger AG, Basel

Introduction

Rathke's cleft cyst (RCC) was first incidentally reported by Lushka in 1860 as 'an epithelial area in the capsule of the human hypophysis resembling oral mucosa' [1]. The first symptomatic RCC case was described by Goldzieher [2] in 1913. RCCs have been referred to by a variety of names including pituitary cyst, mucoid epithelial cyst, intrasellar epithelial cyst, Rathke's pouch cyst, and colloid cyst of the pituitary [3]. Not until 1934 did Frazier and Alpers [4] propose its contemporary name of tumor of Rathke's cleft.

Most RCCs are microscopic in size, asymptomatic, and of greater histological than clinical significance [5]. They do on rare occasion, however, become large enough to cause compression of structures within and/or adjacent to the sella thus eliciting symptoms primarily but not limited to headache, visual and/or endocrine disturbance. Despite a significant evolution in the

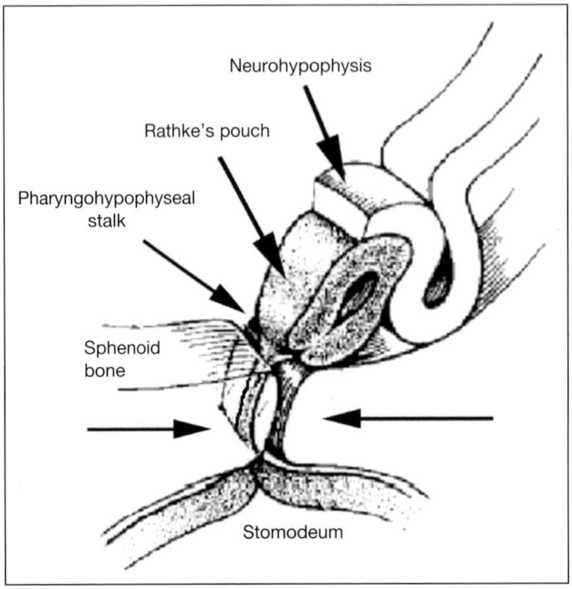

Fig. 1. Schematic depiction of the embryological progenitors of sellar and parasellar structures. Rathke's pouch arises from an outpocketing of stomodeum (ectoderm) and gives rise to the adenohypophysis. The pharyngohypophyseal stalk, which connects the stomodeum and Rathke's pouch, is severed by the sphenoid bone as it grows together (arrows), isolating Rathke's pouch and the neurohypophysis (neuroectoderm) within the sella, the embryological ancestors of the anterior and posterior lobes of the pituitary, respectively; thus all are of ectodermal origin.

management of RCC, several controversies remain regarding the natural history, relationship to craniopharyngioma, recurrence rate, predictive variables, surgical indications and strategies.

Pathogenesis

Several theories regarding the pathogenesis of RCCs have been proposed, including its origination from neuroepithelium [6–8], endoderm [9, 10], and metaplastic anterior pituitary cells [1, 11–13]. The most widely accepted theory of RCC derivation describes its origin from embryological remnants of Rathke's pouch [3, 14–18] (fig. 1).

Around the 24th day of embryonic life, Rathke's pouch arises as a dorsal diverticulum from the stomatodeum and is lined by epithelial cells of ectodermal origin. The infundibulum forms as a downgrowth of neuroepithelium from the diencephalon that subsequently contacts the forming pouch causing occlusion of

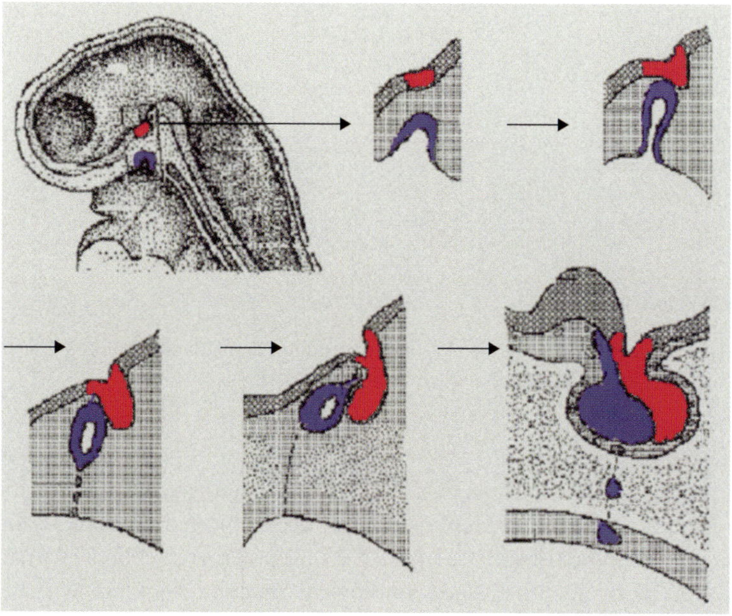

Fig. 2. A schematic depiction of the embryological downgrowth of neuroepithelium from the diencephalon contacting the forming Rathke's pouch which then separates from the oral epithelium while its anterior wall proliferates into the pars distalis and its posterior wall forms the pars intermedia. The residual lumen reduces to a narrow fissure that generally regresses.

its neck at the buccal-pharyngeal junction (fig. 2). The pouch then separates from the oral epithelium and its anterior wall proliferates and develops into the pars distalis. Its posterior wall remains fixed as the poorly defined pars intermedia. The pouch's residual lumen reduces to a narrow fissure termed Rathke's cleft that generally regresses, as is histologically evident in figure 3. The persistence and enlargement of this cleft is thus the origin of the symptomatic RCC.

As the cyst continues to expand and produce its mucinous contents, leakage or hemorrhage may occur. These inflammatory events may stimulate cellular rearrangement and metaplastic transformation resulting in stratified epithelium and histology indistinguishable from that of a craniopharyngioma [19].

Prevalence, Age, Genetics

RCCs account for less than 1% of primary intracranial masses and represent a very small percentage of sellar lesions requiring surgical treatment [20–22]. Nevertheless, their prevalence is higher than these data would suggest,

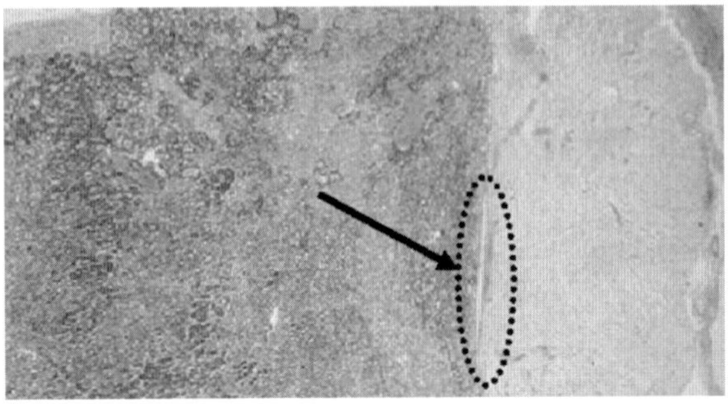

Fig. 3. Histological sample demonstrating a residual remnant of Rathke's pouch (circled) with the pars distalis to its left and pars nervosa to its right.

having been reported in as many as 13–33% of routine autopsy series [1, 3, 13, 21, 23–26]. A marked female predominance has been reported throughout the literature at a rate of approximately 2:1 [3, 23, 27–31], perhaps secondary to an increased awareness of disturbed endocrinological function manifest as menstrual irregularities [28, 31]. Age at presentation varies widely and ranges from 4 to 73 (mean 38) years with the highest frequency occurring in the 6th decade [3, 23, 30, 32]. No racial or genetic predilection exists in the pathogenesis of RCC.

Clinical Presentation

The overwhelming majority of RCCs are asymptomatic. Rarely, a cyst may progressively enlarge and exert compressive effects on the pituitary gland, stalk, optic apparatus, and hypothalamus. Location and resultant symptoms allow patients to be organized into clinical groups: those with suprasellar symptoms, those with hypophyseal dysfunction, those with both, and those with neither.

In 1991, Voelker et al. [3] performed a meta-analysis including 147 cases of RCC in which he elucidated the presentation of patients with RCC (table 1). The duration of symptoms at diagnosis ranged from several days to several years (mean 35 months). Both pediatric and adult patients presented with endocrinopathy. Children and adolescents demonstrated early hypopituitarism with retardation of growth and sexual development. Adults more often presented with diabetes insipidus (DI), amenorrhea and galactorrhea secondary to pituitary stalk and posterior lobe compression with obstruction of prolactin-inhibiting factor (dopamine) transport from the hypothalamus to the anterior pituitary [32–34]. The second most common symptom was of visual disturbances in both acuity and perimetry. Static perimetry most often revealed bitemporal hemianopsia but

Table 1. Comparison of historic and contemporary series: clinical presentation and symptomatology (%)

Reference and year	Headache	Visual dysfunction	Anterior pituitary hypofunction	Hyper-prolactinemia	Diabetes insipidus
Voelker et al. [3], 1991	49	56	69	7	13
Eguchi et al. [102], 1994	N/A	47	100	21	21
el-Mahdy and Powell [28], 1998	46	46	50	29	14
Shin et al. [31], 1999	65	38	81	46	4
Benveniste et al. [38], 2004	71	20	55	42	5
Kim et al. [35], 2004	81	47	30	25	13
Weiss [39], 2004	N/A	49	53	28	0
Frank et al. [86], 2005	14	23	41	18	5
Kanter et al. [36] 2004	86	37	60	22	10

N/A = Data not available.

reports of unilateral temporal hemianopsia, bilateral superior quadrantanopsia, and homonymous hemianopsia are not uncommon. Headache was reported as the third leading complaint, most frequently located in the frontal region.

Contemporary series published in the last 20 years have revealed these same principal signs and symptoms except with varying orders of incidence [28, 29, 35–38] (table 1). This is perhaps related to the introduction, accessibility, diminished expense and threshold in obtaining advanced neuroimaging. In these more recent studies, headache is more frequently the principal complaint, occurring in as many as 70–85% of patients [35, 36, 38, 39]. Although most commonly chronic, some are episodic in nature, perhaps suggesting an intermittent inflammatory reaction to leakage of cyst contents. A third variant is of a sudden onset, severe headache, often related to a hemorrhagic event within the cyst (noted in 11–21% of cases), with or without leakage of its contents [28, 35, 38, 40]. The mean duration of headache at diagnosis is roughly 12 months [35, 38].

Endocrinopathy has decreased in incidence upon presentation, occurring in 30–60% of patients. Symptoms may vary depending upon one's gender and menopausal status [28, 38]. Men most often experience symptoms related to hypogonadism including decreased libido, body hair, and fatigue [28, 31, 38]. Premenopausal women often suffer from menstrual irregularities, galactorrhea and polyuria (DI). Postmenopausal women describe symptoms attributable to panhypopituitarism such as fatigue, mental status changes and constitutional symptoms.

Visual dysfunction has also decreased in both incidence and severity, occurring in 14–37% of cases. We hypothesize that visual symptoms, often reflecting more advanced disease, will continue to decline secondary to a progressively more enlightened, internet-savvy public seeking medical attention earlier and receiving efficient definitive diagnosis and treatment at seasoned neuroendocrine centers. Indeed, early reports revealed symptom duration of an average 3 years with lesions of 15–40 mm and more than two thirds with suprasellar extension, while more recent series report average symptom duration of 12 months, nearly half contained within the sella, and an average size of 8–20 mm [3, 29, 36].

Atypical presentations in patients with RCCs include pituitary apoplexy [28, 41–43], hypophysitis [44–46], aseptic meningitis [26], intracystic abscess [47–49], sphenoid sinusitis [50], precocious puberty [51], empty sella syndrome [52], and micropenis secondary to intrauterine pituitary impairment [53].

Neuroradiological Evaluation

In the pre-CT era, preoperative imaging provided limited information regarding the diagnosis of RCC. Plain skull radiography was obtained in patients presenting with symptoms of presumed sellar origin. The majority of these early films revealed abnormal sellas ranging from 'slight asymmetry of the floor' to its 'massive erosion', some with notable calcifications [15, 54, 55] (fig. 4). Cerebral angiograms demonstrated avascular masses with elevation of proximal anterior cerebral vasculature.

The arrival of the CT scan in 1974 marked a new era in medical imaging and diagnosis. RCCs were more accurately described: round, lobulated or dumbbell-shaped, intra- and suprasellar masses with cystic fluid densities usually mimicking that of cerebrospinal fluid (CSF) [3, 56]. Over time, clinicians began recognizing the variable appearances of RCCs [57]. Reports of mixed density lesions with iso-, hypo- and hyperdense foci arose throughout the literature [30, 31, 35, 57–60]. These variations were presumed in part due to cholesterol crystals and varying mucopolysaccharide concentrations within the cyst [58–60]. Additionally, CT imaging exposed sizeable extensions into the anterior and middle cranial fossa and resultant pathology such as hydrocephalus.

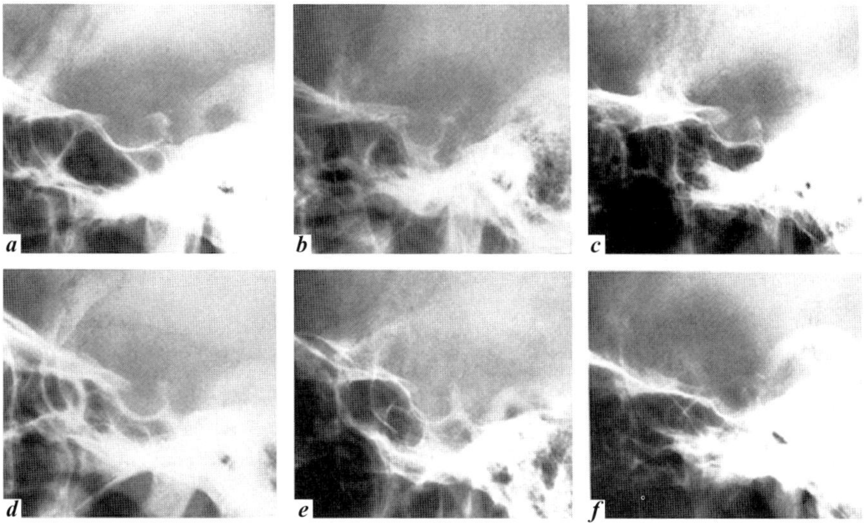

Fig. 4. Structural changes of the sella turcica associated with Rathke's cleft cysts. ***a*** Enlargement in the anteroposterior diameter of the sella. ***b, e*** Double sellar floors. ***c***, ***d***, ***f*** Ballooning and bony erosion is seen. With permission from Oka et al. [54].

Contrast medium added yet another descriptive dimension, as depicted in figure 5, with approximately one quarter revealing ring-like or capsular enhancement secondary to cyst fluid extravasation and inflammation of adjacent structures [35].

The variable appearance on CT is paralleled with MRI (table 2). Studies correlating MRI characteristics with tumor biology have yielded interesting results. Explanted tissue cultures from fragments of Rathke's cyst epithelium have developed into macrocysts lined with epithelium from an accumulation of mucous material and desquamated cells. It is postulated that the number and activity of these cells determines the biochemical nature of the cystic contents and hence its MR appearance [18, 57, 58]. Cysts with CSF-like intensities may suggest more benign lesions with histological and chemical analyses revealing a single-cell epithelial lining and a low protein concentration within the cyst (fig. 6) [58]. Those with hyperintense contents on both T1- and T2-weighted images may contain excess mucopolysaccharides (fig. 7) [60–62]; Shin et al. [31] noted that all hyperintense cysts in their series contained a protein concentration of >90 g/l. Those displaying hyperintense T1-weighted contents with hypointense T2-weighted contents may represent blood products within the capsule [63]. These cysts were also more likely to produce symptoms earlier, when the cysts

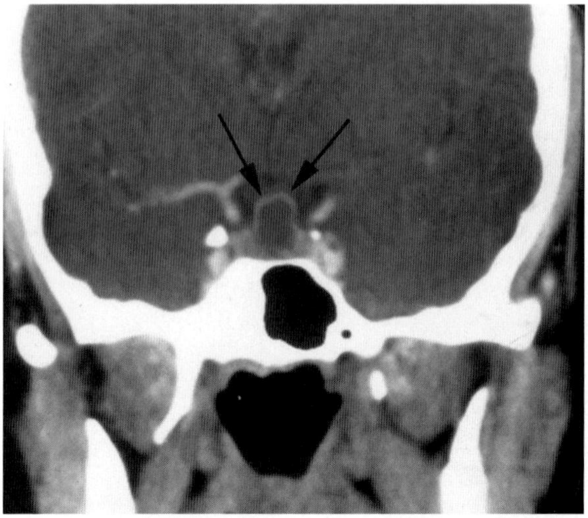

Fig. 5. Coronal sellar computed tomographic (CT) scan of a Rathke's cleft cyst with large suprasellar extension and curvilinear ring enhancement (arrows) following contrast administration.

Table 2. Magnetic resonance imaging signal characteristic variability of Rathke's cleft cysts

Signal intensity		Enhanced, %	Cases, %
T1	T2		
Hypo	Hyper	6	24
Hypo	Iso	4	4
Hypo	Hypo	2	4
Hyper	Hyper	6	26
Hyper	Iso	0	6
Hyper	Hypo	4	22
Mixed	Hyper	6	14
Total		28	100

Hypo = Hypointense; Hyper = hyperintense; Iso = isointense. From Kim et al. [35].

were smaller than their low-intensity counterparts [57]. Cysts with a heterogeneous radiographic appearance more commonly exhibited a cyst wall that was several layers thick making it histologically difficult to distinguish from a craniopharyngioma [58]. A corollary between contrast enhancement and squamous

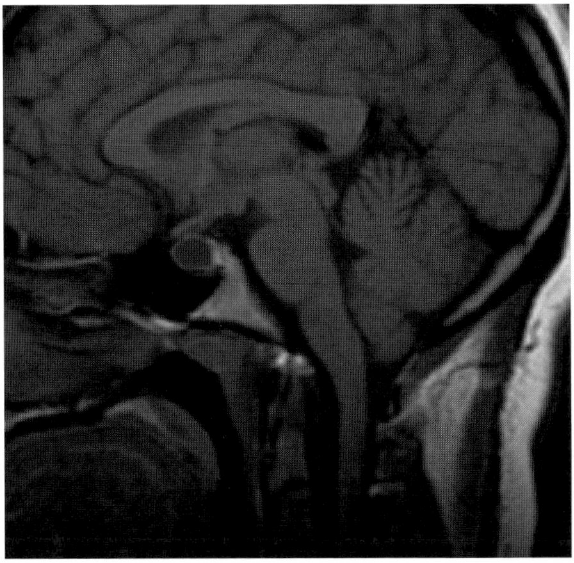

Fig. 6. T1-weighted sagittal MRI demonstrating a well-defined, CSF-like hypointense Rathke's cleft cyst within the sella turcica. Note the high signal intensity of the posterior pituitary (normal) draped over the dorsal aspect of the cyst.

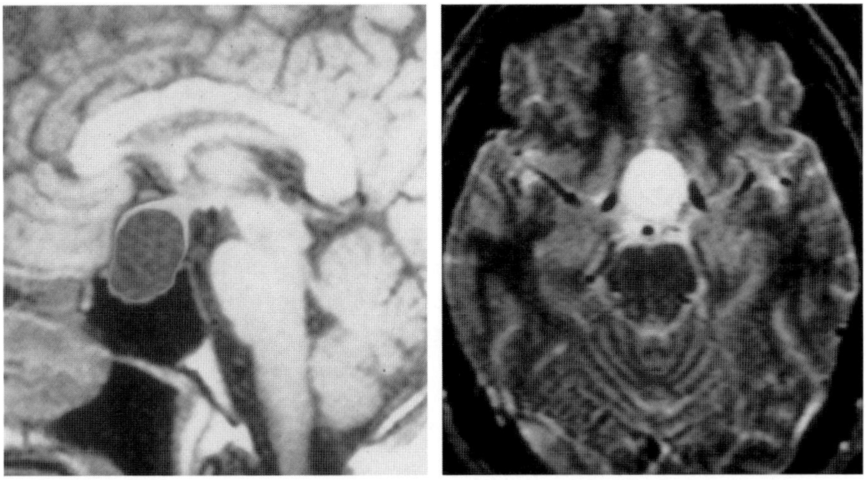

Fig. 7. Magnetic resonance images of an intrasellar cyst with suprasellar extension displaying high signal intensity on T1- and T2-weighted images. Note the peripheral enhancement and superiorly displaced optic apparatus.

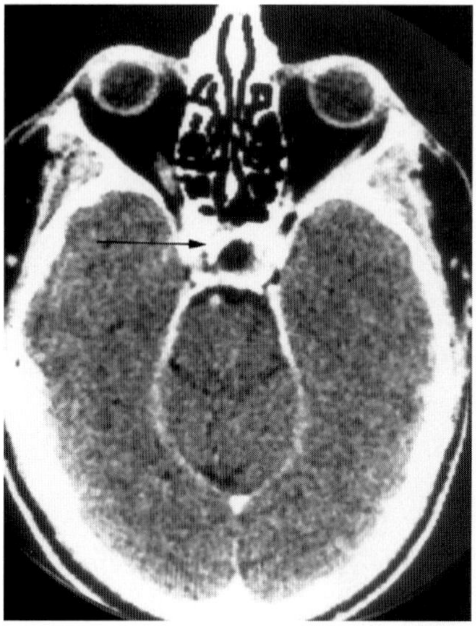

Fig. 8. Axial sellar computed tomographic scan after contrast administration showing Rathke's cleft cyst with patchy wall enhancement and a small calcified nodule (arrow), perhaps indicative of a biologically more aggressive lesion.

epithelium on histological examination was discovered as well, both characteristics predictive of tumor recurrence in univariate and multivariate analyses [35].

In the evaluation process, MRI is the modality of choice for assessing RCCs [56, 60]. Thin section sagittal and coronal sections should be obtained through the sella to delineate the cyst's relationship to the optic nerves, chiasm, hypothalamus, carotid arteries and cavernous sinuses. Adjunct CT adds limited information with the exception of identifying calcifications (fig. 8) or associated bony remodeling, often more indicative of a craniopharyngioma. Of note, a subtle clue to diagnosis may lie in this modality as calcifications associated with RCC seem to adopt a curvilinear shape whereas those found in craniopharyngiomas tend to be more floccular or nodular in shape [56]. That said, there remains no uniform radiological finding or characteristic specific to RCC and the differential diagnosis with other sellar and suprasellar lesions almost always remains in doubt. Far too often, even with radiographic data of cyst location, size, CT density and MR intensity, these lesions are misdiagnosed, and often mismanaged.

Location: Intrasellar vs. Suprasellar

Although the trend in earlier detection may ultimately lead toward discovery of smaller lesions, most published series to date report treatment of intrasellar cysts with varying degrees of suprasellar extension [13, 28, 35, 38, 40, 54, 64, 65]. Approximately one third to as many as one half are found still contained within the confines of the sella. A small number are found exclusively in the suprasellar region [13, 31, 32, 36, 38, 65–67], likely a result of pouch remnants within the pars tuberalis above the diaphragm giving rise to the cystic components [64].

Biochemical Analysis

Biochemical abnormalities secondary to hypothalamic, adenohypophyseal, neurohypophyseal, and infundibular compression within the sellar and suprasellar compartments result in varying degrees of hypopituitarism, hyperprolactinemia and consequent endocrinopathies. Roughly one to two thirds of patients harboring RCCs experience endocrinological dysfunction. Comprehensive biochemical assays often reveal these and additionally expose other, yet undetected irregularities.

The most common biochemical irregularity associated with RCC is consistently hyperprolactinemia, followed by hypocortisolism, hypothyroidism, hypogonadism, and growth hormone deficiency. Approximately 10–15% of assays reveal hypopituitarism, having two or more of the above-mentioned abnormalities [35]. These indices may in part be biased by the fact that the majority of patients are premenopausal women, as men most often experience gonadal deficiency and decreased libido. It is therefore not surprising that when the genders are divided, a threefold burden of gonadal dysfunction exists in men over similarly aged women with RCCs [36, 38].

Pituitary insufficiencies such as hypocortisolemia and hypothyroidism must be recognized and treated prior to surgery to minimize the risk of intra- and postoperative complications. DI occurs in patients with RCCs as much as ten times more often than in other benign pituitary lesions because of the inflammatory and infiltrative characteristics of the cyst and its contents. Its existence may necessitate anesthetic or fluid adjustments throughout the disease course. It is therefore imperative that all patients receive a complete endocrinological evaluation examining the entire hypothalamic-pituitary-end organ axis as well as serum and urine electrolyte concentrations before any intervention (table 3).

A stress dose of glucocorticoid is commonly administered intraoperatively, following which postoperative adrenal sufficiency tests will indicate if further cortisol replacement therapy is warranted. If so, a short-acting oral steroid (e.g. hydrocortisone) is used to minimize endogenous ACTH suppression during the recovery period. Gonadal steroids and growth hormone replacement therapy require routine evaluation in both short- and long-term follow-up.

Hormone/electrolyte
Prolactin
Growth hormone
Follicle-stimulating hormone
Luteinizing hormone
Thyroid-stimulating hormone
Free thyroxine
Adrenocorticotropic hormone
Insulin-like growth factor-1
Cortisol (morning and evening levels)
Serum and urine sodium
Urine specific gravity

Table 3. A complete biochemical analysis of the entire hypothalamic-pituitary-end organ axis as well as serum and urine electrolyte concentrations are evaluated pre- and postoperatively as insufficiencies such as hypocortisolism, hypothyroidism, and diabetes insipidus must be recognized and treated prior to surgical intervention

Growth hormone levels are best assessed in response to an insulin-induced hypoglycemic trial.

Ophthalmological Assessment

Visual dysfunction occurs in roughly one third of patients with RCCs. These most commonly present as diminished acuity, quadrant- or hemianopsias, but reports of cranial nerve dysfunction and diplopia from RCC do exist [28]. All patients should undergo formal preoperative fundoscopic, tangent screen, and perimetry testing pre- and postoperatively. Visual field, acuity, and cranial nerve assessments will serve as baselines for comparison examinations and an objective measure of operative success or failure.

Differential Diagnosis

Given the continuum of epithelial-lined cystic lesions [67], distinction among them (i.e. RCC, craniopharyngioma, arachnoid cyst, pituitary adenoma) remains a difficult challenge [61, 68]. Their signs, symptoms, biochemical and radiographic features often mimic one another, confusing the predictive prognosis and treatment strategy employed by the physicians that treat them [15, 31, 35, 69, 70]. For instance, the presence of hyperprolactinemia often leads to inappropriate medical therapy and a delay in effective surgical management.

Table 4. A comprehensive statistical analysis of distinguishing signs and symptoms characteristic of Rathke's cleft cysts (RCCs), craniopharyngiomas (CRs), and arachnoid cysts (ACs)

Signs/symptoms	RCC %	CR %	AC %
Endocrine			
Amenorrhea	24	64	0
Lethargy	62	62	20
Impotence/decreased libido	67	45	50
Hyperprolactinemia (>20 μg/l)	46	38	20
Reduced secondary sexual features	23	29	0
Somnolence	12	24	0
Gynecomastia	11	18	0
Galactorrhea	35	18	0
Diabetes insipidus	4	10	0
Oligomenorrhea	24	9	0
Neurologic			
Headache	65	62	62
Dizziness	8	10	20
Seizures	0	2	0
Ophthalmologic			
Visual field defects	38	67	0
Psychiatric			
Memory dysfunction, dementia, personality changes, depression	0	33	0

From Shin et al. [31].

To help elucidate distinguishing features, Shin et al. [31] performed a comprehensive systematic analysis of the aforementioned disease entities (table 4). Patients with arachnoid cysts tend to be older at initial diagnosis [31, 71] and very rarely present with greater than one pituitary hormonal axis impairment, in comparison to roughly two thirds of those with either craniopharyngioma (67%) or RCC (62%). Patients with craniopharyngiomas more often presented with panhypopituitarism (95%), neurologic deficits (67%), ophthalmologic complaints (67%) and psychiatric manifestations (33–50%) [31, 72]. Craniopharyngiomas tend to be greater in size [31, 73] and more often are purely suprasellar (67%), 10% having no intrasellar component in comparison to the few suprasellar RCC and arachnoid cyst case reports.

Purely cystic lesions were more likely to be RCC (88%) or arachnoid cysts (100%) than craniopharyngiomas (38%) whereas those with calcifications or a

Table 5. CT and MRI characteristics of Rathke's cleft cysts (RCC) and craniopharyngiomas (CR)

	RCC %	CR %
CT imaging		
Calcification	13	87
Enhancement	56	60
Precontrast density		
Hypodense	79	55
Isodense	21	45
Hyperdense	0	0
MR imaging		
T1-weighted images		
Hypodense	50	33
Isodense	7	50
Hyperdense	42	17
T2-weighted images		
Hypodense	50	92
Isodense	29	0
Hyperdense	21	8

From Shin et al. [31].

solid component on neuroimaging were more commonly craniopharyngiomas (87%) than RCCs (13%) or arachnoid cysts (0%) [31]. Table 5 illustrates the distinguishing, but all too often overlapping imaging characteristics of RCC and craniopharyngiomas. Ultimately, those with craniopharyngiomas are least likely to improve in any pituitary axis and most often require hormone replacement [31]. In addition, nearly two thirds of craniopharyngiomas will recur in comparison to less than 20% of RCCs or arachnoid cysts.

These key features and others, although variable as noted, may help to improve the type and aggressiveness of treatment strategy. A combination of clinical, biochemical, and neuroimaging features must be concurrently evaluated when formulating a presumptive diagnosis.

Gross Morphologic Features

RCCs are most commonly well-circumscribed, smoothly contoured lesions containing thick yellow mucinous fluid [74]. That said, enumerable reports

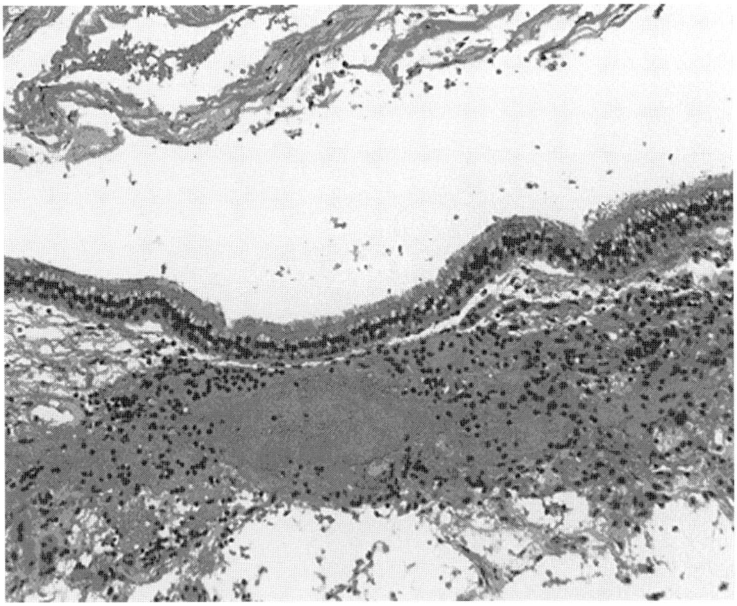

Fig. 9. A histological HE sampling of a Rathke's cleft cyst at low magnification revealing a cystic structure composed of a thin layer of supporting mesenchymal tissue lined by a single layer of ciliated columnar epithelium.

exist on thick, fibrous cyst walls with color variations of blue, gray, white, yellow, pink, red, tan, green, and transparent. Cyst contents are predominantly thick and gelatinous, but watery or serous reports are not infrequent. The fluid may be white, clear, yellow, gray, green or motor oil-like with protein levels ranging from 80 to 1,500 mg/dl [3]. Contents may appear indistinguishable from pus, leading to the misdiagnosis of a sterile abscess [75]. True abscesses in association with RCCs, occurring most commonly via hematogenous spread, have been described [31, 47–49].

Histopathological Features

RCCs typically have fibrous, vascularized connective tissue stroma with a single-layered cuboidal or columnar, ciliated epithelium (fig. 9). Cystic contents are a relatively homogeneous protein-rich, mucinous fluid frequently containing mixed debris of hemosiderin pigments, eosinophils and macrophages (inflammatory infiltrates). Aberrations, such as the focal nests of squamous cells, are hypothesized to occur from metaplasia of the epithelium [76] which has gained

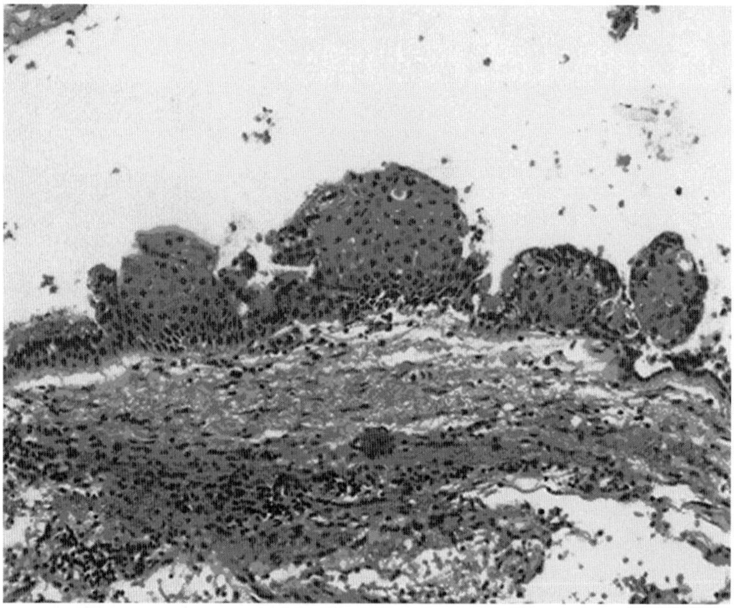

Fig. 10. An area of cyst epithelium reveals clusters of squamous metaplasia, possibly a result of intermittent inflammatory or hemorrhagic injury within the cyst.

popularity as a feature provoking conversion of an asymptomatic lesion to a symptomatic one (fig. 10) [74]. Ikeda et al. [74] suggested that incidental, asymptomatic lesions possess a simple, well-differentiated, hormone-producing cellular layer, while symptomatic cysts consist of a pseudostratified squamous epithelium intermingled with mucous-secreting goblet cells that have lost immunoreactivity for hormone production yet have a significantly amplified proliferation index.

A definitive histopathological distinction between craniopharyngiomas and RCCs can be difficult. Craniopharyngioma, an entity previously distinguished histologically from RCC by its stratified squamous epithelium has been described with epithelial linings of ciliated columnar and goblet cells [54, 77, 78]. Comprehensive reviews between these two entities, as depicted in table 6, reveal significant overlap in multiple histopathological characteristics [31, 35]. An array of classification caveats lead to considerable controversy in diagnosis and management.

Pathological characteristics that had previously denoted 'higher grade' disease, such as chronic or intermittent inflammatory changes in the cyst wall or adjacent pituitary tissue, calcifications, cholesterol crystals, or hemosiderin pigmentation were regularly found in lesions diagnosed as RCCs [31, 46, 74,

Table 6. Histopathological features of Rathke's cleft cysts (RCC) and craniopharyngiomas (CR)

Epithelial lining	RCC %	CR %
Stratified squamous	12	76
Interlacing squamous bands	0	19
Simple columnar[a]	27	5
Pseudostratified columnar[a]	23	0
Simple cuboidal[a]	27	0
Transitional	4	0
Ciliated[a]	69	5
Cholesterol clefts	23	43
Calcification	0	43
Necrotic debris and fibrosis	15	38
Keratin nodules	4	33
Chronic inflammation	0	19
Foreign body giant cells	12	13
Hemosiderin	4	24
Goblet cells	4	0

[a]Favoring diagnosis of RCC ($p < 0.01$).
From Shin et al. [31].

77, 79, 80]. Immunohistochemical analysis also revealed a disparity in epithelial cell structure; some appearing less differentiated and more aggressive while others were granulated, differentiated hormone-producing and benign [40].

It is theorized that transitional forms of RCC emerged from frequent hemorrhage and inflammation within the cyst causing squamous metaplasia, content turbidity and increased viscosity. After several regenerations, the squamous epithelium with its higher proliferation index dominates the cyst wall altering its once smooth, transparent appearance to a thick, opaque, irregular wall. In time, cyst content is predominantly cellular debris and hemorrhagic remnants, resembling that of the typical papillary craniopharyngioma.

As overlapping histopathological and structural characteristics have persisted, clinicians have cautiously accepted the notion that RCCs and craniopharyngiomas represent a spectrum of disease, beginning with the aforementioned simple, typical RCCs and ending with those that are effectively without distinction from craniopharyngiomas [15, 58, 67, 75] (fig. 11). As such, the simple, 'typical' RCCs may in fact be the exception as opposed to the rule.

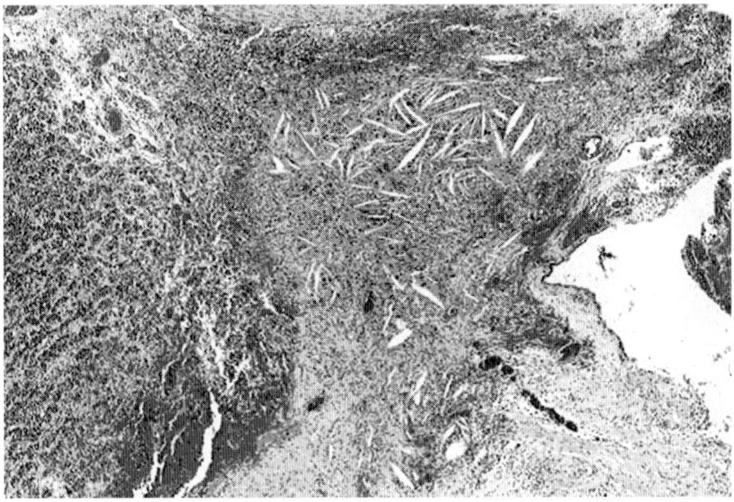

Fig. 11. HE stain reveals prominent cholesterol collections associated with multinucleated giant cells, non-caseating granulomatous inflammation, hemosiderin-laden macrophages, disruption of the epithelial lining, and hemorrhage into the cyst lumen; histology more commonly seen in craniopharyngiomas than in Rathke's cleft cysts.

Concurrent Pituitary Adenomas

The coincident discovery of pituitary adenomas existing concurrently with RCC have been reported in the literature [28, 31, 35, 81–84]. A retrospective analysis by Sumida et al. [82] revealed an incidence of concomitant disease in 3.5% of pituitary adenomas and 11% of RCCs. The cells from which pituitary adenomas develop form by proliferation of the anterior wall of Rathke's pouch, thus sharing a common ancestry with those that lead to the development of RCC (see Pathogenesis Section) [84]. Others advocate that stalk distortion by the growing RCC may stimulate activity in prolactin-secreting cells thus provoking adenoma formation [85]. When coexisting lesions are present, symptoms are almost invariably thought due to the adenoma. Whatever the cause, concurrent lesions have been successfully treated by the same surgical principles as RCC, the critical issue being complete removal of all adenomatous tissue and not simply resection of cystic elements. Some suggest that the adenoma be treated with primary importance as the cyst is likely coincidental and of minimal clinical relevance [81].

Surgical Indications

Surgery for patients with visual impairment or endocrinological dysfunction needs no debate, whereas surgical indications in cysts found either incidentally, with transient symptoms, or in association with headache, remain controversial. Kim et al. [35] evaluated 53 patients, 36% reporting headache as their only preoperative complaint, of which 95% achieved complete postoperative resolution. Our experience and that of others support these findings with greater than 80% consistently achieving headache resolution [3, 31, 36, 38, 86]. It is consequently our recommendation that intractable headache alone is in fact a reasonable surgical indication when a corresponding lesion is noted on neuroimaging and all other structural and functional causes have appropriately been ruled out.

Surgical Management

RCCs were initially treated by craniotomy (predominantly by a right frontal flap) until the transsphenoidal (TS) route became the primary approach in the mid-1970s [87]. Further prompting the switch to the less invasive TS approach was the finding that cystic contents released into the subarachnoid space during craniotomy lead to aseptic meningitis [26, 88]. Occasionally though, RCCs are found in an entirely suprasellar location. In such instances, an extended TS approach may be considered by an experienced TS surgeon with microscopic and endoscopic capacities. At present, craniotomy is generally reserved for firm lesions with significant suprasellar or parasellar extension inaccessible by the TS route [30, 89].

TS surgery can be accomplished by either a sublabial or endonasal approach (fig. 12), the latter of which avoids resection of the anterior nasal spine of the maxilla thereby reducing postoperative nasal and dental complications as well as patient discomfort and healing times. That said, some lesions require increased superior and lateral visualization for complete resection and complication avoidance thus necessitating the advantages provided by the sublabial approach. This approach is also employed in children and others with petite nares unable to accommodate the nasal speculum. Some have avoided the more invasive sublabial incision by utilizing angled endoscopes for extended visualization of the supra- and parasellar territories [86, 90, 91].

Historically, as proposed by Fager and Carter [15] in 1966 and supported by multiple experts thereafter [3, 23, 28–30, 37, 64], the most common surgical strategy for RCC consists of liberal fenestration and biopsy of the cyst wall with complete cyst content evacuation. As large contemporary series with advanced imaging technologies and follow-up data have emerged, it is now

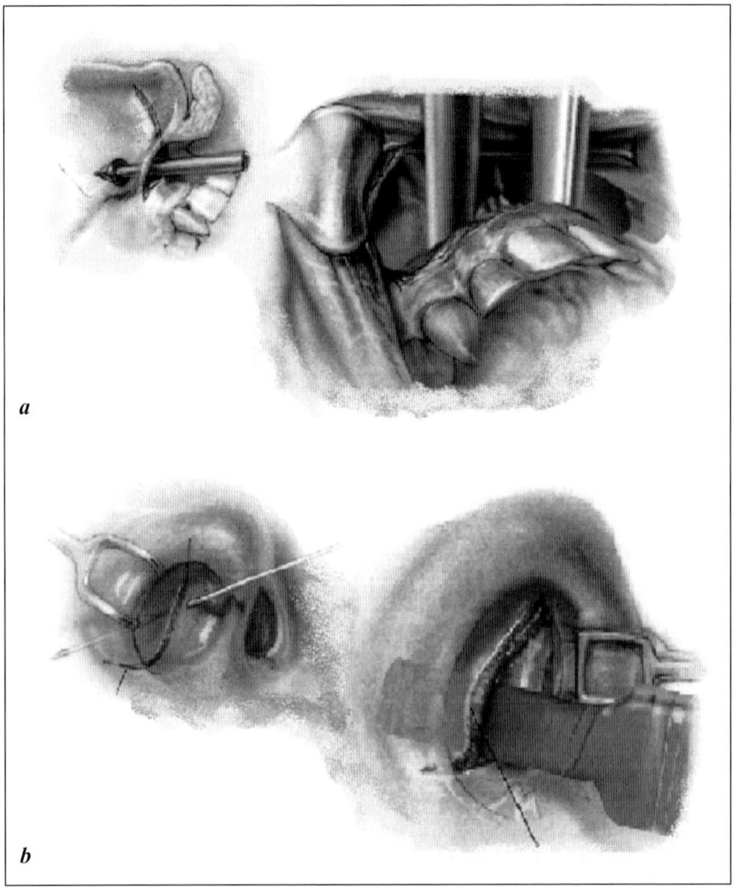

Fig. 12. Sublabial (*a*) and endonasal (*b*) transsphenoidal approaches. The endonasal approach avoids resection of the anterior nasal spine of the maxilla but limits the extended superior and lateral visualization afforded by the sublabial approach.

evident that two surgical philosophies regarding the management of these complicated lesions exists. The first coincides with the historical approach of cyst wall opening and drainage. Some have modified this approach to include marsupialization of the cyst into the sphenoid sinus, leaving the floor of the sella unreconstructed to promote cyst drainage and prolonged decompression. Others resect all non-adherent cyst capsule and coagulate the remnant margins [39]. Those implementing this comparatively conservative strategy have obtained remarkable results with immediate symptom resolution and minimal iatrogenic pituitary dysfunction. That said, nearly half of the postoperative MRIs reveal a small residual cyst [38] that is predictive of progressive regrowth and a trend toward symptom recurrence [18, 20, 30, 38, 40, 92–95].

A second surgical philosophy, emphasized in 1976 by Eisenberg et al. [96] and adopted by the senior author after considerable experience with a relatively low recurrence rate, is that of aggressive cyst wall resection. This approach invariably leads to a greater risk of CSF leak and iatrogenic hypophyseal injury, balanced by the expectation of reducing residual cysts and symptomatic recurrence. All recurrences reported in two independent centers were found in the groups receiving simple decompression and cyst wall biopsy while none of those having undergone total resection relapsed [35, 38]. These findings are supported by the authors' experience, revealing double the recurrence rate when total cyst wall resection was not achieved [36]. Regardless of surgical philosophy, given the variety of descriptions of cyst contents and intraoperative misdiagnoses, it is imperative that tissue biopsy of the cyst wall be performed [35].

Recent advances in endoscopic technique and fiber optic technology have led to its sole or combined use with the microscopic approach with comparable results [22, 86, 90]. The early benefits realized from the endoscopic procedure relate to its nearly negligible anatomic disturbance, such that intra-nasal packing and suturing are avoided, leaving patients with minimal postoperative discomfort [22]. Given this minimalist approach, damage to the pituitary stalk is reduced as well, possibly allowing for more radical resections with improved preservation of this habitually traumatized structure.

Another disparity among surgeons is with regards to the packing and reconstruction of the sella. When no CSF leak is encountered, many leave the fossa floor open without reconstruction allowing any remnant cyst to drain into the sphenoid air sinus [28]. Definitive data do not yet exist, but it is the experience of the authors and others that physiologic closure will usually occur regardless of these precautionary measures. Furthermore, there does not appear to be any increase in the recurrence rate of those receiving sellar packing and floor reconstruction secondary to intraoperative CSF leaks [36, 38]. These data therefore do not discourage our favoring the more aggressive surgical approach as intraoperative CSF leaks and packed sellas do not appear to significantly alter outcomes.

If arachnoid perforation occurs yielding an intraoperative CSF leak, a periumbilical fat graft is used to pack the sella and the sellar floor is reconstructed with autologous bone or a synthetic macropore plate as is illustrated in figure 13. This approach generally suffices, but if a severe leak is apparent, a lumbar drain may be inserted for an average 2–5 days postoperatively. The development of CSF fistula formation is rare but if encountered prompts either prolonged lumbar drainage, or more definitively, reoperation with repacking of the sella and possibly an intranasal mucosal transposition.

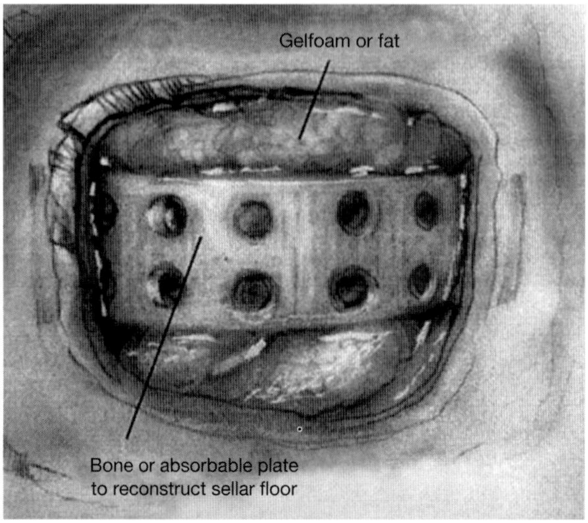

Fig. 13. If an intraoperative CSF leak occurs, a peri-umbilical fat graft and gelfoam are used to pack the sella and the floor is reconstructed with autologous bone or a synthetic macropore plate.

In the absence of a CSF leak, some authors advocate rinsing the evacuated tumor bed with absolute alcohol to destroy microscopic rests of residual epithelial cells [30, 38, 39]. No definitive data exist to support this practice, and there are case reports of sudden blindness, anosmia and cranial nerve palsies from leakage of alcohol from the cyst. It is therefore recommended that this practice be abandoned as its risks currently outweigh any evidence of benefit.

Multiple factors ultimately determine the extent of surgical resection, including the nature and extent of cyst contents, integrity and strength of cyst wall, inflammatory involvement, and adherence to the pituitary gland, stalk and other intracranial structures [75]. It is the authors' philosophy to perform a radical cyst removal whenever possible without inflicting unnecessary damage upon adjacent sellar and suprasellar structures. As such, nearly 100 TS procedures for RCCs have been performed at our center with excellent long-term results and minimal sequelae. Conversely, other exceptionally experienced TS surgeons opt for biopsy, drainage and simple decompression of cystic contents [35, 38, 39, 86], resulting in slightly higher recurrence rates but fewer iatrogenic related hypophyseal impairments. Two poles of surgical opinion thus exist, with most centers falling somewhere in between with regard to presentation, surgical management and outcome. It is, however, agreed upon that each case be individualized with regard to the patient, anatomy, and biology of the specific tumor.

Adjuvant Therapies

Scant evidence exists for the use of high-dose steroids in the treatment of RCCs with the possible exception in those associated with hypophysitis; its pathophysiology is unclear, but presumably relates to the secretion and/or absorption of cyst fluid [45]. Additionally, sporadic reports of radiation therapy or radiosurgery-induced RCC involution do exist [97], but its role in any treatment protocol remains limited at this time.

Outcomes

As is depicted in table 7, most series reveal dramatic improvements in headache, visual dysfunction and symptoms attributable to elevated prolactin levels, while those of hypopituitarism and DI remain less amenable to intervention.

In general, an extraordinary 85–95% of those with headache achieve resolution of symptoms regardless of the surgical philosophy adopted [3, 35, 36, 38]. Those with headache as the sole surgical indication have achieved excellent postoperative remissions providing support for it as a marker for intervention. Exceptional results have also been obtained with regard to recovery of visual function [98] with improvement ranging between 60 and 100% (table 7).

Endocrine symptoms have been less successfully dealt with and iatrogenic dysfunction remains a real danger, especially with more aggressive cyst wall resection of inflamed, adherent tumors. Accordingly, improvement in anterior pituitary function occurs in 15–70% of patients. The most remarkable improvements occur in those patients with menstrual irregularities and galactorrhea, whereas minimal recovery occurs in those with preoperative panhypopituitarism [29, 33, 35, 36, 38, 40, 99, 100]. It has been suggested that inflammation from the RCC may extend into the adjacent pituitary tissue, overwhelm it, and cause irreparable damage [19]. This theory is challenged by studies of benign pituitary macroadenomas (without inflammatory changes) with resultant panhypopituitarism, also yielding low rates of postoperative pituitary function recovery [101].

Specific hormonal anomalies resistant to surgical correction are hypothyroidism and hypocortisolemia, both improving in only one fifth of patients [35, 39]. We found that approximately one third of patients remain without improvement in anterior pituitary symptoms and as many as 10% may develop new dysfunction secondary to the surgical procedure itself. Others have reported a

Table 7. Following transsphenoidal surgery for RCC, most series reveal dramatic improvements in headache, visual dysfunction and symptoms attributable to elevated prolactin levels while those of hypopituitarism and diabetes insipidus remain less amenable to surgical intervention

Reference and year	% revealing improvement in				
	headache	visual dysfunction	anterior pituitary hypofunction	hyperprolactinemia	diabetes insipidus
Voelker et al. [3], 1991	88	85	12	90	0
Eguchi et al. [102], 1994	N/A	89	69	N/A	0
el-Mahdy and Powell [28], 1998	70	67	15	63	25
Shin et al. [31], 1999	82	70	61	67	0
Benveniste et al. [38], 2004	91	96	28	N/A	0
Kim et al. [35], 2004	93	64	63	77	29
Weiss [39], 2004	N/A	98	69	100	0
Frank et al. [86], 2005	100	100	N/A	100	0
Kanter et al. [36], 2004	85	86	70	83	50

N/A = Data not available.

significantly higher incidence of anterior pituitary dysfunction following more aggressive resections [38]. All in all, the premise stated years prior by el-Mahdy and Powell [28] remains: patients with the poorest preoperative status have the poorest recovery rates.

DI remains in a category by itself in regard to the rarity of postoperative resolution [28, 29, 31, 33, 35, 38, 39, 99, 100, 102]. We, remarkably achieved resolution in 50% of patients with preexisting DI [36]. Conversely, nearly one fifth of patients free of DI preoperatively developed a water imbalance following surgery requiring persistent desmopressin replacement therapy [36, 39]. Iatrogenic DI remains a common problem within the field as many attribute its occurrence to overly aggressive cyst wall resections. We consequently stratified into groups those receiving total resections versus simple drainage and biopsy following which the incidence diverged insignificantly (21 vs. 17%, respectively) [36]; others have confirmed these findings [35]. Accordingly, an individualized risk/benefit analysis must always be performed as the neurosurgical care team and patient formulate the operative plan.

Mortality associated with RCCs and their treatment is exceptionally rare and more often related to anomalous vascular complications encountered at resection than to tumor biology.

Complications

Postoperative CSF rhinorrhea is rare following TS RCC resections, occurring in less than 3% of patients [30, 38, 39]. As previously described, a conservative approach with lumbar drainage may be attempted, or more definitive surgical repair may be done, with repacking of the sella and sphenoid sinus utilizing various synthetic bonding agents, glues and plating systems. On exceptionally rare occasions, a CSF fistula may persist despite the most valiant efforts, and an intranasal mucosal transposition may be required.

Meningitis is also an infrequent consequence of RCC resections, although it may occur in conjunction with a persistent CSF leak [28, 30, 36, 38, 39]. If this is the case, broad-spectrum intravenous antibiotics must be administered without delay following which previously obtained CSF cultures can later narrow the species coverage. Treatment is continued for at least 3 weeks. Aseptic meningitis, from leakage of cyst contents at craniotomy can be treated with short-term steroids; its self-limiting course is usually short lived.

Iatrogenic pituitary injury with resultant hypopituitarism, especially DI, remains a prominent problem following TS RCC resections [28, 36]. Comprehensive biochemical and metabolic assays must be routinely performed to identify postoperative hormone deficiencies so that expeditious replacement therapy can be initiated. This is extremely important in the recovering patient as adequate hormone levels are required to maintain energy and muscle strength, minimize adipose mass, and regulate serum lipid levels.

Recurrence and Its Treatment

Numerous studies have implicated multiple factors predisposing a patient to recurrence. These include MRI enhancement [35, 61, 68, 70], extent of cyst wall resection [35, 36], residual cyst on postoperative MRI, squamous metaplasia and inflammatory changes (primarily macrophage infiltration) [9, 18, 35, 38, 40, 92]. These features are likely interrelated as cyst secretions produce inflammatory changes that induce the transformation of squamous metaplasia [19]. This then is indicative of a more aggressive lesion that may in turn re-encapsulate and undergo progressive re-accumulation of cystic fluid and ultimately symptom recurrence [38, 40].

Recurrence rates vary widely and depend upon numerous factors including surgical philosophy and technique, length of follow-up, and imaging evaluation. Recurrence rates of zero to greater than 30% have been reported, with Shin et al. [31] reporting recurrence-free survival of 85 and 81% at 5 and 20 years, respectively [3, 20, 28, 30, 31, 35, 37, 39]. Interpreting these rates is complicated, as those performing total resections may report recurrence when a residual cyst appears on postoperative imaging while others report recurrence only if the cyst regrowth is accompanied by symptom recurrence. Those who perform simple drainage procedures often report recurrence only if the habitually present postoperative residual cyst increases in size, some with symptoms, and some without. A conventional definition for recurrence should be adopted.

Given the considerable number of asymptomatic lesions noted incidentally on neuroimaging or at chance autopsy, some suggest that the same criteria utilized to determine initial surgical indication be used to define and treat recurrence: a visible lesion on neuroimaging with associated symptomatology. This viewpoint is supported by evidence of high residual cyst rates but very few resulting in symptom recurrence [28, 38, 39]. Furthermore, when reoperations were performed in these cases, surgical specimens revealed identical histopathology to the cysts previously removed [28, 38, 39]. Conversely, several reports of cysts containing benign simple cuboidal epithelium at initial resection have at reoperation revealed histological properties typical of papillary craniopharyngiomas [35, 40]. We fear that the aforementioned conservative approach may allow recurrent lesions without recurrent symptoms to grow, extend, invade, dedifferentiate and potentially advance along the hypothesized disease spectrum to a more aggressive status, decreasing the opportunity for successful symptom resolution with repeat intervention. We therefore recommend that judicious follow-up occur in previously symptomatic patients, with a low threshold for repeat intervention, even if symptoms have not yet recurred.

Following discharge, follow-up should consist of routine clinical and biochemical evaluations performed by experienced neuroendocrine specialists including a neurosurgeon, endocrinologist, and neuro-ophthalmologist at intervals of roughly 6 weeks postoperatively and annually thereafter. Repeat imaging should be performed with each visit starting at the 3-month check-up and annually for the first several years, following which the neurosurgeon may liberalize scheduled assessments depending upon individualized patient preference and indication.

If necessary, TS surgery remains the gold standard in the treatment of recurrent disease abiding by the same surgical principles as the initial procedure with the exception of including advanced computer-based operative guidance systems to aid in sellar localization, which may be indistinct and distorted from the initial procedure [36]. Clinical, neurological, and endocrinological outcomes have been reported as comparable to those of the initial surgery without a significant increase in risks, complications, or patient discomfort [38].

Conclusions

RCCs are usually benign, cystic lesions of the sella, eliciting symptoms primarily of headache, visual and/or endocrine disturbance. Its natural history, classification, surgical management, and recurrence rate have been topics of controversy for many years. RCCs exist along a spectrum from simple clinically benign cysts to clinically aggressive lesions that behave similar to craniopharyngiomas. Simple cyst drainage causes few endocrinological complications but is associated with higher recurrence rates. To reduce recurrence, we have advocated an aggressive cyst wall resection recognizing the increased incidence of pituitary dysfunction. Our experience with these lesions is growing, as is our ability to minimize their burden on society with prompt recognition and expeditious management. Compulsive follow-up with MRI, biochemical analysis and neuro-ophthalmological assessment remains an essential element in these cases as predictable recurrence rates exist in these otherwise benign lesions.

References

1 Shanklin WM: The incidence and distribution of cilia in the human pituitary with a description of microfollicular cysts derived from Rathke's cleft. Acta Anat 1951;11:361–382.
2 Goldzieher M: Ueber Sektionsbefunde bei Diabetes insipidus. Vern Dtsch Ges Pathol 1913;16: 281–287.
3 Voelker JL, Campbell RL, Muller J: Clinical, radiographic, and pathological features of symptomatic Rathke's cleft cysts. J Neurosurg 1991;74:535–544.
4 Frazier CH, Alpers BJ: Tumors of Rathke's cleft (hitherto called tumors of Rathke's pouch). Arch Neurol Pyschiatry 1934;32:973–984.
5 Berry RG, Schlezinger NS: Rathke-cleft cysts. AMA Arch Neurol 1959;1:62–72.
6 Concha S, Hamilton BP, Millan JC, et al: Symptomatic Rathke's cleft cyst with amyloid stroma. J Neurol Neurosurg Psychiatry 1975;38:782–786.
7 Leech RW, Olafson RA: Epithelial cysts of the neuraxis. Presentation of three cases and a review of the origins and classification. Arch Pathol Lab Med 1977;101:196–202.
8 Shuangshoti S, Netsky MG, Nashold BS Jr: Epithelial cysts related to sella turcica. Proposed origin from neuroepithelium. Arch Pathol 1970;90:444–450.
9 Matsushima T, Fukui M, Fujii K, et al: Epithelial cells in symptomatic Rathke's cleft cysts. A light- and electron-microscopic study. Surg Neurol 1988;30:197–203.
10 Palma L, Celli P: Suprasellar epithelial cyst: case report. J Neurosurg 1983;58:763–765.
11 Asa S: Atlas of Tumor Pathology, fasc 22. Washington, Armed Forces Institute of Pathology, 1998.
12 Naiken VS, Tellem M, Meranze DR: Pituitary cyst of Rathke's cleft origin with hypopituitarism. J Neurosurg 1961;18:703–708.
13 Rasmussen AT: Ciliated epithelium and mucus-secreting cells in the human hypophysis. Anat Rec 1929;41:273–283.
14 Eisenberg HM, Weiner RL: Benign pituitary cysts; in Wilkins RH, Rengachary SS (eds): Neurosurgery. Highstown, McGraw-Hill, 1985, pp 932–934.
15 Fager CA, Carter H: Intrasellar epithelial cysts. J Neurosurg 1966;24:77–81.
16 Northfield DWC: Rathke-pouch tumors. Brain 1957;80:293–311.
17 Smith RA, Bucy PC: Pituitary cyst lined with a single layer of columnar epithelium. J Neurosurg 1953;10:540–543.

18 Yoshida J, Kobayashi T, Kageyama N, et al: Symptomatic Rathke's cleft cyst. Morphological study with light and electron microscopy and tissue culture. J Neurosurg 1977;47:451–458.
19 Hama A, Arita K, Nishisaka T, et al: Changes in the epithelium of Rathke cleft cyst asociated with inflammation. J Neurosurg 2002;96:209–216.
20 Mukherjee JJ, Islam N, Kaltsas G, et al: Clinical, radiological, and pathological features of patients with Rathke's cleft cysts: tumors that may recur. J Clin Endocrinol Metab 1997;82:2357–2362.
21 Teramoto A, Hirakawa K, Sanno N, et al: Incidental pituitary lesions in 1000 unselected autopsy specimens. Radiology 1994;193:161–164.
22 Zada G, Kelly DF, Cohan P, et al: Endonasal transsphenoidal approach for pituitary adenomas and other sellar lesions: an assessment of efficacy, safety, and patient impressions. J Neurosurg 2003;98: 350–358.
23 Baskin DS, Wilson CB: Transsphenoidal treatment of non-neoplastic intrasellar cysts. J Neurosurg 1984;60:8–13.
24 Bayoumi ML: Rathke's cleft and its cysts. Edinburgh Med J 1948;55:745–749.
25 Gillman T: The incidence of ciliated epithelium and mucous cells in the normal Bantu pituitary. S Afr J Med Sci 1940;5:30–40.
26 Steinberg GK, Koenig GH, Golden JB: Symptomatic Rathke's cleft cysts. Report of two cases. J Neurosurg 1982;56:290–295.
27 Agnetti V, Carreras M, Rocca A, et al: Epithelial cysts related to the Rathke's cleft. J Neurosurg Sci 1974;18:65–69.
28 el-Mahdy W, Powell M: Transsphenoidal management of 28 symptomatic Rathke's cleft cysts, with special reference to visual and hormonal recovery. Neurosurgery 1998;42:7–16.
29 Isono M, Kamida T, Kobayashi H, et al: Clinical features of symptomatic Rathek's cleft cysts. Clin Neurol Neurosurg 2001;103:96–100.
30 Ross DA, Norman D, Wilson CD: Radiologic characteristics and results of surgical management of Rathke's cysts in 43 patients. Neurosurgery 1992;30:173–179.
31 Shin JL, Asa SL, Woodhouse LJ, et al: Cystic lesions of the pituitary: clinicopathological features distinguishing craniopharyngioma, Rathke's cleft cyst, and arachnoid cyst. J Clin Endocrinol Metab 1999;84:3972–3982.
32 Tolis G, Somma M, Van Campenhout J, et al: Prolactin secretion in sixty-five patients with galactorrhea. Am J Obstec Gynecol 1974;118:91–101.
33 Wenzel M, Salcman M, Kristt DA, et al: Pituitary hyposecretion and hypersecretion produced by a Rathke's cleft cyst presenting as a noncystic hypothalamic mass. Neurosurgery 1989;24:424–428.
34 Woodruff WW Jr, Heinz ER, Djang WT, et al: Hyperprolactinemia: an unusual manifestation of suprasellar cystic lesions. AJNR Am J Neuroradiol 1987;8:113–116.
35 Kim JE, Kim JH, Kim OL, Paek SH, Kim DG, Chi JG, Jung HW: Surgical treatment of symptomatic Rathke's cleft cyst: clinical features and results with special attention to recurrence. J Neurosurg 2004;100:33–40.
36 Kanter AS, Diallo AO, Vance ML, Laws ER: Rathke's cleft cysts: a single center's experience. American Association of Neurological Surgery Conference, 2004.
37 Kasperbauer JL, Orvidas LJ, Atkinson JLD, et al: Rathke cleft cyst: diagnostic and therapeutic considerations. Laryngoscope 2002;112:1836–1839.
38 Benveniste RJ, King WA, Walsh J, Lee JS, Naidich TP, Post KD: Surgery for Rathke cleft cysts: technical considerations and outcome. J Neurosurg 2004;101:577–584.
39 Aho CJ, Liu C, Zelman V, Couldwell WT, Weiss MH: Surgical outcomes in 118 patients with Rathke's cleft cysts. J Neurosurg 2005;102:189–193.
40 Ikeda H, Yoshimoto T: Clinicopathological study of Rathke's cleft cysts. Clin Neuropathol 2002;21:82–91.
41 Nishioka H, Ito H, Miki T, et al: Rathke's cleft cyst with pituitary apoplexy: case report. Neuroradiology 1999;41:832–834.
42 Onesti ST, Wisniewski T, Post KD: Pituitary hemorrhage into a Rathke's cleft cyst. Neurosurgery 1990;27:644–646.
43 Pawar SJ, Sharma RR, Lad SD, et al: Rathke's cleft cyst presenting as pituitary apoplexy. J Clin Neurosci 2002;9:76–79.

44 Albini CH, MacGillivray MH, Fisher JE: Triad of hypopituitarism, granulomatous hypophysitis, and ruptured Rathke's cleft cyst. Neurosurgery 1988;22:133–136.
45 Daikokuya H, Inoue Y, Nemoto Y, et al: Rathke's cleft cyst associated with hypophysitis. Neuroradiology 2000;42:532–534.
46 Wearne MJ, Barber PC, Johnson AP: Symptomatic Rathke's cleft cyst with hypophysitis. Br J Neurosurg 1995;9:799–803.
47 Bognar L, Szeifert GT, Fedorcsak I, et al: Abscess formation in Rathke's cleft cyst. Acta Neurochir (Wien) 1992;117:70–72.
48 Obenchain TG, Becker DP: Abscess formation in Rathke's cleft cyst – case report. J Neurosurg 1972;36:359–362.
49 Sonntag VK, Plenge KL, Balis MS, et al: Surgical treatment of an abscess in a Rathke's cleft cyst. Surg Neurol 1983;20:152–156.
50 Nader R, Frenkiel S, Mohr, et al: Rahtke's cleft cyst presenting as sphenoid sinusitis. Otolaryngol Head Neck Surg 2001;124:174–179.
51 Monzavi R, Kelly DF, Geffner ME: Rathke's cleft cyst in two girls with precocious puberty. J Pediatr Endocrinol Metab 2004;17:781–785.
52 Baldini M, Mosca L, Princi L: The empty sella syndrome secondary to Rathke's cleft cyst. Acta Neurochir 1980;53:69–78.
53 Setian N, Aguiar CH, Galvao JA, et al: Rathke's cleft cyst as a cause of growth hormone deficiency and micropenis. Childs Nerv Syst 1999;15:271–273.
54 Oka H, Suwa T, Yada K, et al: Radiological study of symptomatic Rathke's cleft cysts. Neurosurgery 1994;35:632–637.
55 Verkijk A, Bots GTAM: An intrasellar cyst with both Rathke's cleft and epidermoid characteristics. Acta Neurochir 1980;51:203–207.
56 Nakasu Y, Isozumi S, Nakasu S, et al: Rathke's cleft cyst: computed tomographic scan and magnetic resonance imaging. Acta Neurochir 1990;103:99–104.
57 Saeki N, Hoshi S, Sunada S, et al: Rathke's cleft cyst with large frontal extension: unusual shape and pathomechanism of its formation. J Clin Neurosci 2000;7:452–454.
58 Kucharczyk W, Peck WW, Kelly WM, et al: Rathke cleft cysts: CT, MR imaging, and pathologic features. Radiology 1987;165:491–495.
59 Maggio WW, Brookeman JR, Persing JA, Jane JA: Rathke's cleft cyst: computed tomographic and magnetic resonance imaging appearances. Neurosurgery 1987;21:60–62.
60 Nemoto Y, Inoue Y, Fukuda T, et al: MR appearance of Rathke's cleft cysts. Neuroradiology 1988;30:155–159.
61 Byun WM, Kim OL, Kim DS: MR imaging findings of Rathke's cleft cysts: significance of intracystic nodules. Am J Neuroradiol 2000;21:485–488.
62 Hayashi Y, Tachibana O, Muramatsu N, et al: Rathke cleft cyst: MR and biomedical analysis of cyst content. J Comput Assist Tomog 1999;23:34–38.
63 Wagle VG, Nelson D, Rossi A, et al: Magnetic resonance imaging of symptomatic Rathke's cleft cyst: report of a case. Neurosurgery 1989;24:276–278.
64 Barrow DL, Spector RH, Takei Y, et al: Symptomatic Rathke's cleft cysts located entirely in the suprasellar region: review of diagnosis management, and pathogenesis. Neurosurgery 1985;16: 766–772.
65 Itoh J, Usui K: An entirely suprasellar symptomatic Rathke's cleft cyst: case report. Neurosurgery 1992;30:581–585.
66 Rout D, Das L, Rao VR, et al: Symptomatic Rathke's cleft cysts. Surg Neurol 1983;19:42–49.
67 Harrison MJ, Morgello A, Post KD: Epithelial cystic lesions of the sellar and parasellar region: a continuum of ectodermal derivatives? J Neurosurg 1994;80:1018–1025.
68 Hua F, Asato R, Miki Y, et al: Differentiation of suprasellar nonneoplastic cysts from cystic neoplasms by Gd-DTPA MRI. J Comput Assist Tomogr 1992:16:744–749.
69 Banna M: Craniopharyngioma: based on 160 cases. Br J Radiol 1976;49:206–223.
70 Sumida M, Uozumi T, Mukada K, et al: Rathke cleft cysts: correlation of enhanced MR and surgical findings. AJNR Am J Neuroradiol 1994;15:525–532.
71 Meyer FB, Laws ER: Intrasellar arachnoids cysts. Surg Neurol 1987;28:105–110.

72 Adamson TE, Kleihues P, Yasargil MG: Correlation of clinical and pathological features in surgically treated craniopharyngiomas. J Neurosurg 1990;73:12–17.
73 Fahlbusch R, Paulus W, Huk W, et al: Surgical treatment of craniopharyngiomas: experience with 168 patients. J Neurosurg 1999;90:237–250.
74 Ikeda H, Yoshimoto T, Suzuki J: Immunohistochemical study of Rathke's cleft cyst. Acta Neuropathol 1988;77:33–38.
75 Laws ER, Kanter AS: Rathke cleft cysts. J Neurosurg 2004;101:571–572.
76 Hunter IJ: Squamous metaplasia of cells of the anterior pituitary gland. J Pathol Bacteriol 1955;69:141–145.
77 Matsushima T, Fukui M, Ohta M, et al: Ciliated and goblet cells in craniopharyngioma. Light and electron microscopic studies at surgery and autopsy. Acta Neuropathol 1980;50:199–205.
78 Goodrich JT, Post KD, Duffy P: Ciliated craniopharyngioma. Surg Neurol 1985;24:105–111.
79 Adelman L, Post KD: Calcification in Rathke's cleft cyst. J Neurosurg 1977;47:641.
80 Nakasu Y, Nakasu S, Nakajima M, et al: Atypical Rathke's cleft cyst associated with ossification. AJNR Am J Neuroradiol 1999;20:1287–1289.
81 Nishio S, Mizuno J, Barrow DL, et al: Pituitary tumors composed of adenohypophyseal adenoma and Rathke's cleft cyst elements: a clinicopathological study. Neurosurgery 1987;21:371–377.
82 Sumida M, Migita T, Tominaga A, et al: Concomitant pituitary adenoma and Rathke's cleft cyst. Neuroradiology 2001;43:755–759.
83 Swanson SE, Chandler WE, Latack J, et al: Symptomatic Rathke's cleft cyst with pituitary adenoma: case report. Neurosurgery 1985;17:657–659.
84 Troukoudes KM, Walfish PG, Holgate RC, et al: Sellar enlargement with hyperprolactinemia and a Rathke's pouch cyst. JAMA 1978;240:471–473.
85 Turski PA, Newton TH, Horten BH: Sellar contour: anatomic polytomographic correlation. AJR Am J Roentgenol 1981;2:213–216.
86 Frank G, Sciarretta V, Mazzatenta D, et al: Transsphenoidal endoscopic approach in the treatment of Rathke's cleft cyst. Neurosurgery 2005;56:124–129.
87 Hardy J, Vezina JL: Transphenoidal neurosurgery of intracranial neoplasm. Adv Neurol 1976;15:261–274.
88 Shimoji T, Shinohara A, Shinizu A, et al: Rathke's cleft cysts. Surg Neurol 1984;21:295–310.
89 Day JD: Surgical approaches to the suprasellar and parasellar tumors. Neurosurg Clin North Am 2003;14:109–122.
90 Alfieri A, Schettino R, Tarfani A, et al: Endoscopic endonasal removal of an intra-suprasellar Rathke's cleft cyst: case report and surgical considerations. Minim Invasive Neurosurg 2002;45: 47–51.
91 Koren I, Hadar T, Rappaport ZH, et al: Endoscopic transnasal transsphenoidal microsurgery versus sublabial approach for the treatment of pituitary tumors: endonasal complication. Laryngoscope 1999;109:1838–1840.
92 Iraci G, Giordano R, Gerosa M, et al: Ocular involvement in recurrent cyst of Rathke's cleft: case report. Ann Ophthalmol 1979;11:94–98.
93 Marcincin RP, Gennarelli TA: Recurrence of symptomatic pituitary cysts following transsphenoidal drainage. Surg Neurol 1982;18:448–451.
94 Raskind R, Brown HA, Mathis J: Recurrent cyst of the pituitary: 26-year follow-up from first decompression. J Neurosurg 1968;28:595–599.
95 Yamamoto M, Jimbo M, Ide M, et al: Recurrence of symptomatic Rathke's cleft cyst: a case report. Surg Neurol 1993;39:263–268.
96 Eisenberg HM, Sarwar M, Schlocher S Jr: Symptomatic Rathke's cleft cysts. J Neurosurg 1976;45:585–588.
97 Moringlane JR, Alexander C, Kirsch CM: Successful low-dose intradavitary irradiation of a Rathke's cleft cyst with colloidal rhenium-186. Minim Invasive Neurosurg 2001;44:218–220.
98 Rao GP, Blyth CPJ, Jeffreys RV: Ophthalmic manifestations of Rathke's cleft cysts. Am J Ophthalmol 1995;119:86–91.

99 Landolt AM, Zachmann M: Results of transsphenoidal extirpation of craniopharyngioma and Rathke's cysts. Neurosurgery 1991;28:410–415.
100 Rottenburg GT, Chong WK, Powell MP, et al: Cyst formation of the craniopharyngeal duct. Clin Radiol 1994;49:126–129.
101 Nelson AT Jr, Tucker HS Jr, Becker DP: Residual anterior pituitary function following transsphenoidal excision of pituitary macroadenomas. J Neurosurg 1984;61:577–580.
102 Eguchi K, Uozumi T, Arita K, et al: Pituitary function in patients with Rathke's cleft cyst: significance of surgical management. Endocr J 1994;41:535–540.

Adam S. Kanter, MD
Department of Neurological Surgery, Health Sciences Center
University of Virginia, PO Box 800212
Charlottesville, VA 22908 (USA)
Tel. +1 434 924 2203, Fax +1 434 924 9656, E-Mail ask9z@hscmail.mcc.virginia.edu

Laws ER Jr, Sheehan JP (eds): Pituitary Surgery – A Modern Approach.
Front Horm Res. Basel, Karger, 2006, vol 34, pp 158–184

Treatment of Cushing's Disease: A Retrospective Clinical Study of the Latest 100 Cases

Bernd M. Hofmann, Rudolf Fahlbusch

Department of Neurosurgery, University of Erlangen–Nuremberg, Erlangen, Germany

Abstract

We evaluate the current role of microsurgery for Cushing's disease (CD) and the efficacy of adjuvant treatment modalities. The standard treatment for primary CD remains transsphenoidal surgery followed by adjuvant therapy in cases with persisting hypercortisolism. Moderately severe cases are treated with radiotherapy, while in the very severe adrenalectomy is performed. In our series of primary CD (March 1997 to September 2004, mean observation period 18.8 months) adenomas were confirmed intraoperatively in 84.0% of the cases. Remission was achieved in 75.0% and recurrence was observed in 4.8% of the patients. Complications occurred in 2.0% of the cases and all resolved without resulting in permanent morbidity. In the literature, the rates of intraoperative confirmation of an adenoma vary between 59.1 and 100%, remission rates between 42 and 100%, and recurrence rates between 3.0 and 63.2% depending on the experience of the surgeon and on the definition of remission. These rates have not improved significantly over the years. In experienced hands selective adenomectomy remains the least damaging and most effective treatment modality since it results in rapid clinical improvement if performed successfully. Therefore, it remains the treatment of choice. Patients not cured by surgery alone benefited from a combination of adjuvant treatment tailored to their specific needs using medications, radiation and/or adrenalectomy. In this fashion, we achieved normalization of cortisol levels in 79% and improvement in another 18% of the patients. We expect these rates to increase further once patients treated with radiotherapy begin to experience its full effect within the next few years.

Copyright © 2006 S. Karger AG, Basel

Introduction

Within pituitary surgery Cushing's disease (CD) takes a special place. The differential diagnosis of central CD is based on sophisticated dynamic

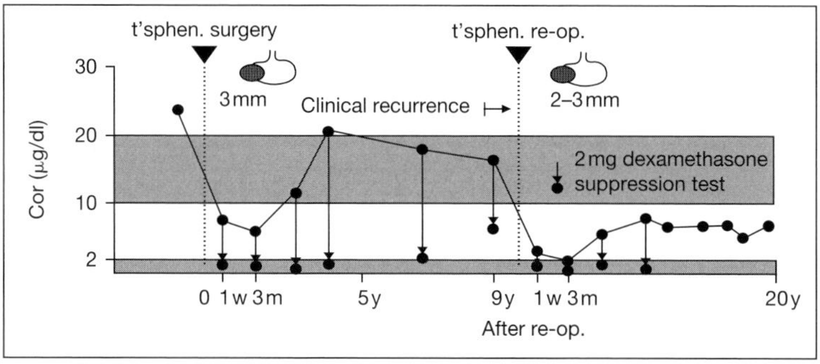

Fig. 1. Long-term follow-up after successful (repeated) microneurosurgery in Cushing's disease.

endocrinological tests on which the indication for surgery is based. Selective microsurgical adenomectomy is considered the first treatment option but recently some authors have propagated extensive resection of the anterior lobe, although this results in more endocrine deficits and more complications. Since the first selective adenomectomy for CD was introduced by us 35 years ago [1], we have developed the impression that even in the hand of experienced endocrine surgeons no convincing improvement in remission rates has been achieved. Nevertheless, long intervals of endocrine and clinical remission have been observed following (even repeated) microneurosurgery (fig. 1). The inhomogeneous definition of remission of hypercortisolism and its still not fully understood pathophysiology might be reasons for this. It remains unclear if technical progress (e.g. endoscopy, neuronavigation, intraoperative MRI) is helpful in the treatment of this particular disease. Following the increasing importance of focused radiotherapy this treatment option is again being discussed as an alternative.

In several microsurgical studies [2–30] the rates of confirmation of an adenoma during surgery vary between 59.1 and 100%, remission rates between 42 and 100% and recurrence rates between 3.0 and 63.2%. Complications are reported in up to 27% of the cases with a maximum mortality rate of 3.6%. New endocrine deficits are observed in up to 88% of the patients.

The aim of this paper is to demonstrate the current role of microsurgery in primary CD and to compare its results with the effects of other treatment modalities. This leads to the definition of new (combined) treatment strategies. For this purpose we will first demonstrate the modern diagnostic procedures and the results of multimodal treatment strategies on the basis of a consecutive series of the latest 100 patients we have treated. Our results will be compared with the literature, and the efforts to improve the operative results will be discussed based on our many years of experience.

Current Diagnosis of Cushing's Disease

The classical phenotypical symptoms can be impressive or even absent. Often the disease is only suspected after diabetes mellitus or hypertension is observed and is difficult to treat successfully.

Dynamic endocrine function tests lead to the diagnosis of the disease: a fasting morning basal cortisol level of >2 μg/dl after administering 2 mg dexamethasone (DEXA; 2-mg DEXA suppression test) at 10.00 p.m. the previous day leads to the diagnosis of Cushing's syndrome. The pituitary origin of the disease is proven by suppression of the cortisol level to <50% of the original value after administration of 8–32 mg DEXA [31, 32]. Furthermore, the function of the anterior pituitary lobe is assessed by determining serum levels of prolactin, TSH, thyronine, thyroxine, LH, FSH, estradiol or testosterone, and ACTH plasma levels as well as cortisol serum levels before and after ACTH stimulation following an overnight fast.

A thin-layer MRI scan (2–3 mm) of the sellar region including T_1 and T_2 coronal and sagittal planes is performed to confirm a sellar tumor. When no adenoma is visible on MRI and the pituitary origin of the disease is in doubt, an inferior petrosal sinus sampling (IPSS) combined with a selective catheterization of the abdominal and thoracic veins is performed and ACTH and cortisol plasma levels are determined. By using these tests, an adrenal origin of the hypercortisolism or ectopic or paraneoplastic ACTH production can be ruled out. Furthermore they yield indirect evidence of the precise intrasellar location of the tumor. This is important for choosing the side on which to perform hemihypophysectomy in case no adenoma is found during sella exploration. In this test a larger than twofold central to peripheral gradient of ACTH levels (larger than threefold after CRH stimulation) is highly sensitive for the diagnosis of a pituitary adenoma and a more than 1.4-fold interpetrosal gradient is indicative of the lateral tumor localization [33]. Recently, its value in predicting the exact intrasellar tumor location has been discussed controversially [33–36]. In about 15% of the patients, technical problems with catheterization occur (e.g. the presence of a unilateral sinus only), and in about one third the prediction of a pituitary adenoma is false (i.e. a false-positive result).

An elevated free urinary cortisol (>300 μg/24 h) [37] or an abolished diurnal rhythm of cortisol secretion (normally exhibiting a maximum in the morning and at 8.00 p.m. the value is <50% of the morning value) are indicative of CD as well, and might be of use in uncertain cases.

A single CRH test (0–60 min) is used less often but is still of diagnostic value. Patients suffering from ectopic Cushing's syndrome may show no increase in cortisol and ACTH after administering CRH and, in the case of an adrenal tumor, ACTH levels may be within the lower normal range [38].

Preoperative and Operative Treatment

Since the advent of modern anesthesiology methods preoperative treatment to improve the patients' clinical status prior to surgery is necessary only if exceptionally severe metabolic changes caused by their hypercortisolism, such as hypokalemia or diabetes mellitus, hypertension or severely symptomatic osteoporosis are present. Ketoconazol is still the drug of choice; it exerts its effect by blocking corticosteroid synthesis in the liver at the level of cytochrome P-450 enzyme. By administering 600–800 mg/day at least a temporary decrease in cortisol plasma levels can be achieved until the development of adverse hepatic side effects preclude further use of the drug [39].

The transsphenoidal approach to the sella turcica, either by a sublabial paraseptal, a pernasal paraseptal or a direct pernasal route, has become the surgical standard. After opening the sphenoid sinus and removing the mucosa the sellar floor is opened using a diamond drill and the endosteum is opened with a pair of scissors. In case an adenoma is visible on MRI, a selective adenomectomy is performed by incising the pituitary body near the suspected tumor pole and removing the adenoma with ring curettes or suction. Furthermore, a small rim of the surrounding tissue is removed to ensure complete resection.

In case there is focally invasive tumor growth into the cavernous sinus and especially when a pseudocapsule is visible, tumor resection can be continued by carefully opening the medial wall of the cavernous sinus and then total tumor removal from the sinus can be attempted. Bleeding from smaller injuries to the cavernous sinus can be handled by an experienced surgeon. Larger scale tumor invasion of the cavernous sinus reaching the passing carotid arteries precludes further resection in this area. Tumor remnants have to be left within the cavernous sinus, leading to subtotal tumor resection.

If no tumor is found on MRI, sellar exploration is performed. Meticulously, systematic incisions into the pituitary body are carried out approximately 1–2 mm apart while the surgeon is looking for tissue suspicious for an adenoma. Once all adenomatous tissue has been removed, the whole pituitary body as well as the extraglandular space is explored in order to not miss any tumor. In the case of a negative exploration in the presence of an interpetrosal ACTH concentration gradient confirmed by preoperative sampling, a hemihypophysectomy of the putative side harboring the adenoma is performed [33]. Complete hypophysectomy is considered as an obsolete operation today. Five to 7 days perioperatively, antibiotics (usually clindamycin) and low-dose heparin (5,000 IU three times/day) are given. Postoperatively the patient may be kept in the intensive care unit overnight in order to treat the expected effects of hypocortisolism (e.g. hypotension) following successful tumor removal.

Histopathological work-up consists of normal HE staining of the specimen as well as immunohistochemical staining for pituitary hormones. Furthermore, a cell explant culture can be performed to document ACTH expression.

Definition of Outcome and Cure

Postoperatively, an early basal cortisol level is determined the day following surgery (if necessary also the day thereafter) and replacement of corticosteroids is started if the cortisol levels are below the normal range. This is considered one criterion of remission. One week and about 3 months postoperatively dynamic endocrine function tests are repeated to confirm remission of the disease as well as to detect possible new endocrine deficits. The patient is defined as in endocrinological remission if the fasting basal cortisol level following 2 mg DEXA is <2 μg/dl. This may occur immediately or in a delayed fashion (1–3 months) following surgery.

Current Treatment after Initial Diagnosis of Cushing's Disease: A Clinical Study of Our Latest 100 Cases

To illustrate our current treatment regimen the latest 100 consecutive patients suffering from CD who underwent pituitary microsurgery at the Neurosurgical Department of the University of Erlangen–Nuremberg, Germany, will be analyzed. The results will be compared to the literature and to those reported for alternative treatment regimens.

Patients

From March 1, 1997 until September 30, 2004, a total of 100 patients suffering from primary CD underwent initial surgical treatment.

In 98 patients the primary diagnosis of CD was made prior to admission to our hospital and confirmed by us prior to surgery (table 1). In 1 of these patients, the preoperative work-up was incomplete. In another patient, the biochemical data obtained preoperatively were inconsistent. Subsequently, surgical exploration of the sella was performed. Five patients were treated with ketoconazol, preoperatively. In the 2 remaining of the 100 cases there were no clinical signs for hypercortisolism but later histological work-up revealed an ACTH-producing pituitary adenoma.

There was a female preponderance of 77:23 (3.3:1) and an age range at the time of surgery of 5–77 (mean 40.7) years. The age range of the female patients was 5–77 (mean 42.5) years and that of the male patients 9–60 (mean 33.4) years.

Endocrinological Work-Up

Preoperatively basal cortisol levels ranged between 2.9 and 100.2 (mean 25.5) μg/dl. Excluding 5 patients (2 harbored silent ACTH-secreting tumors, 2 were diagnosed at an external hospital by high-dose DEXA or SPS, and 1 patient with an incomplete preoperative work-up), the

Table 1. Pre- and postoperative findings in 100 patients

Patient collective	100	
Female/male	77/23	3.3/1
Age	5–77 years	
Preoperative endocrine function		
Basal cortisol	2.9–100.2 μg/dl	mean 25.5 μg/dl
ACTH		
Cortisol follow-up, 2 mg DEXA	2.3–61.2 μg/dl	mean 19.2 μg/dl
Petrosal sinus sample	50	
Unilateral catheterization only	3	
Gradient right	21 (44.7%)	
Gradient left	21 (44.7%)	
No gradient	5 (10.6%)	
Imaging	100	
Adenoma visibile	15 macro, 35 micro	
Indirect sign of adenoma	8	
No adenoma found	42	
Operation		
Ketoconazol pretreatment	5	
Transsphenoidal	99	
Transcranial	1	
Macroadenoma	15	
Microadenoma	69	
Histological work-up		
Adenoma	76 (90.5%)	
Hyperplasia	2 (2.4%)	
None/normal pituitary	5 (5.9%)	
Crooke cells	1 (1.2%)	
Postoperative endocrine function		
Cortisol <5 μg/dl	47	
Cortisol <9 μg/dl	7	
Cortisol ≤21 μg/dl	24	
Cortisol >21 μg/dl	22	
Cortisol follow-up, 2 mg DEXA		
Normal	65	
Pathological	34	

preoperative cortisol levels following 2 mg DEXA, ranged between 2.3 and 61.2 (mean 19.2) μg/dl. Except for 1 case in which the central origin of Cushing's syndrome was not certain, all patients met the criteria for the diagnosis of CD following high-dose DEXA suppression testing. The postoperative observation period was between 3 and 86 (mean 18.8) months.

Radiological Results

An MRI scan (Siemens Somatom Sonata®, 1.5 T) was performed in all 100 patients at the study hospital. In these MRI scans, there was clear evidence

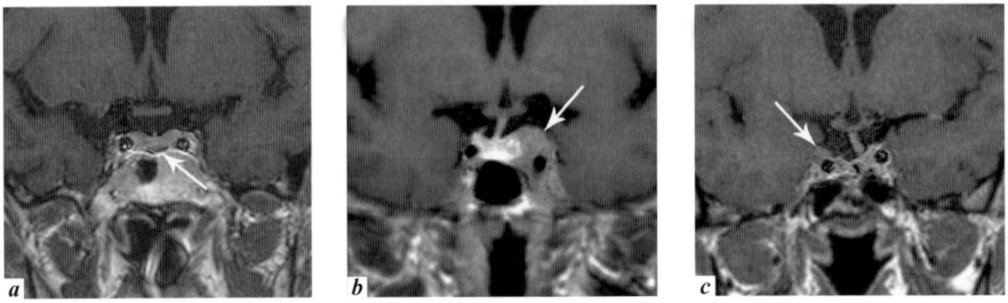

Fig. 2. Radiological findings in Cushing's disease. ***a*** Intrasellar microadenoma. ***b*** Invasion into the cavernous sinus. ***c*** Invasive tumor remnant in the cavernous sinus, scheduled for radiosurgery.

of a macroadenoma in 15 and a microadenoma in 35 cases who, taken together, represent 50% of the patients. Assuming that a microadenoma was also present in all patients with negative MRI scans, there was a prevalence of 15% for macro- and 85% for microadenoma (fig. 2a). These findings correspond to those in the literature which report macroadenomas in 9–20% of the cases [3, 4, 7].

Indirect evidence of an adenoma, such as a deviated pituitary stalk, an increase in intrasellar volume or erosion of a subjacent part of the sellar floor, was found in 8 patients. In 42 patients no evidence of a tumor was visible on the MRI scan.

An IPSS was performed in 53 patients. A significant gradient between central and peripheral ACTH levels were found in 50 of these cases (94.3%). Furthermore in 2 patients a gradient was found but was not significant. Catheterization of both inferior petrosal sinuses was possible in 47 cases. An interpetrosal gradient towards the right sinus was found in 21 (44.7%), towards the left sinus in 21 (44.7%), and no gradient was found in 5 cases (10.6%).

Operative Results

In 84 of 100 patients who underwent primary surgery a tumor was found and (selective) adenomectomy was attempted. No tumor was found in 16 of 100 patients, and sella exploration (n = 9) or hemihypophysectomy (n = 7) were carried out (fig. 3).

Analysis of the Postoperative Outcome

In the following, the surgical results are presented and analyzed on the basis of the various pre- and intraoperative findings.

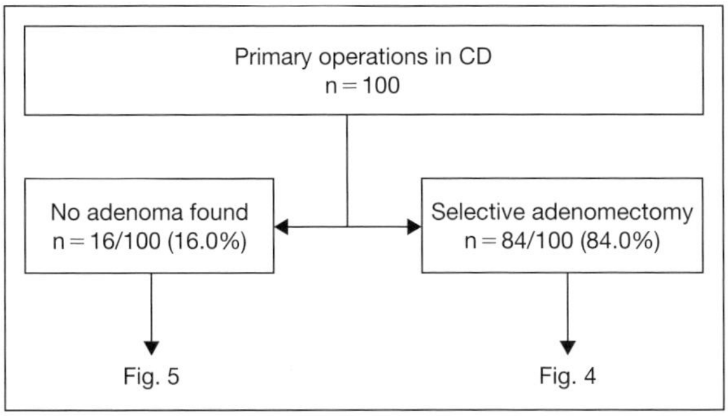

Fig. 3. Findings during primary operation.

In 84 of 100 patients an adenoma was found during transsphenoidal surgery leading to a selective adenomectomy (fig. 4a). Tumor size ranged from 1.2 to 26.0 (mean 6.7) mm according to the surgeon's impression. Invasive tumor growth was found in 11 patients. In 2 of these, the tumor was only focally invasive allowing its removal from the cavernous sinus.

63 of 84 patients (75.0%) showed early remission following transsphenoidal adenomectomy and recurrence was observed in only 3 of them (4.8%). The mean observation period of these 3 patients was 18.8 (range 3–86) months. For them, remission was either achieved by radiotherapy alone, successful re-operation at another center, and unsuccessful re-operation succeeded by radiotherapy, respectively. In summary, long-term remission was observed in 60 of 63 cases (95.2%) following selective adenomectomy alone and in 100% following surgery succeeded by augmentative treatment.

The persistence rate of the disease was 25.0% (21/84) requiring further treatment as described below.

Histological work-up (table 1) confirmed a pituitary adenoma in 76 of 84 cases (90.5%). Expression of ACTH was proven by immunohistochemistry in all except one of the specimens which was too small for precise examination. Follicular hyperplasia was found in 2 cases (2.4%). No tumor or only normal pituitary tissue (at the tumor margin) was found in 5 cases (5.9%). In 1 case (1.2%) Crooke cells were found within the normal pituitary tissue, which is an indirect sign for the presence of an ACTH-producing adenoma [40].

As invasiveness into the cavernous sinus (fig. 2b) can be regarded as a negative predictor of total tumor removal as well as the elimination of hypercortisolism, the results after selective adenomectomy of noninvasive tumors are better (fig. 4b). Their tumor size was between 1.7 and 25.0 (mean 6.0) mm and showed no significant difference compared to the total patient collective. The

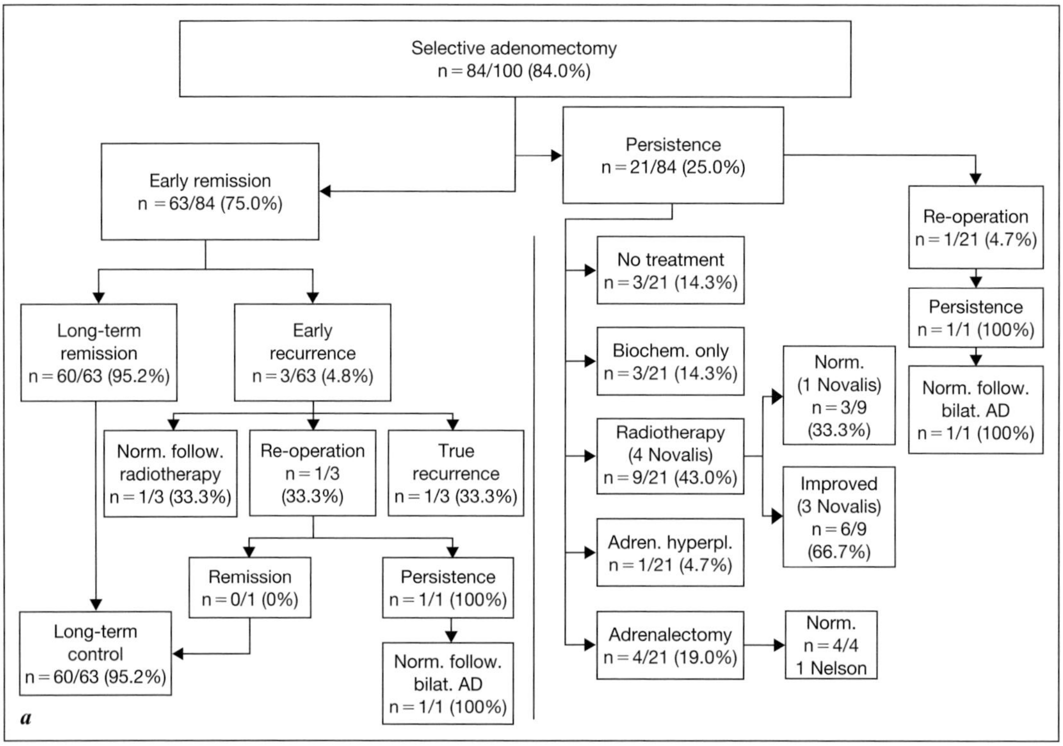

Fig. 4. ***a*** Outcome after selective adenomectomy in Cushing's disease. ***b*** Outcome after selective adenomectomy in Cushing's disease in patients with noninvasive tumors.

remission rate in these patients was 82.2% (60/73) while the recurrence rate was 5.0% (3/60) resulting in a long-term remission rate of 95.0% (57/60). Persistence of the disease occurred in 17.8% (13/73).

The remission rate is correlated to the tumor size after selective adenomectomy. It is substantially higher after surgery for microadenoma compared to macroadenoma. 56 of 69 patients (81.2%) suffering from a microadenoma were in remission following transsphenoidal surgery whereas only 7 of 15 patients (46.7%) suffering from a macroadenoma were in remission.

During primary transsphenoidal surgery in patients suffering from CD no adenoma was found in 16 of 100 patients (fig. 5). In 9 of these 16 patients (56.2%) exploration of the sella contents was performed but no adenoma was found and hypercortisolism persisted. A hemihypophysectomy was not carried out in these patients either because no convincing gradient could be obtained during IPSS or because a small volume of the pituitary gland made it impossible

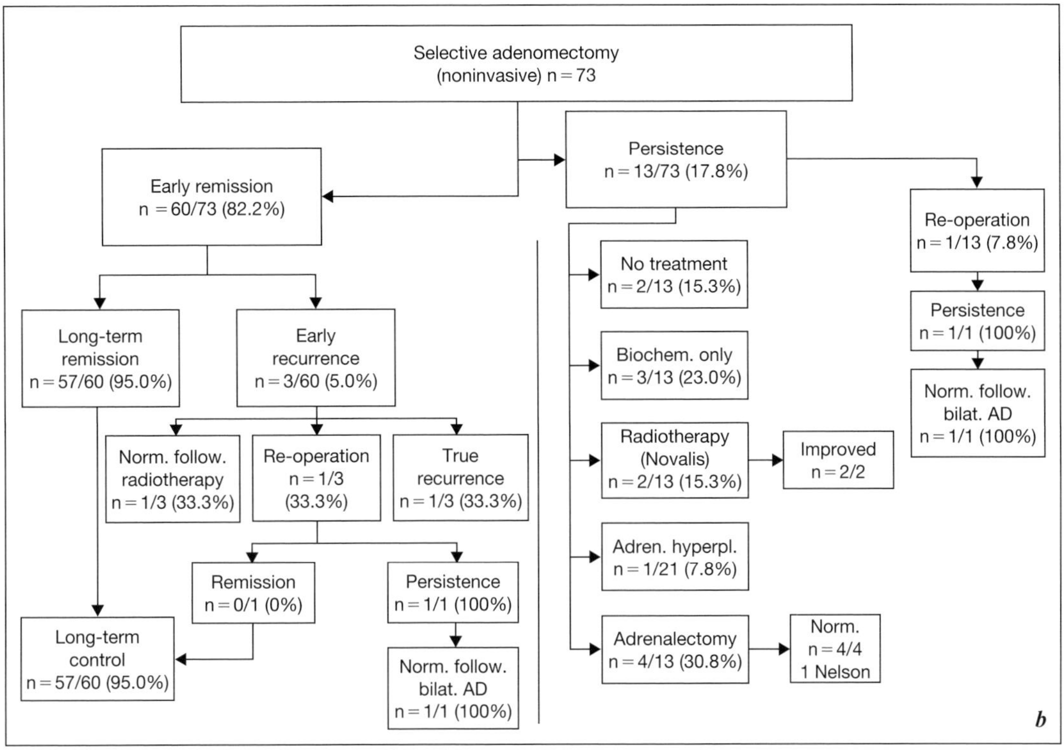

to perform the procedure. In the remaining 7 of 16 patients (43.8%) partial hypophysectomy was performed. Early and long-term remission was observed in 3 of them (42.9%). One patient underwent additional radiotherapy. Persistence of the disease after surgery was observed in 4 of 7 patients (57.1%). The mean observation period was 18.4 (3–76) months. Augmentative treatment of these patients was performed according to the guidelines as described below.

Postoperative assessment of endocrine function in the whole series, including the cases in which sella exploration was negative, revealed the following results. 44 of the 100 patients met remission criteria immediately postoperatively and 22 more met them after 3 months, leading to a total remission rate of 66%. One patient left the hospital without undergoing endocrinological testing. The mean cortisol level of all the other patients following DEXA was 6.4 (range 0.1–49.7) μg/dl and in those patients meeting remission criteria, it ranged between 0.1 and 2.1 (mean 1.0) μg/dl. One patient was believed to be cured despite a slightly elevated cortisol level (2.1 μg/dl) because he showed clear

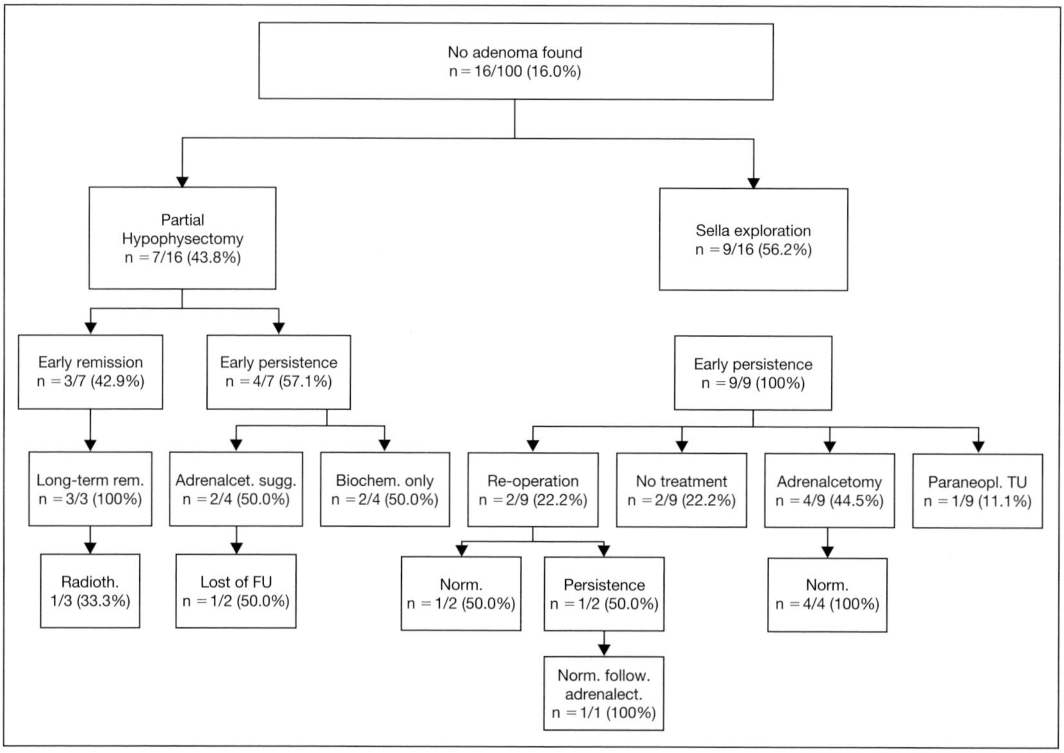

Fig. 5. Outcome when no tumor was found during operation.

evidence of clinical remission and, on further follow-up, his cortisol level was <2.0 μg/dl following 2 mg DEXA (table 1).

Basal cortisol levels 1 week after surgery were between 0.2 and 64.4 (mean 12.6) μg/dl. In 54 patients the level ranged between 0.2 and 8.9 (mean 2.2) μg/dl. At least temporarily in these patients it became necessary to start substitution therapy by administering hydrocortisone, 25 mg/day (table 1). 47 of these 54 patients exhibited tertiary adrenal insufficiency with postoperative basal cortisol levels of <5.0 (range 0.2–4.9, mean 1.5) μg/dl and were considered to be cured of CD. The insufficiency was due to the long-term suppression of normal ACTH-producing cells within the pituitary by ACTH oversecretion from tumor cells [41].

The mean observation period in all 100 patients was 18.8 (range 3–86) months.

In the present series, preoperative bilateral blood sampling from both inferior petrosal sinuses was possible in 47 patients. In 42 of these patients a significant gradient to one side was observed, but in only 27 of these 42 cases (64.3%) was a tumor found on the corresponding side. These numbers are comparable to other series published in the literature [34, 35]. Hence, hemihypophysectomy after negative sella exploration does not guarantee a remission even if performed on the side suggested by preoperative IPSS.

In this series no mortality occurred. The morbidity includes two complications (complication rate 2%). One patient suffered from a deep vein thrombosis and another one from a mesenteric infarction which both resolved after administration of heparin. There was no new endocrine deficit other than corticotrope insufficiency; permanent hypocortisolism was found in 3 patients (3.0%), following selective adenomectomy in 2 and following hemihypophysectomy in 1. In 1 of the patients it persisted for a follow-up period of more than 3 years. This probably is related more to a long history of preexisting disease and the resulting permanent suppression of anterior pituitary function rather than to surgery.

Additional Treatment and Outcome in Persisting Hypercortisolism

In 21 cases the hypercortisolism persisted following primary transsphenoidal surgery and intended selective adenomectomy (fig. 4a).

In 1 of these patients (4.7%) unilateral adrenalectomy was performed because of accompanying adrenal hyperplasia and the patient improved. In 1 case (4.7%) transsphenoidal re-operation was performed after an incomplete transcranial resection to remove the remaining intrasellar parts of the tumor. When this failed to achieve normalization, bilateral adrenalectomy was carried out.

Radiotherapy was performed in 9 patients after surgery did not result in normal cortisol levels (9/21, 43.0%). In 4 cases linear accelerator (LINAC) radiosurgery using the NOVALIS® system was performed for small circumscribed generally invasive tumor remnants in the lateral cavernous sinus (fig. 2c). Before the advent of radiosurgery or because the tumor remnants were large or too close to the optic system, the 5 remaining cases where treated with conventional co-planar radiotherapy. Normalization of ACTH and cortisol levels was achieved in 3 of 9 cases (33.3%). One of these had undergone radiosurgery. In the remaining 6 patients (3 treated with radiosurgery) cortisol levels improved but the observation period to date has been very short.

Because there were neither visible pituitary tumor remnants nor any circumstantial evidence of them on the MRI scans adrenalectomy was performed in 4 of 21 patients (19.0%). In all of them, hypocortisolism was achieved. One patient developed a Nelson tumor which necessitated radiotherapy of the sella.

In another 3 patients, there were only biochemical but no clinical signs of CD. These patients are being observed closely but do not require any treatment. The last 3 patients exhibit only mild symptoms of the disease and are of advanced age and, therefore, not subject to any treatment but rather observation at short intervals.

A negative surgical exposure of the sella took place in 9 patients whose hypercortisolism subsequently persisted (fig. 5). In 1 (11.1%) of them further diagnostic tests revealed a paraneoplastic tumor which was then removed. Despite no clear evidence of a pituitary origin of the disease, this patient demanded sella exploration. In 2 of these patients (22.2%) no further treatment was necessary as symptoms of their disease were only mild and they were of advanced age. Four patients (44.5%) were normalized following adrenalectomy and 1 patient (11.1%) underwent re-operation followed by adrenalectomy due to failure of the former procedure. Another patient (11.1%) was in remission following re-operation.

Following partial hypophysectomy in 3 patients normocortisolism was observed, but hypercortisolism persisted in 4 patients (fig. 5). In 2 of the latter, there were only biochemical but no clinical signs of persistence of CD, so that no further treatment became necessary and the patients are being observed to date. Adrenalectomy was suggested for 2 other patients, but 1 of them refuses therapy and 1 has been lost to follow-up.

Combining all treatment methods, a normalization of cortisol levels was achieved in 80 cases. Clinical remission despite biochemical persistence of the disease occurred in 5 patients. Five patients showed only mild symptoms of CD after treatment. An improvement has so far been found in a further 7 cases. In 6 of them normalization of cortisol levels is expected to occur in the near future when the radiotherapy they underwent takes full effect. No change in symptoms was observed in those 2 patients who did not undergo any treatment and the 1 who suffered from paraneoplastic tumor. Nelson syndrome was observed in 1 of 11 adrenalectomized patients but in no patient who underwent combined treatment with adrenalectomy and radiotherapy.

Current Value of Surgical Treatment in Cushing's Disease

A review of the literature over the last decades yielded 31 series ranging from 9 [42] to 668 [4] patients treated. These include single-surgeon as well as multicenter studies. Some studies examined only adults or children, while others combined both groups. Some series give an overview on the treatment of Cushing's syndrome in general. Others focus on the treatment of pituitary adenomas. Their great variety makes them difficult to compare. In the following, an overview on the rates of confirmation of an adenoma, remission and recurrence rates as well as complication rates will be given and some studies of interest will be discussed. Only studies examining more than 20 patients have been considered.

The rates of confirmation of an adenoma during surgery are reported in 20 modern series published between 1985 and 2004. They range from 59.1 to 94.1% [2, 6–12, 15, 16, 18–21, 27–29, 43, 44]. Rates vary depending on whether the surgeon's impression of tumor removal only or also histological results were taken into account (90.0 vs. 66.7%) [15]. In one series, the surgeon intraoperatively had the impression that a tumor was present in 90% of the cases, albeit this was not confirmed with a pathological work-up [25]. These results were comparable to those of our series. It is obvious that there is a difference in the rates of intraoperative confirmation of an adenoma depending on whether those of microadenomas only, or those of both micro- and macroadenomas are examined (73.5 vs.82.4%) [7]. Furthermore, technical advances have not resulted in a significant improvement. In another series with a 100% adenoma finding rate, the impression of the surgeon only was considered [2].

Remission rates are reported in 25 series and range from 42.0 to 98.2% [2–4, 6–13, 15, 16, 18–21, 25–30, 43–45], with a majority reported between 70 and 90%. There is no change in remission rates over the years but they are strongly dependent on the remission criteria used. The remission rate depends on whether an adenoma is found intraoperatively and on what kind of surgical procedure is done. There was a higher remission rate when an adenoma was found intraoperatively than whenhemihypophysectomy was performed following negative exploration of the sella (69.2 vs. 62.5%) [12]. Furthermore, the remission rate is dependent on the surgeon's experience, which should correlate to the number of operations in his/her series. This relationship may be compromised when a surgeon has to deal with a selected patient collective consisting of more complicated cases. Comparing micro- and macroadenomas, there is a better remission rate found in the former group (88.0 vs. 33.3% [7], 92.6 vs. 66.7% [28]). The remission rate after surgery for recurrent tumors is lower than that after surgery of primary ones [26, 45]. The remission rate in children is about 70% [12, 18]. In a multicenter study, which might represent a good cross-section with regard to patient collective and individual surgeon abilities, the remission rate is 76.3% [4].

Recurrence rates are reported in 17 series and range from 3.4 to 50% [2, 4, 6, 8–10, 13, 16, 18, 20, 21, 25–28, 43, 44]. The rate quoted in 1 series was believed to be biased because no distinction was made between primary and recurrent disease [11]. The time between operation and recurrence ranged between 16 months and 10 years during a mean follow-up period of 3 months to 7 years. The remission rate was <5% in 2 series, <10 and 15%, respectively, in 4 series each, <20% in 1 series, <25% in 2 series, and >25% in 4 series. There was no reduction in the recurrence rates over the years. As expected, the incidence of recurrent disease increases with the length of the observation period.

The recurrence rate seems to be higher (50%) [6] and the appearance of recurrent disease takes place earlier [3] after primary resection of macroadenomas than of microadenomas. It might be higher in children which is shown in a series [18] examining children only (41.2%), and is supported by another series examining a collective of children and adults (26.9%) [10]. In the European multicenter study the recurrence rate was 12.7% [4].

Mortality and morbidity were reported in 14 series. The mortality rate was 0% in 10 series and 1.7 up to 8.4% in the others [2–4, 9, 10, 15, 16, 20, 23, 26, 29, 30, 44]. A mortality rate of 8.4% was reported in a large series [19] reviewing early pituitary surgery. In the more recent series no mortality was reported.

Hypocortisolism after surgery is a good prognostic factor predicting a lower risk of recurrence. It may persist due to adrenal insufficiency caused by long-term suppression of normal pituitary tissue. Persistent hypocortisolism was reported in 5 series with an incidence ranging from 1.7 to 44.4%. After hemihypophysectomy the incidence was reported to be 33.3% [2, 20, 26, 29, 30]. As their CD is cured, this side effect is generally well accepted by the patients and they are subsequently placed on replacement therapy.

Other persisting endocrine deficits are reported in 0–71% of all treated cases [2–4, 7, 9, 10, 15, 16, 18, 20, 23, 26, 30, 44]. In about half of the series they are reported to occur in <1 of 5 cases but even in some newer series, their incidence exceeds 25%. The reason for this might be injury to the normal pituitary during aggressive tumor removal performed to achieve cure of the disease. On closer examination, the high incidence of rates of endocrine deficits are found either in older or in smaller series. This leads to the assumption that the experience of the surgeon plays a major role in sparing the normal pituitary tissue.

Morbidity rates ranged between 0 and 53% [2, 4, 9, 10, 15, 16, 19, 20, 23, 26, 29, 30, 44] with the exception of a 65% rate reported in a series examining macroadenomas only [3]. In a multicenter study it was 14.5% [4].

No morbidity at all was found in 3 series, the rate was <5% in 3 series, <10% in 1 and <15% in 3 series. Thus, in 10 of 14 series the morbidity rate was <15%. Among the other series there were 2 each with a morbidity rate of below and above 50%.

There seems to be no correlation between morbidity rates and the number of patients examined or the length of time that has passed since the study was performed.

Major complications reported were CSF leakage, meningitis, sinusitis, deep vein thrombosis and pulmonary embolism, visual deficits, cranial nerve palsies, wound healing problems, and perforations of the nasal septum.

Intraoperative Prediction of the Operative Results

It is of major interest to determine the outcome of an operation intraoperatively, and this was the aim of a number of studies, but so far all methods tried seem to have failed in CD. Intraoperative MRI scans using 0.2 or 1.5 T scanners are helpful in larger and/or invasive pituitary adenomas. The extent of the resection can be determined intraoperatively and in case there is some accessible tumor left it can be removed during a second look [46, 47]. Considering a spatial resolution in MRI of 3 mm [48] and the small tumor size mostly found in CD, it is easy to understand that intraoperative control of the resection does not make sense in those cases.

Another attempt to determine the remission of endocrine hypersecretion was to measure the intraoperative decline of excess hormone levels. As shown in an unpublished series by the authors, this is possible in patients suffering from acromegaly and prolactinomas, but remains difficult in patients with ACTH hypersecretion. There might be too much interference with pituitary function resulting from stress in the immediate pre- and postoperative period and during anesthesia as the normal ACTH-producing cells may not be totally suppressed by hypercortisolism. This may lead to elevated intraoperative cortisol levels in spite of complete adenoma removal. Furthermore increased ACTH levels may result from the variability of the secretion pattern within the adenomas and from manipulation of the tumor. These findings are in accordance with the literature [49, 50].

Another attempt was made by Flitsch et al. [51] to differentiate between adenomatous tissue and normal anterior lobe during surgery in order to facilitate total tumor resection. Homogenization of biopsies was performed by ultrasound and ACTH levels were determined. An ACTH level of >300 ng/100 mg was considered evidence of adenomatous tissue. But this method, also, could not guarantee that all parts of, e.g., an invasive or dumbbell-shaped adenoma were removed.

Progress in Microsurgical Treatment of Cushing's Disease

By comparing the present study with the literature as well as the first series of 100 cases published by the senior author in 1986 [14], the rate of intraoperative confirmation of an adenoma (84.0%) is above the median of all published rates but not as good as in the senior author's previous study (96%). The remission rate remained almost unchanged (present 75%/previous 74%) and lies within range given in the literature. The recurrence rate is low (4.8%) compared to the literature and has improved slightly since 1986 (5%). The lower rate of intraoperative confirmation of an adenoma might be due to the increasing number of diagnostically challenging patients referred to our specialized center nowadays. The remission rate has not changed since 1986, similar to the other series in the literature. This may be a consequence of the relatively large number of patients in our series with very small tumors that are difficult to detect on the one hand, and with macroadenomas, which are difficult to resect completely on the other. Unfortunately, these disadvantages cannot yet be overcome by

Table 2. Characteristics of different treatment options

	Operation	Radiotherapy	Gamma-knife radiosurgery	LINAC radiosurgery	Adrenalectomy	Medical treatment
Remission rate	70–90%	46–80%	50–83% (100%)	80%	100%	90%
	combined 55–86%					
General complications	15%	4%	CD 2.3% Others: 1.9–8.0%	0	19%	–/–
Endocrine deficits	1.7–44% Subnormal cortisol: 20%	85%	CD 16% Others: 1.9–33%	30%	–/–	–/–
Disadvantages	–/–	–/–	(Limited to tumor volume)	(Limited to tumor volume)	Nelson syndrome, replacement therapy	Temporary effect as long as on treatment

technological progress. The mortality rate alone has improved over the years, which may be due to better anesthesia and intensive care.

Role of Additional Treatment

To evaluate the role of adjuvant treatment modalities a brief overview of their results and complications as cited in the literature is given and compared to our latest experiences (table 2).

For medical treatment inhibiting steroid synthesis, drugs like aminoglutethimide, metyrapone, trilostane and mitotane were used, but the only one currently administered is ketoconazol [52]. Using the latter in one large series [39] examining 34 patients, normalization of cortisol levels was observed in 88.2%. The main side effects seen were skin rash, liver toxicity, gastrointestinal symptoms or aggravation of a preexisting gynecomastia.

Long-term control of hypercortisolism using ketoconazol without any significant side effects was described in another 2 series [53, 54] and reported even during pregnancy [55].

Recently, another agent used to treat diabetes has raised hopes: the PPAR-γ ligand rosiglitazone. Improvement was observed in 6 of 14 patients (42.9%) treated with this drug [56], but these results could not be reproduced. We observed a partial improvement in cortisol levels after suppression with 2 mg DEXA but no significant decrease in the clinical symptoms in 2 of 3 patients. One of 3 patients suffering from a Nelson tumor showed a significant decrease in ACTH levels following treatment with rosiglitazone [Kreutzer J, Fahlbusch R, unpublished results].

Another therapeutic strategy was investigated after the discovery of D_2-receptor expression and inhibition of ACTH secretion in ACTH-producing pituitary tumors following their activation. Administration of the D_2-receptor ligand, cabergoline, led to a 50% or more decrease in urinary free cortisol in 60% of the patients examined [57].

The first radiotherapy applied was the conventional co-planar, three-field external fractionated radiation using a linear accelerator to deliver doses between 0.18 and 0.2 Gy per fraction up to a total dose of 45–50 Gy. In the series of patients suffering from CD who were undergoing conventional radiotherapy as their sole treatment, remission rates of 46% were observed but recurrence occurred in 45.5% of them [58]. Other series reported remission rates of 66 and 80% after 9 and 12 months, respectively, in children [59] and 100% in adults [60]. About 40 months after medical pretreatment the remission rate following conventional radiotherapy was between 36.8 [61] and 92.9% [62]. When radiotherapy was administered following incomplete surgical removal of the adenoma, the remission rate was 70% [63] in adults and 100% in children [64]. Combined with additional medical pretreatment a remission rate of 83.3% [65] was achieved in this situation.

Comparing the results of radiotherapy following incomplete adenoma removal and radiotherapy alone, there is a slight difference in favor of combined treatment. The remission rate is 55.6 vs. 52%, respectively [66]. Regarding complications, insufficiency of one pituitary axis is reported in 8.3–80% of the cases when radiotherapy is applied alone or in combination with medical treatment [59, 62]. According to one series, when radiotherapy is combined with microsurgery the incidence of panhypopituitarism is 3.3%, and deficits for one or more hormones are reported in 7.1–86% [63–65] of the cases. Yet in two series no hormonal insufficiencies were observed at all [61, 66]. While some authors [61, 66] did not describe any such complications, the reported incidence rate of new neurological deficits is up to 4.2% [58]. No significant difference regarding any combination of treatment options has been found.

In the series studying treatment with gamma-knife surgery alone in patients suffering from CD, the remission rates vary between 16.7 and 100% and an improvement in endocrine status was observed in 50–58.3% of the cases [67–70]. Taking patients with CD only from series examining all pituitary tumors, gamma-knife surgery alone or in combination with microsurgery leads to remission rates between 35% in the largest series [71] of 20 patients and 100% in series [72–76] examining less than 10 patients. An improved endocrine status was observed in 25–75% of the cases following an observation period of 2–30 years. It made no difference whether any other pretreatment took place [77–79]. Following adrenalectomy tumor control and therefore prevention of the development of a Nelson tumor was achieved in 81.8% of the cases [80]. Only in 1 series were complications following gamma-knife radiosurgery in CD reported: 2 years after surgery, new insufficiencies mainly regarding TSH-secretion were observed in 16% of the cases and a new visual deficit in 1 patient (2.3%) [77]. In the larger series examining different types of pituitary adenomas insufficiency rates vary between 1.9 and 33% and complication rates between 1.9 and 8.0% [74, 75, 78, 79]. In one series including 53 patients no insufficiency or complication were reported [73].

LINAC radiosurgery applied after unsuccessful microsurgery led to an improvement in endocrine hyperfunction in 88.5% and of clinical signs in 79.2% of the cases within 1 year. Pituitary insufficiency was observed in 29.2% of the patients (TSH 16.7%, gonadotropins 4.2%, panhypopituitarism 8.3%) but no other radiation-related complications were seen [81].

Comparing the different radiotherapeutic treatment options both gamma-knife and LINAC radiosurgery are highly effective treatments resulting in rates of endocrine normalization between 50 and 100% regardless of whether applied alone or in combination with other treatment options. Their disadvantage is that they are restricted to tumors of smaller size. Conventional radiotherapy is slightly less effective but can also be applied to larger tumors. Nevertheless its results were better when preceded by surgical reduction of the tumor mass.

The incidence rate of pituitary insufficiencies seemed to be higher in conventional radiotherapy (up to 85%, depending on the series) than in radiosurgery (up to 15%). Neurological complications are observed in up to 4% of the cases following conventional radiotherapy and up to 0.6% following radiosurgery alone or up to 8.0% following a combined treatment consisting of microsurgery followed by radiosurgery. The higher rate of neurological complications after combined treatment may be related to subclinical injury caused by surgery which is then aggravated by the radiosurgery or to the more unfavorable location and larger size of the tumors subjected to this treatment regimen.

Conventional radiotherapy is expected to take effect 2–5 years after treatment, while radiosurgery seems to show first effects already 1 year following treatment.

Finally, adrenalectomy is performed to achieve an immediate termination of hypercortisolism. Nagesser et al. [82] reported remnants of the adrenal gland in 27.0% resulting in a remission rate of 95.0% of the patients only and a recurrence in 4.8%. In more recent series [83–86] (the largest with 82 patients) open adrenalectomy is associated with a morbidity rate ranging between 0 and 17% and a mortality rate ranging between 0 and 2.6%. As another complication, in 9% of the patients acute steroid deficiency was observed and 60% complain of chronic fatigue which was difficult to treat with replacement therapy [87]. About 46% of the patients developed Nelson syndrome and in half of them pituitary surgery became necessary because of a Nelson tumor causing visual deficits. Complications of the open procedure quoted in the literature were hemorrhage and shock, cardiac arrhythmia, cholecystitis, pancreatitis, subphrenic abscess, septicemia, pulmonary infections and embolism, wound healing complications, pneumothorax, deep vein thrombosis and problems caused by scar tissue formation.

Beginning in the mid 1990s, laparoscopic adrenalectomy became the standard treatment. It is associated with a morbidity rate ranging between 3 and 25%. The highest morbidity rate was seen in a small series following hypophysectomies that did not result in normalization of cortisol levels [88–90]. Major complications were injury of the urethra, fever and hematoma, herniation of peritoneal contents, atrial fibrillation, puncture of the kidney and anemia. In total, laparoscopic adrenalectomy is associated with fewer complications and a faster postoperative recovery of the patients. In both modalities one has to keep in mind that postoperative substitution of mineralo- and glucocorticoids is essential to the patients' welfare. Adequate substitution therapy helps to avoid Nelson syndrome which can also be presented by radiation of the sella.

Current Standard of Treatment for Cushing's Disease

As the remission rate following microsurgery is as high as that following radiosurgery, surgery remains the treatment of choice. It may lead to an immediate normalization of cortisol levels or at least to a decrease in tumor volume which allows smaller isodoses if radiation therapy becomes necessary. Regarding complication rates, microsurgery if performed by experienced hands is comparable to radiotherapy and has a lower complication rate than adrenalectomy. When endocrine deficits are compared, microsurgery shows the best results. The remission rate following adrenalectomy may be higher than that following surgery but it is associated with a higher complication rate and the disadvantages of lifelong replacement therapy as well as the risk of developing a Nelson syndrome. Medical treatment using ketoconazol seems to be as effective as surgery but carries the disadvantage of lifelong treatment and possible side effects.

In case of an unsuccessful operation because of tumor invasion into the cavernous sinus and especially following re-operation, radiotherapy has to be performed next. This is essential in cases of so-called 'silent secreting adenomas', which tend to grow more aggressively [91].

Small tumor remnants are best treated by stereotactic radiosurgery using a linear accelerator or gamma-knife to provide a sufficient margin of safety when their distance to the optic chiasm is great enough. Larger tumor remnants and/or remnants located beneath the optic chiasm still require 3d-conformal radiotherapy. Women of childbearing age should have completed their family planning before the full effect of radiotherapy is reached which, in rare cases, leads to pituitary insufficiency. It has to be discussed whether medical treatment or adrenalectomy represents an alternative to radiotherapy in this special case. On the other hand, the advent of radiosurgery with its lower risk for insufficiency seems to make this discussion superfluous.

Adrenalectomy is performed only in cases of severe disease to achieve immediate normalization of the hypercortisolemic state. Care has to be taken to provide sufficient replacement therapy in order to prevent accelerated growth of the remaining pituitary adenoma which otherwise would be promoted by the lack of a feedback mechanism. In case of a significant growth of the pituitary tumor remnants or an increase in plasma ACTH levels, 3d-conformal radiotherapy of the sella or radiosurgery of the tumor bed has to be carried out to prevent Nelson syndrome.

Medical treatment, mainly using ketoconazol, is of particular importance during the preoperative phase to improve the patient's clinical condition and, in the postoperative phase, to ride out the period until the radiotherapy takes effect.

Observation is possible in older patients only exhibiting mild symptoms and in patients with only biochemical signs of the disease.

Besides choosing the right additional treatment, its timing plays an important role. As in 21 of 66 cases (31.8%) a delayed normalization of hypercortisolism was found in our series we do not support the idea of Knappe and Luedecke [17] to perform an early re-operation in cases of a persisting hypercortisolism just 1 week after initial surgery in order to achieve normalization. Except for severe cases with known or suspected residual tumor after surgery, we believe additional treatment should be started about 3 months following surgery after another assessment of the patient's endocrine status.

Treatment of Recurrences

Management of recurrent CD is much more difficult and definitely belongs in the hands of experienced endocrine neurosurgeons. In case of a true endocrine recurrence based on a pathological 2 mg DEXA, re-operation is the treatment of choice even if there is no visible tumor on MRI. Petrosal sinus sampling is not found to be helpful prior to or during operations for recurrent disease. As the tumor is always found in the same location as during the initial operation, re-operation can take place after diagnosis of a recurrence without obtaining any further imaging studies [92] if detailed data about the primary operation are available. If these data are not available, meticulously dissection of the pituitary gland may be necessary in order to find a small recurrent tumor. Additional treatment consisting of radiotherapy has to follow to avoid further growth of possible tumor remnants resulting in a recurrence. Moreover, in the presence of a severe disease, adrenalectomy should be performed and concomitant medical treatment should be administered.

Conclusion

CD which remains difficult to diagnose is a severe and life-threatening illness that requires both interdisciplinary diagnostic work-up and treatment. An early diagnosis and the optimal choice of the order of treatment modalities have a great influence on the patient's outcome and quality of life after the onset of the illness. Microneurosurgery in CD remains the treatment of choice even though results following the use of adjuvant treatment modalities have improved and they have become effective alternative measures for the treatment of persistent or recurrent disease. Their use has to be tailored exactly to an individual patient's condition.

Acknowledgement

We wish to thank Dr. Kreutzer and Dr. Hlavac, Department of Neurosurgery, University of Erlangen–Nuremberg, and Prof. Buchfelder, Department of Neurosurgery, University of Göttingen, for providing data; Prof. Huk, Department of Neuroradiology, University of Erlangen–Nuremberg, for providing MRI, angiography and IPSS; Prof. Grabenbauer and Prof. Sauer, Department of Radiotherapy, University of Erlangen–Nuremberg, for performing radiotherapy; Prof. Hohenberger, Surgical Department, University of Erlangen–Nuremberg, for performing most of the adrenalectomies, and Prof. Blümcke, Prof. Paulus, Prof. Plate and Dr. Buslei, Department of Neuropathology, University of Erlangen–Nuremberg, and Prof. Saeger, Neuropathologist, Marienhospital, Hamburg, for the histopathological work-up and for providing data. Furthermore, we are grateful to the members of the 'Neuroendokrinologischer Arbeitskreis' and to the many neuroendocrinologists for admitting and treating the patients.

Finally, we are grateful to Dr. Anker, Department of Neurosurgery, University of Erlangen–Nuremberg, for revising the manuscript, and Mr. F. Bittner for providing illustrations.

References

1 Fahlbusch R, Marguth F: Changes in indication and operative technique for surgery of hormonally active pituitary adenomas. Langenbecks Arch Chir 1983;361:561–567.

2 Bakiri F, Tatai S, Aouli R, Semrouni M, Derome PJ, Chitour F, Benmiloud M: Treatment of Cushing's disease by transsphenoidal, pituitary microsurgery: prognosis factors and long-term follow-up. J Endocrinol Invest 1996;19:572–580.

3 Blevins LS Jr, Christy JH, Khajavi M, Tindall GT: Outcomes of therapy for Cushing's disease due to adrenocorticotropin-secreting pituitary macroadenomas. J Clin Endocrinol Metab 1998;83:63–67.
4 Bochicchio D, Losa M, Buchfelder M: Factors influencing the immediate and late outcome of Cushing's disease treated by transsphenoidal surgery: a retrospective study by the European Cushing's disease survey group. J Clin Endocrinol Metab 1995;80:3114–3120.
5 Buchfelder M, Fahlbusch R: Neurosurgical treatment of Cushing's disease in children and adolescents. Acta Neurochir Suppl (Wien) 1985;35:101–105.
6 Cannavò S, Almoto B, Dall'asta C, Corsello S, Lovicu RM, DeMenis E, Trimarchi F, Ambrosi B: Long-term results of treatment in patients with ACTH-secreting pituitary macroadenomas. Eur J Endocrinol 2003;149:195–200.
7 Chandler WF, Schteingart DE, Lloyd RV, McKeever PE, Ibarra-Perrez G: Surgical treatment of Cushing's disease. J Neurosurg 1987;66:204–212.
8 Chen JCT, Amar AP, Choi SH, Singer P, Couldwell WT, Weiss MH: Transsphenoidal microsurgical treatment of Cushing disease: postoperative assessment of surgical efficacy by application of an overnight low-dose dexamethasone suppression test. J Neurosurg 2003;98:967–973.
9 Chee GH, Mathias DB, James RA, Kendall-Taylor P: Transsphenoidal pituitary surgery in Cushing's disease: can we predict outcome? Clin Endocrinol 2001;54:617–626.
10 Devoe DJ, Miller WL, Conte FA, Kaplan SL, Grumbach MM, Rosenthal SM, Wilson CB, Gitelman SE: Long-term outcome in children and adolescents after transsphenoidal surgery for Cushing's disease. J Clin Endocrinol Metab 1997;82:3196–3202.
11 Dickerman RD, Oldfield EH: Basis of persistent and recurrent Cushing disease: an analysis of findings and repeated surgery. J Neurosurg 2002;97:1343–1349.
12 Dyer EH, Civit T, Visot A, Delalande O, Derome PJ: Transsphenoidal surgery for pituitary adenomas in children. Neurosurgery 1994;34:207–212.
13 Erem C, Algun E, Ozbey N, Azezli A, Aral F, Orhan Y, Molvalilar S, Sencer E: Clinical laboratory findings and results of therapy in 55 patients with Cushing's syndrome. J Endocrinol Invest 2003;26:65–72.
14 Fahlbusch R, Buchfelder M, Müller OA: Transsphenoidal surgery for Cushing's disease. J R Soc Med 1986;79:262–269.
15 Guilhaume B, Bertagna X, Thomsen M, Bricaire C, Vila-Porcile E, Olivier L, Racadot J, Derome P, Lautat MH, Girard F, Bricaire H, Luton JP: Transsphenoidal pituitary surgery for the treatment of Cushing's disease: results in 64 patients and long-term follow-up studies. J Clin Endocrinol Metab 1988;66:1056–1064.
16 Hoybye C, Grenback E, Thorén M, Hulting AL, Lundblad L, van Holst H, Änggard A: Transsphenoidal surgery in Cushing's disease: 10 years of experience in 34 consecutive cases. J Neurosurg 2004;100:634–638.
17 Knappe UJ, Luedecke DK: Persistent and recurrent hypercortisolism after transsphenoidal surgery for Cushing's disease. Acta Neurochir Suppl (Wien) 1996;65:31–34.
18 Leinung MC, Kane LA, Scheithauer BW, Carpenter PC, Laws Jr ER, Zimmermann D: Long term follow-up of transsphenoidal surgery for the treatment of Cushing's disease in childhood. J Clin Endocrinol Metab 1995;80:2475–2479.
19 Mampalam TJ, Tyrrell JB, Wilson CB: Transsphenoidal microsurgery for Cushing's disease: a report of 216 cases. Ann Intern Med 1988;109:487–493.
20 Nagesser SK, van Seters AP, Kievit J, Hermans J, van Dulken H, Krans HM, van de Velde CJ: Treatment of pituitary-dependent Cushing's syndrome: long-term results of unilateral adrenalectomy followed by external pituitary irradiation compared with transsphenoidal pituitary surgery. Clin Endocrinol 2000;52:427–435.
21 Nakane T, Kuwayama A, Watanabe M, Takahashi T, Kato T, Ichihara K, Kageyama N: Long term results of transsphenoidal adenomectomy in patients with Cushing's disease. Neurosurgery 1987;21:218–222.
22 Savage MO, Lienhardt A, Lebrethon MC, Johnston LB, Huebner A, Grossman AB, Afshar F, Plowman PN, Besser GM: Cushing's disease in childhood: presentation, investigation, treatment and long-term outcome. Hormone Res 2001;55(suppl 1):24–30.
23 Semple PL, Laws ER Jr: Complications in a contemporary series of patients who underwent transsphenoidal surgery for Cushing's disease. J Neurosurg 1999;91:175–179.

24 Semple PL, Vance ML, Findling JW, Laws ER Jr: Transsphenoidal surgery for Cushing's disease: outcome in patients with abnormal magnetic resonance imaging scan. Neurosurgery 2000;46: 553–559.
25 Sheehan JM, Lopes MB, Sheehan JP, Ellegala DB, Webb KM, Laws ER Jr: Results of transsphenoidal surgery for Cushing's disease in patients with no histologically confirmed tumor. Neurosurgery 2000;47:33–39.
26 Shimon I, Ram Z, Cohen ZR, Hadani M: Transsphenoidal surgery for Cushing's disease: endocrinological follow-up monitoring of 82 patients. Neurosurgery 2002;51:57–62.
27 Sonino N, Zielezny M, Fava GA, Fallo F, Boscaro M: Risk factors and long-term outcome in pituitary-dependent Cushing's disease. J Clin Endocrinol Metab 1996;81:2647–2652.
28 Stévenaert A, Perrin G, Martin D, Beckers A: Maladie de Cushing et adénome corticotrophe: résultats de la microchirurgie hypophysaire. Neurochirurgie 2002;48:234–265.
29 Tindall GT, Herring CJ, Clark RV, Adams DA, Watts NB: Cushing's disease: results of transsphenoidal microsurgery with emphasis on surgical failures. J Neurosurg 1990;72:363–369.
30 Trainer PJ, Lawrie HS, Verhelst J, Howlett TA, Lowe DG, Grossman AB, Savage MO, Afshar F, Besser GM: Transsphenoidal resection in Cushing's disease: undetectable serum cortisol as the definition of successful treatment. Clin Endocrinol 1993;38:73–78.
31 Liddle GW: Tests of pituitary-adrenal suppression in the diagnosis of Cushing's syndrome. J Clin Endocrinol Metab 1960;20:1539–1560.
32 Tyrrell JB, Findling JW, Aaron DC: An overnight high dose dexamethasone suppression test for rapid differential diagnosis of Cushing's syndrome. Ann Intern Med 1986;104:180–186.
33 Oldfield EH, Chrousos GP, Schulte HM, Schaaf M, McKeever PE, Krudy AG, Cutler GB Jr, Loriaux DL, Doppman JL: Preoperative lateralization of ACTH-secreting pituitary microadenomas by bilateral and simultaneous inferior petrosal venous sinus sampling. N Engl J Med 1985;312:100–103.
34 Colao A, Faggiano A, Pivonello R, Giraldi FP, Cavagnini F, Lombardi G: Inferior petrosal sinus sampling in the differential diagnosis of Cushing syndrome: results of an Italian multicenter study. Eur J Endocrinol 2001;144:499–507.
35 DeHerder WW, Uitterlinden P, Pietermann H: Pituitary tumour localisation in patients with Cushing's disease by magnetic resonance imaging. Is there a place for petrosal sinus sampling? Clin Endocrinol 1994;40:87–92.
36 Doppman JL, Oldfield EH, Krudy AG: Petrosal sinus sampling for Cushing's syndrome: anatomical and technical considerations. Radiology 1984;150:99–103.
37 Vidal Trecan G, Laudat MH, Thomopoulos P, Luton JP, Bricaire H: Urinary free corticoids: an evaluation of their usefulness in the diagnosis of Cushing's syndrome. Acta Endocrinol (Copenh) 1983;103:110–115.
38 Chrousos GP, Schulte HM, Oldfield EH, Gold PW, Cutler GB Jr, Loriaux DL: The corticotropin-releasing factor stimulation test. An aid in the evaluation of patients with Cushing's syndrome. N Engl J Med 1984;310:622–626.
39 Sonino N, Boscaro M, Paoletta A, Mantero F, Ziliotto D: Ketoconazole treatment in Cushing's syndrome: experience in 34 patients. Clin Endocrinol 1991;35:347–352.
40 Martin R, Cetin Y, Fehm HL, Fahlbusch R, Voigt KH: Multiple cellular forms of corticotrophs in surgically removed pituitary adenomas and periadenomatous tissue in Cushing's disease. Am J Pathol 1982;106:332–341.
41 Fitzgerald PA, Aron CD, Findling JW, Brooks RM, Wilson CB, Tyrrell JB: Cushing's disease: transient secondary adrenal insufficiency after selective removal of pituitary tumours. Evidence for an pituitary origin. J Clin Endocrinol Metab 1982;27:481–490.
42 Weber A, Trainer PJ, Grossman AB, Afsahr F, Medbak S, Perry LA, Plowman PN, Rees LH, Besser GM, Savage MO: Investigation, management and therapeutic outcome in 12 cases of childhood and adolescent Cushing's syndrome. Clin Endocrinol 1995;43:19–28.
43 Tagliaferri M, Berselli ME, Loli P: Transsphenoidal microsurgery for Cushing's disease. Acta Endocrinol (Copenh) 1986;113:5–11.
44 Knappe UJ, Luedecke DK: Transnasal microsurgery in children and adolescents with Cushing's disease. Neurosurgery 1996;39:484–493.
45 Friedman RB, Oldfield EH, Nieman LK, Chroussos GP, Doppman JL, Cutker GB, Loriaux DL: Repeat transsphenoidal surgery for Cushing's disease. J Neurosurg 1989;71:520–527.

46 Martin CH, Schwartz R, Jolesz F, Black PM: Transsphenoidal resection of pituitary adenomas in an intraoperative MRI unit. Pituitary 1999;2:155–162.
47 Fahlbusch R, Ganslandt O, Buchfelder M, Schott W, Nimsky C: Intraoperative magnetic resonance imaging during transsphenoidal surgery. J Neurosurg 2001;95:381–390.
48 Buchfelder M, Nistor R, Fahlbusch R, Huk WJ: The accuracy of CT and MR evaluation of the sella turcica for detection of adrenocorticotropic hormone-secreting adenomas in Cushing disease. Am J Neuroradiol 1993;14:1183–1190.
49 Luedecke DK: Intraoperative measurement of adrenocorticotropic hormone in peripituitary blood in Cushing's disease. Neurosurgery 1989;24:201–205.
50 Czirjak S, Bezzegh A, Gal A, Racz K: Intra- and postoperative plasma ACTH concentrations in patients with Cushing's disease cured by transsphenoidal pituitary surgery. Acta Neurochir (Wien) 2002;144:971–977.
51 Flitsch J, Knappe UJ, Luedecke DK: Direct intraoperative micromethod for hormone measurements of pituitary tissue in Cushing's disease. Surg Neurol 1999;52:585–591.
52 Nieman LK: Medical treatment of Cushing's disease. Pituitary 2002;5:77–82.
53 Berwaerts JJ, Verhelst JA, Verhaert GC, Verhaegen AA, Abs RE: Corticotropin-dependent Cushing's syndrome in older people: presentation of five cases and therapeutical use of ketoconazole. J Am Geriatr Soc 1998;46:880–884.
54 Chou SC, Lin JD: Long-term effects of ketoconazole in the treatment of residual or recurrent Cushing's disease. Endocr J 2000;47:401–406.
55 Berwaerts JJ, Verhelst JA, Mahler C, Abs RE: Cushing's syndrome in pregnancy treated by ketoconazole: case report and review of the literature. Gynecol Endocrinol 1999;13:175–182.
56 Ambrosi B, Dall'asta C, Cannavò S, Libè R, Vigo T, Epaminonda P, Chiodini I, Ferrero S, Trimarchi F, Arosio M, Beck-Peccoz P: Effects of chronic administration of PPAR-γ ligand rosiglitazone in Cushing's disease. Eur J Endocrinol 2004;151:173–178.
57 Pivonello R, Ferone D, de Herder W, Kros J, de Caro M, Arvigo M, Annunziato L, Lombardi G, Colao A, Hofland L, Lamberts S: Dopamine receptor expression and function in corticotroph pituitary tumors. J Clin Endocrinol Metab 2004;89:2452–2462.
58 Littley MD, Shalet SM, Beardwell CG, Ahmed SR, Sutton ML: Long-term follow-up of low-dose external pituitary irradiation for Cushing's disease. Clin Endocrinol 1990;33:445–455.
59 Jennings AS, Liddle GW, Orth DN: Results of treating childhood Cushing's disease with pituitary irradiation. N Engl J Med 1977;3:957–962.
60 Grigsby PW, Stokes S, Marks JE, Simpson JR: Prognostic factors and results of radiotherapy alone in the management of pituitary adenomas. Int J Radiat Oncol Biol Phys 1988;15:1103–1110.
61 Ahmed SR, Shalet SM, Beardwell CG, Sutton ML: Treatment of Cushing's disease with low dose radiation therapy. Br Med J (Clin Res Ed) 1984;289:643–646.
62 Ross WM, Evered DC, Hunter P, Benaim M, Cook D, Hall R: Treatment of Cushing's disease with adrenal blocking drugs and megavoltage therapy of the pituitary. Clin Radiol 1979;30:149–153.
63 Vicente A, Estrada J, de la Cuerda C, Astigarra B, Marazuela M, Blanco C, Lucas T, Barcelo B: Results of external pituitary irradiation after unsuccessful transsphenoidal surgery in Cushing's disease. Acta Endocrinol (Copenh) 1991;125:470–474.
64 Storr HL, Plowman PN, Caroll PV, Francois I, Krassas GE, Afsahr F, Besser GM, Grossman AB, Savage MO: Clinical and endocrine response to pituitary radiotherapy in pediatric Cushing's disease: an effective second-line treatment. J Clin Endocrinol Metab 2003;88:34–37.
65 Estrada J, Boronat M, Mielgo M, Magallon R, Millan I, Diez S, Lucas T, Barcelo B: The long-term outcome of pituitary irradiation after unsuccessful transsphenoidal surgery in Cushing's disease. N Engl J Med 1997;336:172–177.
66 Howlett TA, Plowman PN, Wass JAH, Rees LH, Jones AE, Besser GM: Megavoltage pituitary irradiation in the management of Cushing's disease and Nelson's Syndrome: long term follow-up. Clin Endocrinol (Oxf) 1989;31:309–323.
67 Izawa M, Hayashi M, Nakaya K, Satoh H, Ochiai T, Hori T, Takakura K: Gamma knife radiosurgery for pituitary adenomas. J Neurosurg 2000;93(suppl 3):19–22.

68 Rahn T, Thorén M, Hall K, Backlund EO: Stereotactic radiosurgery in Cushing's syndrome: acute radiation effects. Surg Neurol 1980;14:85–92.
69 Vladyka V, Liscak R, Simonova G, Chytka T, Novotny J Jr, Vymaza J, Marek J, Hana V, Vavros D: Radiosurgical treatment of hypophyseal adenomas with gamma knife: results in a group of 163 patients during a 5-year period (in Czech). Cas Lek Cesk 2000;139:757–766.
70 Hoybye C, Grenback E, Rahn T, Degerblad M, Thorén M, Hulting AL: Adrenocorticotropic hormone-producing pituitary tumors: 12- to 22-year follow-up after treatment with stereotactic radiosurgery. Neurosurgery 2001;49:284–292.
71 Kobayashi T, Kida Y, Mori Y: Gamma knife radiosurgery in the treatment of Cushing disease: long term results. J Neurosurg 2002;97(suppl 5):422–428.
72 Inoue HK, Kohga H, Hirato M, Sasaki T, Ishihara J, Shibazaki T, Ohye C, Andou Y: Pituitary adenomas treated by microsurgery with or without gamma knife surgery: experience in 122 cases. Stereotact Funct Neurosurg 1999;72(suppl 1):125–131.
73 Kim SH, Huh R, Chang JW, Park YG, Chung SS: Gamma knife radiosurgery for functioning pituitary adenoma. Stereotact Funct Neurosurg 1999;72(suppl 1):101–110.
74 Lim YJ, Leem W, Kim TS, Rhee BA, Kim GK: Four year's experiences in the treatment of pituitary adenomas with gamma knife radiosurgery. Stereotact Funct Neurosurg 1998;70 (suppl 1):95–109.
75 Morange-Ramos I, Regis J, Dufour H, Andrieu JM, Grisoli F, Jaquet P, Peragut JC: Short-term endocrinological results after gamma-knife surgery of pituitary adenomas. Stereotact Funct Neurosurg 1998;70(suppl 1):127–138.
76 Pan L, Zhang N, Wang E, Wang B, Xu W: Pituitary adenomas: the effect of gamma knife radiosurgery on tumor growth and endocrinopathies. Stereotact Funct Neurosurg 1998;70(suppl 1):119–126.
77 Sheehan JM, Vance ML, Sheehan JP, Ellegala DB, Laws ER Jr: Radiosurgery for Cushing's disease after failed transsphenoidal surgery. J Neurosurg 2000;93:738–742.
78 Pollock BE, Kondziolka D, Lunsford LD, Flickinger JC: Stereotactic radiosurgery for pituitary adenomas: imaging, visual and endocrine results. Acta Neurochir Suppl 1994;62:33–38.
79 Martinez R, Bravo G, Burzaco J, Rey G: Pituitary tumors and gamma knife surgery. Clinical experience with more than two years of follow-up. Stereotact Funct Neurosurg 1998;70(suppl 1):127–138.
80 Pollock BE, Young WF Jr: Stereotactic radiosurgery for patients with ACTH-producing pituitary adenomas after prior adrenalectomy. Int J Radiat Oncol Biol Phys 2002;54:839–841.
81 Yoon SC, Suh TS, Jang HS, Chung SM, Kim YS, Ryu MR, Choi KH, Son HY, Kim MC, Shinn KS: Clinical results of 24 pituitary macroadenomas with LINAC-based stereotactic radiosurgery. Int J Radiat Oncol Biol Phys 1998;41:849–853.
82 Nagesser SK, van Seters AP, Kievit J, Hermans J, Krans HM, van de Velde CJ: Long-term results of total adrenalectomy for Cushing's disease. World J Surg 2000;24:108–113.
83 McCance DR, Russell CFJ, Kennedy TL, Hadden DR, Kennedy L, Atkinson AB: Bilateral adrenalectomy: low mortality and morbidity in Cushing's disease. Clin Endocrinol 1993;39:315–321.
84 Chapuis Y, Pitre J, Conti F, Abboud B, Pras-Jude N, Luton JP: Role and operative risk of bilateral adrenalectomy in hypercortisolism. World J Surg 1996;20:775–780.
85 van Herden JA, Young WF Jr, Grant CS, Carpenter PC: Adrenal surgery for hypercortisolism – surgical aspects. Surgery 1995;117:446–472.
86 Zeiger MA, Fraker DL, Pass HI, Nieman LK, Cutler GB Jr, Chrousos GP, Norton JA: Effective reversibility of the signs and symptoms of hypercortisolism by bilateral adrenalectomy. Surgery 1993;114:1183–1143.
87 O'Riordan DS, Farley DR, Young WF Jr, Grant CS, van Herden JA: Long-term outcome of bilateral adrenalectomy in patients with Cushing's syndrome. Surgery 1994;116:1088–1093.
88 Bax TW, Marcus DR, Galloway GQ, Swanstrom LL, Sheppard BC: Laparoscopic bilateral adrenalectomy following failed hypophysectomy. Surg Endosc 1996;10:1150–1153.
89 Walz MK, Peitgen K, Hoermann R, Giebler RM, Mann K, Eigler FW: Posterior retroperitoneoscopy as a new minimally invasive approach for adrenalectomy: results of 30 adrenalectomies in 27 patients. World J Surg 1996;20:769–774.

90 Brunt LM, Moley JF, Doherty GM, Lairmore TC, DeBenedetti MK, Quasebarth MA: Outcome analysis in patients undergoing laparoscopic adrenalectomy for hormonally active adrenal tumors. Surgery 2001;130:629–635.
91 Scheithauer BW, Jaap AJ, Horvath E, Kovacs K, Lloyd RV, Meyer FB, Laws ER Jr, Young WF Jr: Clinically silent corticotroph tumors of the pituitary gland. Neurosurgery 2000;47:723–730.
92 Hofmann BM, Hlavac M, Kreutzer J, Grabenbauer G, Fahlbusch R: Management of recurrent Cushing's disease. In preparation, 2005.

Bernd M. Hofmann, MD
Department of Neurosurgery, University of Erlangen–Nuremberg
Schwabachanlage 6
DE–91054 Erlangen (Germany)
Tel. +49 9131 8533001, Fax +49 9131 8534569
E-Mail hofmann@nch.imed.uni-erlangen.de

Laws ER Jr, Sheehan JP (eds): Pituitary Surgery – A Modern Approach.
Front Horm Res. Basel, Karger, 2006, vol 34, pp 185–205

Stereotactic Radiosurgery for Pituitary Adenomas: A Review of the Literature and Our Experience

Jason P. Sheehan, Jay Jagannathan, Nader Pouratian, Ladislau Steiner

Lars Leksell Gamma Knife Center, Department of Neurological Surgery, Health Sciences Center, University of Virginia, Charlottesville, Va., USA

Abstract

Pituitary adenomas are not just one of the most common intracranial tumors but also one of the most difficult to cure. Neurosurgeons have adapted their tools to include precise ionizing radiation in the form of the gamma knife to treat pituitary adenomas. The use of the gamma knife in the management of pituitary adenomas following microsurgery or in selected cases as a primary treatment is safe. The combined application of transsphenoidal surgery and Gamma Knife surgery is beneficial in many difficult cases. However in some patients, optimal control of tumor growth and normalization of hypersecretory states are not achieved. Innovative improvements in operative and radiosurgical techniques are required to avoid pituitary insufficiency and to reduce the number of the cases in which optimal radiosurgery is not feasible because of close tumor proximity to the optic pathways.

Copyright © 2006 S. Karger AG, Basel

Introduction

Pituitary adenomas represent between 10 and 20% of all primary brain tumors [1, 2]. Epidemiological studies have demonstrated that nearly 20% of the general population has a pituitary adenoma [1]. Pituitary adenomas are broadly classified into two groups. The first category of tumor is those that secrete excess amounts of normal pituitary hormones and, consequently, present with a variety of clinical syndromes depending upon hormones secreted. The most common of these is the prolactinoma which causes Forbes-Albright syndrome (consisting of amenorrhea-galactorrhea in women and impotence and infertility in men). The second most common secretory pituitary adenoma is the growth hormone-secreting variant in which patients present with acromegaly in adults and gigantism when the hormone is secreted before closure of the epiphyseal plates [3]. Corticotropin-secreting tumors are another type of secretory pituitary adenoma, producing Cushing's disease or, if bilateral adrenalectomies have been performed, Nelson's syndrome [4, 5].

The second category of pituitary adenomas is comprised of tumors without endocrine hypersecretion, although they may have immunoreactivity to one or more of the pituitary hormones. These nonsecretory adenomas represent between 18 and 30% of all pituitary tumors [6]. These so-called nonfunctioning or null cell pituitary adenomas progressively enlarge in the pituitary fossa and may even extend outside the confines of the sella turcica. Like secretory adenomas, nonsecretory adenomas may cause symptoms related to a mass effect whereby the optic nerves and chiasm are compressed, resulting in characteristic bitemporal visual field loss. Those with nonsecretory adenomas can also have hypopituitarism as a result of compression of the normal functioning pituitary gland.

The type of adenoma, size at diagnosis, vicinity to the optic pathways, and the tendency to infiltrate surrounding structures (e.g. cavernous sinus) determine the goals and strategy of their treatment. For both types of pituitary adenomas, recurrence as a result of tumor invasion into surrounding structures (e.g. the dura or cavernous sinus) or incomplete tumor resection is quite common. The presence of residual tumor is not uncommon in adenomas with either a suprasellar component or cavernous sinus involvement, and the incidence of recurrence has been shown to correlate with dural tumor invasion [7, 8]. Long-term tumor control rates after microsurgery alone vary from 50 to 80% [1, 2, 9–11]. Radiosurgery can be administered postoperatively as adjuvant therapy to inhibit recurrent growth or, later, when clinical symptoms, laboratory results, or radiographic signs indicate recurrence. It may also be utilized postoperatively to treat known residual tumor following incomplete resection.

In 1951, stereotactic radiosurgery was described by Leksell [12] as the 'closed skull destruction of an intracranial target using ionizing radiation'. In 1968, Leksell treated the first pituitary adenoma patient with the Gamma Knife®. Since that time, stereotactic radiosurgery has been utilized in more than 20,000 patients to control tumor growth and normalize hormonal production from pituitary adenomas. At the same time, great attention and effort in the field of stereotactic radiosurgery have been placed on the preservation of surrounding neuronal, vascular, and hormonal structures. We assess the results to date of radiosurgical treatment for pituitary adenomas and the role of gamma knife surgery in the treatment armamentarium.

Radiosurgical Techniques

Radiosurgery is performed using the gamma knife, a linear accelerator-based system, or proton beams produced by cyclotrons. Gamma knife surgery usually involves multiple isocenters of different beam diameter to achieve a dose plan that conforms to the irregular three-dimensional volumes of most mass lesions. The total number of isocenters varies depending upon the size, shape, and number of lesions. The recent version of the gamma knife (model C) combines advances in dose planning with robotic engineering and obviates the need to set coordinates manually for each isocenter [13]. The soon to be released gamma knife 4C integrates additional neuroimaging modalities (e.g. SPECT and PET) into planning software.

In linear accelerator (LINAC)-based radiosurgery, multiple radiation arcs are utilized to crossfire photon beams at a target defined in stereotactic space [14]. Most of the presently functioning systems use non-dynamic techniques in which the patient couch is set at an angle and the arc is moved around its radius to deliver radiation that enters the skull through various nodal points. Numerous techniques have been developed to enhance conformality of dose planning and delivery using LINAC-based systems. These include beam shaping and intensity modulation. Newer developments include the introduction of jaws, noncircular, and mini- and micro-leaf collimators. The conformal beam can be delivered with the micromultileaf collimator or conformal blocks.

Proton beam radiosurgery offers a theoretical advantage because of the quantum wave properties of protons to reduce dose delivered to tissue surrounding the target [15]. In practice, this advantage has not been rigorously demonstrated. Moreover, cyclotrons required to produce a proton beam are only available at a limited number of centers due to financial and logistical constraints.

The effective delivery of radiation to a target requires clear and accurate imaging of that target. Over the past 20 years, significant advances in neuroimaging have increased the efficacy and safety of radiosurgical treatment of pituitary lesions. In the pre-MRI era, CT was utilized routinely. However, now it is generally reserved for patients who cannot undergo an MRI (e.g. a patient with a pacemaker). Tumor localization for dose planning is more accurately achieved with enhanced coronal MR than with CT imaging [16]. An MRI sequence consisting of post-contrast, thin-slice (e.g. 1 mm) volume acquisition is typically utilized to define the tumor within the sellar region. In patients with previous surgery, fat suppression techniques can prove useful for differentiating tumor from surgical fat grafts. For hormonally active lesions, if the tumor is unable to be localized on imaging studies, radiosurgery may still be successful in achieving hormonal normalization. In this case, the entire sellar region (including the inferior dura) is selected as the radiosurgical target when no definitive tumor can be visualized [5, 17, 18].

As part of the pre-operative work-up, we routinely perform thorough endocrinological testing and a neuro-ophthalmological evaluation. Frame placement at the University of Virginia is done in the main operating room, utilizing standard sterile technique. Monitored anesthesia is performed by a neuro-anesthesiologist, and both intravenous and local anesthetics are typically utilized. This surgical protocol affords optimal frame placement and a pain-free experience for the patient. For pediatric patients, the entire procedure including frame placement, neuroimaging acquisition, and gamma surgery are often performed under general anesthesia.

After frame placement and stereotactic image acquisition, dose planning is performed. Through the strategic selection of isocenters, gamma angle, prescription dose, beam-blocking patterns, and isodose selection, the borders of the tumor can be encompassed and a suitable radiation dose delivered. One must take into account the radiation falloff characteristics unique to the type of unit utilized. Moreover, if fractionated radiation therapy has previously been administered, the dose and timing of that treatment must be considered when selecting the dose for radiosurgery.

Radiosurgical Goals and Outcomes

For patients with pituitary adenomas, radiosurgery is meant to inactivate the tumor cells thereby preventing tumor growth and, for secretory adenomas, normalizing hormonal overproduction. Ideally, these goals are met without damaging the normal pituitary gland and the surrounding vascular and neuronal structures. Radiosurgery should be carried out in such a way so as to avoid delayed, radiation-associated secondary tumor formation.

A total of 35 peer-reviewed studies including 1,621 patients were reviewed [2, 5, 19–52]. Results of these studies are summarized in tables 1–5. We also review our own experience of treating 270 patients with recurrent or residual pituitary adenomas using the gamma knife. All of these 270 pituitary tumors were macroadenomas and locally invasive. Most had been previously treated one or more times by some other modality. Microsurgery alone was used in 90.3%, radiation therapy and microsurgery in 8.2% and radiation therapy alone in 1.5%. Tumor volume ranged from 0.9 to 32 cm^3 with an average volume of 11 cm^3. Tumors were treated with a maximum dose of 6–60 (average 37.5) Gy. Periphery dose ranged from 3 to 28 (average 15) Gy.

Table 1. Radiosurgery for patients with nonfunctioning pituitary adenomas

Reference and year	Radiosurgery unit	Number of patients	Follow-up mean or median months	Margin dose Gy	Growth control %
Martinez et al. [36], 1998	GK	14	36	16	100
Lim et al. [35], 1998	GK	22	26	25	92
Mitsumori et al. [37], 1998	LINAC	7	47	15	100
Witt et al. [48], 1998	GK	24	32	19	94
Yoon et al. [51], 1998	LINAC	8	49	17	96
Hayashi et al. [24], 1999	GK	18	16	20	92
Inoue et al. [27], 1999	GK	18	>24	20	94
Mokry et al. [38], 1999	GK	31	21	14	98
Izawa et al. [28], 2000	GK	23	28	22	94
Shin et al. [47], 2000	GK	3	19	16	100
Feigl et al. [21], 2002	GK	61	55	15	94
Sheehan et al. [46], 2002	GK	42	31	16	98
Wowra and Stummer [50], 2002	GK	30	58	16	93
Petrovich et al. [42], 2003	GK	56	41	15	100
Muramatsu et al. [40], 2003	LINAC	8	30	15	100
Pollock and Carpenter [43], 2003	GK	33	43	16	97
Losa et al. [55], 2004	GK	54	41	17	96

GK = Gamma knife; LINAC = linear accelerator.

Extent of Pituitary Adenoma Growth Control

Most series define tumor control as either an unchanged or decreased volume on follow-up radiological imaging studies. In radiosurgery, tumor growth cessation, not the amount of volume reduction, is still considered a successful treatment. In nearly all published series, stereotactic radiosurgery afforded excellent control of tumor growth (table 1; figs 1–3) [15, 21, 24, 27, 28, 35, 36, 38, 40, 42, 43, 46–48, 50, 51]. Most studies reported a greater than 90% control of tumor size (range 68–100%). A weighted average tumor control rate for all published series detailing such findings and encompassing a total of 1,283 patients was 96%. The lowest value reported for tumor control was 68% by Kim et al. [29]; this number represented the fraction of tumors that had decreased in size. Some series have even demonstrated tumor shrinkage and improvement in visual function following radiosurgery [24, 28, 46, 61, 53–55].

Most pituitary adenomas are slow-growing lesions. As such, it may be misleading to look at series of patients with relatively short follow-up. Eight published series had mean or median patient follow-up periods of 4 or more years. In these studies, tumor control rates varied from 83 to 100% [21, 25, 26, 31, 38, 47, 50, 51].

a 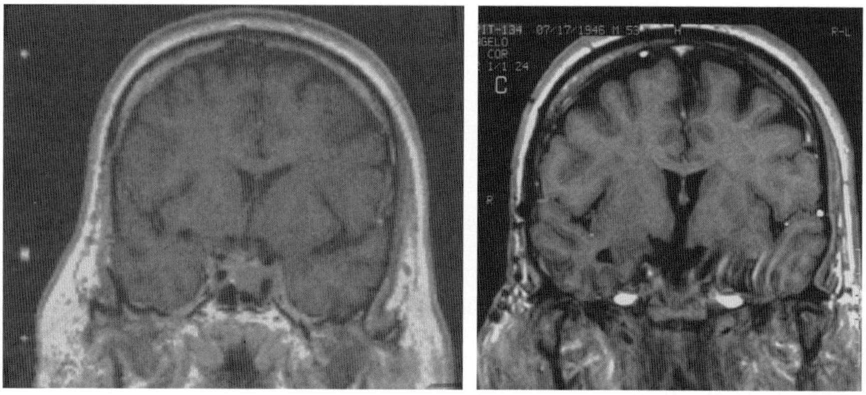 b

Fig. 1. ***a*** Preoperative, coronal T1-weighted MRI with contrast demonstrating a prolactinoma with cavernous sinus invasion on the right and suprasellar extension. This patient had Cushing's disease with a tumor volume of 5.9 cm^3. ***b*** Nine years after radiosurgery, the tumor has decreased markedly to a volume of 0.2 cm^3.

For nonsecretory adenomas at the University of Virginia, we have treated 92 patients, 82 of whom have a radiographic and endocrinological follow-up of a minimum of 6 months and an average of 34 months. Of these, 93% had documented tumor control; 55 (67%) had a decrease in the volume of their tumors and 21 had no change in volume (26%). Six increased in size (7%). New hypopituitarism occurred in 12 patients (15%). The only indication we have to date for treating these tumors is for postoperative residual tumors in order to lower the incidence of tumor progression or progression in spite of previous surgery or radiation therapy.

Cushing's Disease

Cushing's disease, perhaps the most famous of pituitary disorders, was described by Harvey Cushing in 1912 [56]. It was not until 1933 that Cushing first performed neurosurgery to treat a patient with a pituitary adenoma secreting excess ACTH [56]. Over the years, neurosurgeons and endocrinologists have debated the criteria for defining a 'cure' for Cushing's disease. Many favor the use of a 24-hour urine free cortisol (UFC) as the 'gold standard.' However, others have argued for the importance of measuring the morning serum cortisol level. Still others measure ACTH or basal serum cortisol and factor these into the evaluation of endocrinological success or failure in Cushing's disease. In a recent consensus statement by leading endocrinologists, there was no widespread agreement regarding the definition of endocrinological cure, and the

Table 2. Radiosurgery for patients with Cushing's disease

Reference and year	Radiosurgery unit	Number of patients	Follow-up mean or median months	Margin dose Gy	Endocrine cure rate %
Levy et al. [34], 1991	proton/helium beam	64	NR	NR	86
Ganz et al. [23], 1993	GK	4	18	25	50
Martinez et al. [36], 1998	GK	3	36	24	100
Lim et al. [35], 1998	GK	4	26	25	25
Mitsumori et al. [37], 1998	LINAC	5	47	15	40
Morange-Ramos et al. [39], 1998	GK	6	20	28	67
Witt et al. [48], 1998	GK	25	32	19	28
Yoon et al. [51], 1998	LINAC	1	49	17	NR
Hayashi et al. [24], 1999	GK	10	16	24	10
Inoue et al. [27], 1999	GK	3	>24	20	100
Kim et al. [29], 1999	GK	8	27	29	62
Laws and Vance [2], 1999	GK	50	NR	NR	58
Mokry et al. [38], 1999	GK	5	56	17	33
Izawa et al. [28], 2000	GK	12	28	22	17
Sheehan et al. [5], 2000	GK	43	44	20	63
Shin et al. [47], 2000	GK	7	88	32	50
Hoybye et al. [25], 2001	GK	18	204	NR	83
Feigl et al. [21], 2002	GK	4	55	15	NR
Kobayashi et al. [31], 2002	GK	20	64	29	35
Pollock et al. [44], 2002	GK	9	42	20	78
Petrovich et al. [42], 2003	GK	4	41	15	50
Choi et al. [20], 2003	GK	5	42.5	28.5	56

GK = Gamma knife; LINAC = linear accelerator; NR = not reported.

remission rates vary according to the criteria used and the time interval at which they were assessed [57]. Most centers define an endocrinological remission as a UFC in the normal range coupled with the resolution of clinical stigmata or a series of normal postoperative serum cortisol levels obtained throughout the day (range 5.4–10.8 μg/dl or 150–300 nmol/l) [57].

Twenty-two series have reported the results for 314 patients with Cushing's disease treated with radiosurgery (table 2) [2, 5, 20, 21, 23–25, 27–29, 31, 34–39, 42, 44, 47, 48, 51]. The mean radiosurgical margin doses for these series range from 15 to 32 Gy. Nine series utilize the 24-hour urine cortisol collection as part of the criteria for endocrinological evaluation. Unfortunately, another 8 of

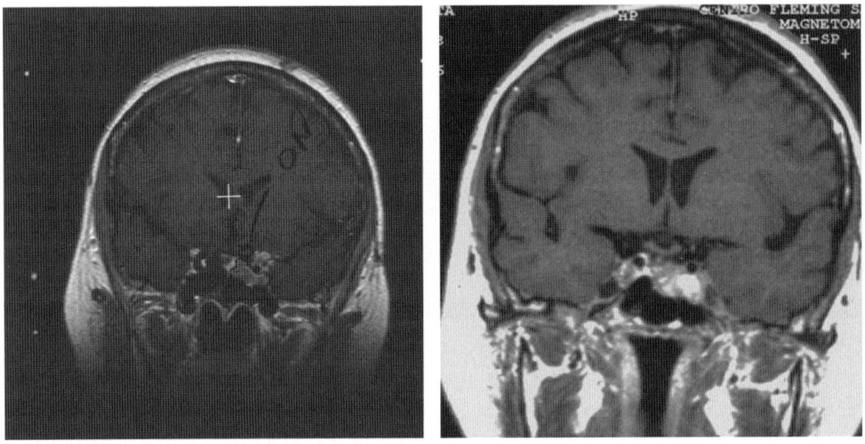

a *b*

Fig. 2. ***a*** This depicts a pituitary adenoma with cavernous sinus involvement in a patient with Cushing's disease. The tumor volume was 3.3 cm^3. ***b*** Six years after Gamma surgery, the patient's Cushing's disease was in remission and his tumor had shrunk to 1.9 cm^3.

these studies do not report the methodology employed to establish endocrinological remission or failure. The others utilize a combination of the aforementioned endocrinological tests. Endocrinological remission rates vary from 10 to 100%. In those series with at least 10 patients and a median follow-up of 2 years, endocrinological remission rates range from 17 to 83%. This latter value was reported by Hoybye et al. [25] and represents the largest single series of Cushing's patients. It is important to note, however, that many of the patients in this series were treated in the pre-CT and MRI era of radiosurgery and had to be treated as often as four times before their Cushing's disease went into remission.

At the University of Virginia, 74 patients with ACTH-secreting tumors underwent 80 gamma knife procedures. These patients all underwent prior microsurgery. Following gamma surgery, imaging follow-up demonstrated a decrease in the size of the tumor in 61 cases (76%), no change in 13 (16%), and an increase in size in 6 (8%; fig. 2). However, since hypercortisolism defines the dangerous character of the ACTH-secreting tumor, the control of endocrine abnormalities is the true measure of tumor control. Normal 24-hour UFC levels were achieved in 46 patients (64%), at an average time of 10.6 (range 1–40) months after treatment. Six of these patients had repeat gamma surgery, with 4 patients achieving another remission. New endocrine deficiencies developed in 18 patients (24%), with growth hormone deficiency being the most commonly found new endocrinopathy. Four patients developed new-onset visual acuity deficits, two of whom had received prior conventional fractionated radiation therapy. Evidence of radiation-induced changes was seen in 3 patients, but only

1 had symptoms attributable to these changes. These findings are notably different from our earlier published results in that more patients went on to develop a recurrence after an initial period of hormonal remission [5].

Acromegaly

Just as the endocrinological criteria for Cushing's disease remain the subject of debate, the criteria for curing acromegaly have also been inconsistent. The most widely accepted guidelines for a remission in acromegaly consist of a GH level of <1 ng/ml in response to a glucose challenge and a normal serum IGF-1 when matched for age and gender [58, 59].

In preparation for radiosurgery, many centers have recommended a temporary cessation of antisecretory medications in the perioperative time period. In 2000, Landolt et al. [60] first reported a significantly lower hormone normalization rate in acromegalic patients who were receiving antisecretory medications at the time of radiosurgery. Since then, this same group as well as others have documented a counterproductive effect of antisecretory medications on the rate of hormonal normalization following radiosurgery [33, 44]. The mechanism by which antisecretory medications lower hormonal normalization rates is unknown, but Landolt et al. [32, 33] have hypothesized that these drugs alter cell cycling and thus potentially decrease tumor cell radiosensitivity. Moreover, the optimal time period to hold antisecretory medications in conjunction with stereotactic radiosurgery is not clear. Landolt and Lomax [33] recommend that dopamine agonists be withheld 2 months prior to radiosurgery. For acromegalics, they recommend altering antisecretory medication administration as early as 4 months prior to radiosurgery and completely halting all antisecretory medications 2 weeks prior to radiosurgery [32]. Although many centers, including ours, have incorporated such methodology into their treatment regimen, the radiosurgical team must weigh the potential risk and benefits of altering antisecretory medication administration. The functional adenoma may be more likely to respond to radiosurgery. However, in the absence of antisecretory medication control, the adenoma may also enlarge thereby increasing the risk of radiosurgery to adjacent structures (e.g. the optic apparatus), necessitating a lower prescription dose, and making effective radiosurgical treatment more difficult.

Twenty-five studies detail the results of radiosurgical treatment for 420 patients with acromegaly (table 3) [2, 19–24, 26–30, 32, 35–42, 44, 48, 51, 52]. The mean radiosurgery margin doses in these series range from 15 to 34 Gy. Seven studies do not report the criteria utilized to define an endocrinological remission. Of the remaining 18 studies, 12 different criteria are employed to define remission. Remission rates following radiosurgery vary from 0 to 100%. In those series with at least 10 patients and a median follow-up of 2 years, endocrinological remission rates range from 20 to 96%. This latter value was

Table 3. Radiosurgery for patients with acromegaly

Reference and year	Radiosurgery unit	Number of patients	Follow-up mean or median months	Margin dose Gy	Endocrine cure rate %
Ganz et al. [23], 1993	GK	4	18	19.5	25
Martinez et al. [36], 1998	GK	7	36	25	71
Landolt et al. [32], 1998	GK	16	NR	25	81
Lim et al. [35], 1998	GK	20	26	25	38
Mitsumori et al. [37], 1998	LINAC	1	47	15	0
Morange-Ramos et al. [39], 1998	GK	15	20	28	20
Witt et al. [48], 1998	GK	20	32	19	20
Yoon et al. [51], 1998	LINAC	2	49	17	50
Hayashi et al. [24], 1999	GK	22	16	24	41
Inoue et al. [27], 1999	GK	12	>24	20	58
Kim et al. [30], 1999	GK	2	12	22	0
Kim et al. [29], 1999	GK	11	27	29	46
Laws and Vance [2], 1999	GK	56	NR	NR	25
Mokry et al. [38], 1999	GK	16	46	16	31
Izawa et al. [28], 2000	GK	29	28	22	41
Shin et al. [47], 2000	GK	6	43	34	67
Zhang et al. [52], 2000	GK	68	34	31	96
Fukuoka et al. [22], 2001	GK	9	42	20	50
Ikeda et al. [26], 2001	GK	17	48	25	82
Feigl et al. [21], 2002	GK	9	55	15	NR
Pollock et al. [44], 2002	GK	26	42	20	42
Attanasio et al. [19], 2003	GK	30	46	20	37
Petrovich et al. [42], 2003	GK	6	41	15	100
Muramatsu et al. [40], 2003	LINAC	4	30	15	50
Choi et al. [20], 2003	GK	12	42.5	28.5	50

GK – Gamma knife; LINAC – linear accelerator; NR – not reported.

reported by Zhang et al. [52] and represents the single largest series with 68 patients. Certainly, some of the wide variation in endocrinological remission rates with acromegaly may be attributed to the myriad of criteria utilized to define a remission. Another confounding variable is the degree to which somatostatin analogs may have been utilized during the time of radiosurgery and subsequent endocrinological evaluation in each of the series.

At the University of Virginia, we have performed 74 gamma knife procedures on 70 patients with growth hormone-secreting adenomas (fig. 3). Reliable endocrine follow-up is available for 38 of these patients. There was

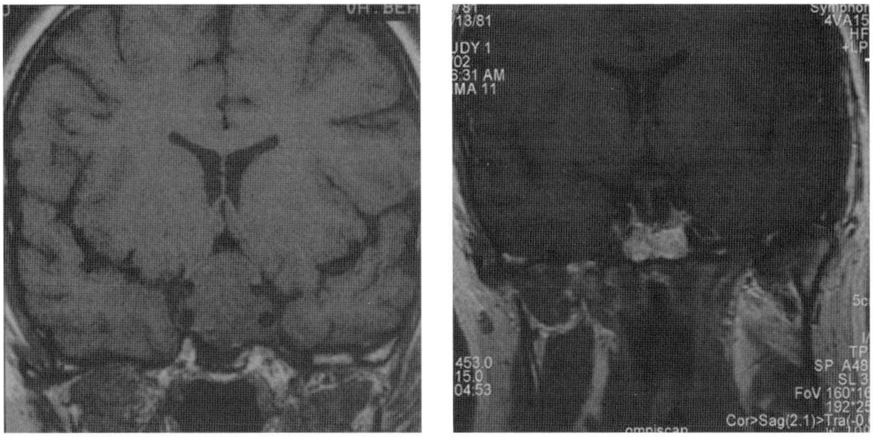

a *b*

Fig. 3. ***a*** This MRI depicts a pituitary adenoma with a volume of 3.4 cm^3 in a patient with acromegaly. ***b*** Eighteen months after radiosurgery, the tumor had decreased in volume to 1.5 cm^3, and the patient's acromegaly remains in remission.

normalization of IGF-1 in 43% of the cases. No patient had an elevation in growth hormone level after gamma surgery. Five patients developed recurrence of their acromegaly after initial remission, with a mean time to recurrence of 47 months. New endocrinological deficiencies developed in 31% of the patients, with hypothyroidism and low testosterone levels being the most common new endocrinopathies.

A decrease in tumor size was seen in 60 cases (81%) and no change in tumor size was seen in 6 cases (8%). Tumor growth was seen after 8 procedures (11%). Four patients developed a new onset of visual acuity deficits; 2 of these patients had received prior conventional fractionated radiation therapy. Three patients developed deterioration in visual fields likely secondary to tumor growth. Evidence of radiographic changes was seen in only 2 patients, neither of whom developed clinical symptomatology.

Prolactinomas

In patients with prolactinomas, the criteria utilized to define endocrinological remission are generally more consistent. Most studies define remission as a normal serum prolactin level for gender in a patient. Twenty-two radiosurgical studies report the results for 393 patients with prolactinomas (table 4) [2, 20, 21, 23, 24, 27–30, 33–37, 39–42, 44, 48, 51]. The mean radiosurgical dose to the tumor margin varied from 13.3 to 33 Gy. Although 8 of these studies do not report the endocrinological criteria defining remission, the remaining studies utilize relatively similar criteria. Remission rates varied from 0 to 84%.

Table 4. Radiosurgery for patients with prolactinomas

Reference and year	Radiosurgery unit	Number of patients	Follow-up mean or median months	Margin dose Gy	Endocrine cure rate %
Levy et al. [34], 1991	proton/helium beam	20	12	NR	60
Ganz et al. [23], 1993	GK	3	18	13.3	0
Martinez et al. [36], 1998	GK	5	36	33	0
Lim et al. [35], 1998	GK	19	26	25	56
Mitsumori et al. [37], 1998	LINAC	4	47	15	0
Witt et al. [48], 1998	GK	12	32	19	0
Yoon et al. [51], 1998	LINAC	11	49	17	84
Hayashi et al. [24], 1999	GK	13	16	24	15
Inoue et al. [27], 1999	GK	2	>24	20	50
Kim et al. [30], 1999	GK	20	12	22	19
Kim et al. [29], 1999	GK	18	27	29	17
Laws and Vance [2], 1999	GK	19	NR	NR	7
Mokry et al. [38], 1999	GK	21	31	14	21
Morange-Ramos et al. [39], 1998	GK	4	20	28	0
Izawa et al. [28], 2000	GK	15	28	22	20
Landolt and Lomax [33], 2000	GK	20	29	25	25
Pan et al. [41], 2000	GK	128	33	32	15
Feigl et al. [21], 2002	GK	18	55	15	NR
Pollock et al. [44], 2002	GK	7	42	20	29
Petrovich et al. [42], 2003	GK	12	41	15	83
Muramatsu et al. [40], 2003	LINAC	1	30	15	0
Choi et al. [20], 2003	GK	21	42.5	28.5	24

GK = Gamma knife; LINAC = linear accelerator; NR = not reported.

In 11 studies with at least 10 patients and a median or mean follow-up of 2 years, the range in remission rates following radiosurgery was just as varied. The largest series by Pan et al. [41] reported a 15% endocrinological remission rate for 128 patients with a median follow-up of 33 months. Although the remission rates for prolactinomas appear to be less than that for Cushing's disease or acromegaly, a substantial number of patients have a reduction but not complete remission of their hyperprolactinemia following radiosurgery. In a similar fashion to acromegaly, widespread differences in the use of antisecretory dopamine agonists at institutions may confound the efficacy of radiosurgery and the subsequent endocrinological assessment of patients with prolactinomas in these series. In addition, Hoybye et al. [25] have demonstrated

Table 5. Radiosurgery for patients with Nelson's syndrome

Reference and year	Radiosurgery unit	Number of patients	Follow-up mean or median months	Margin dose Gy	Endocrine cure rate %
Levy et al. [34], 1991	proton/helium beam	17	NR	NR	NR
Ganz et al. [23], 1993	GK	3	18	NR	0
Wolffenbuttel et al. [49], 1998	GK	1	33	12	0
Laws and Vance [2], 1999	GK	9	NR	NR	11
Kobayashi et al. [31], 2002	GK	6	63	28.7	33
Pollock and Young [45], 2002	GK	11	37	20	36

GK = Gamma knife; NR = not reported.

that radiosurgery may cause an elevation in prolactin levels possibly through injury or irritation of the infundibulum and impaired transport of dopamine to the anterior pituitary. This elevation can last for several years and may falsely lower the reported remission rates for patients with prolactinomas treated with radiosurgery.

Of the 28 prolactin-secreting tumors treated by us at the University of Virginia, 25 have radiographic follow-up of 12 months or more. Ninety-six percent of patients had tumor control after gamma knife surgery and 11 (44%) had a decrease in the size of their tumor (fig. 1). Two tumors had increased in volume on last follow-up (8%). Endocrine follow-up was available in 21 patients. Four of 21 patients (19%) had documented endocrinological remission on the last follow-up.

Nelson's Syndrome

Compared to nonsecretory and other secretory pituitary adenomas, much less information is available about the efficacy of stereotactic radiosurgery for the treatment of Nelson's syndrome. In patients with ACTH-secreting tumors who have undergone bilateral adrenalectomies, these pituitary adenomas tend to result in more aggressive growth rates. As such, endocrinological remission and growth control are critical for Nelson's syndrome.

Six studies detailed the results of stereotactic radiosurgery in 47 patients with Nelson's syndrome (table 5) [2, 23, 31, 34, 45, 49]. The mean tumor margin dose varied from 12 to 28.7 Gy. Unfortunately, only 2 of the studies detailed the endocrinological criteria utilized to define a remission. Remission rates ranged from 0 to 36%. However, tumor growth control rates were more favorable and varied from 82 to 100%.

At the University of Virginia, we have performed gamma surgery on 14 Nelson's patients. All patients had documented tumor growth and hyperpigmentation as well as elevated ACTH levels (mean 840 ng/ml) at the time of radiosurgery. One patient had previously received conventional fractionated radiation therapy, and 2 patients had received prior gamma surgery for Cushing's disease. The mean endocrine follow-up was 33 (range 6–78) months, and the mean radiological follow-up was 31 (range 5–72) months. The median dose to the tumor margin was 25 (range 4–30) Gy. Tumor growth control was achieved in 12 of 14 patients (86%). ACTH levels decreased in 14 patients (81%) with a median decrease of 59% (range −93% to +33%). Five patients (31%) achieved normal ACTH levels with a mean time to remission of 9.4 months after radiosurgery. New endocrinopathies were seen after 5 gamma surgeries (31%), with low growth hormone levels being the most common new hormonal deficit. No patient exhibited radiographic or clinical evidence of damage to the optic apparatus or surrounding brain.

Rates of Endocrine Improvement and Late Recurrence

An ideal treatment would lead to a rapid endocrinological normalization. The rate and time of onset of hormonal improvement and normalization following radiosurgery are difficult to predict. Some series have reported hormonal improvement in as little as 3 months following radiosurgery, whereas others have reported normalization occurring more than 8 years afterwards [5, 47]. Generally, if endocrinological normalization is going to occur following radiosurgery, it usually does so within the first 2 years [2, 5, 45, 52, 61]. Several instances of late recurrence of hormonal oversecretion have been reported despite earlier confirmed remissions [5]. As such, long-term radiological and endocrinological follow-up is recommended for all pituitary patients to detect any possibility of late recurrence and tumor growth.

The effects of treatment volume and dose selection on the rate and extent of hormonal normalization remain the subject of debate. Some investigators have found that radiation dose and treatment volume do not affect the rate or extent of hormonal normalization [30, 62]. Others have found a correlation between hormonal normalization and the following: treatment isodose, maximal dose, margin dose, and the absence of hormone-suppressive medications around the time of radiosurgery [32, 33, 41, 44]. There does not appear to be a correlation between tumor volume response and the endocrinological response following radiosurgery [5, 21, 32]. As most pituitary adenomas are well within the size of lesion that is suitable for stereotactic radiosurgery, dose-volume considerations are not as much of an issue. The dose is usually limited by the proximity of the adenoma to the optic pathways, and current shielding techniques can help to facilitate delivery of higher doses. Since the systemic effects of secretory adenomas can be so devastating to patients, it seems intuitive to deliver a reasonably high dose (≥20 Gy to the margin) to effectuate hormonal normalization and tumor growth control. Nonsecretory pituitary adenomas appear to require a lower radiosurgery treatment dose than secretory adenomas [11, 28, 35, 47, 62]. The lowest effective dose for pituitary adenomas is not known.

Complications following Radiosurgery for Pituitary Adenomas

Cranial Neuropathies following Radiosurgery

In our review of 35 studies encompassing 1,621 patients, there were 16 reported cases of damage to the optic apparatus (~1%). The post-radiosurgical visual apparatus deficits ranged from quadrantanopias to complete visual acuity loss. Radiosurgical doses associated with visual field loss varied from 0.7 to 12 Gy. The tolerable level of radiation to the optic apparatus is still a subject of debate. Some advocate that the optic apparatus can tolerate doses as high as 12–14.1 Gy [54, 64, 65]. Others recommend an upper limit of 8–10 Gy [66, 67]. Small volumes of the optic apparatus exposed to doses of 10 Gy or less may be acceptable in some cases [64, 68]. Both the tolerable absolute dose and volume undoubtedly vary from patient to patient. This degree of variability likely depends upon the extent of damage to the optic apparatus by pituitary adenoma compression, ischemic changes, type and timing of previous interventions (e.g. fractionated radiation therapy and surgery), the patient's age, and the presence or absence of other co-morbidities (e.g. diabetes) [69, 70].

The other consideration for limiting damage to the optic apparatus during radiosurgery is the distance between the optic apparatus and the residual adenoma. A distance of 5 mm between the adenoma and the optic apparatus is desirable, but a distance of as little as 1–2 mm may be acceptable; the dose volume of the optic apparatus may be a better way to determine dose and risk [5, 35, 48, 54]. The tolerable distance is a function of the degree to which a dose plan can be designed to deliver a suitable radiation dose to the adenoma yet spare the optic apparatus. Without achievement of a suitable stereotactic radiosurgery dose plan, alternative treatment modalities (i.e. surgical resection, medical management, or fractionated radiation therapy) should be chosen.

Just as visual dysfunction of the optic apparatus has been described following radiosurgery, so too has improvement in visual function. Improvement in visual acuity and fields has been noted following radiosurgery in some patients with pituitary adenomas and may be a result of tumor shrinkage and optic nerve decompression [24, 28, 46, 51, 53, 54, 71].

The other cranial nerves in the cavernous sinus appear to be much more resistant to injury from radiosurgery. In the 35 studies reviewed, 21 patients had new neuropathies develop in either the oculomotor, trochlear, trigeminal, or abducent nerves, and nearly half of these cranial neuropathies were transient.

Injury to Adjacent Vascular Structures

Injury to the cavernous segment of the carotid artery is rare following radiosurgery. A total of 4 cases have been reported and in only 2 of these cases were the patients symptomatic from carotid artery stenosis [35, 40, 44]. Pollock et al. [44] recommended that the prescription dose should be limited to <50% of the intracavernous carotid artery vessel diameter. Shin et al. [47] recommended restricting the dose to the internal carotid artery to <30 Gy.

Hypopituitarism

The incidence of hypopituitarism after radiosurgery is difficult to determine at present. Reports in the literature for the incidence of post-radiosurgery hypopituitarism vary widely. Well-respected groups have reported a low incidence (0–36%) of pituitary dysfunction following radiosurgery [5, 34, 43, 46, 72]. A long-term study from the Karolinska Institute with a mean follow-up of 17 years indicated a 72% incidence of hypopituitarism [25]. However, many of these patients comprising that study were treated with targeting based upon antiquated imaging techniques and received doses much higher than those used today. Fiegl et al. [21] found that hypopituitarism following radiosurgery correlated with the radiation dose to the pituitary stalk, and Vladyka et al. [73] demonstrated that certain normal adenohypophysis cell types are more susceptible to radiation than others. The difficulty with determining the exact incidence of radiosurgery-induced hypopituitarism stems in part from the fact that many of the patients have already undergone previous surgical resection and some previous fractionated radiotherapy. In addition, pituitary deficiencies may result in part from aging. Thus, it is likely that hypopituitarism in the post-radiosurgical population is multifactorial in etiology and related to radiosurgery as well as age-related changes and prior treatments (e.g. microsurgery and radiotherapy). The methods of endocrinological follow-up are inconsistent and unreliable; the indications for obtaining hormone levels and the time at which they were obtained vary widely from study to study.

Conclusions

Multimodality treatment is often employed to manage patients with pituitary adenomas. Treatment options include medical management, microsurgery, radiosurgery and radiotherapy. Except for prolactinomas, microsurgery remains the primary treatment in surgically fit patients for sellar lesions, particularly when the lesion is demonstrating a mass effect on the optic apparatus or hormonal overproduction. Nevertheless, 20–50% of patients demonstrate recurrence of their adenomas, and adjuvant treatment is recommended for these patients.

Historically, fractionated radiation therapy was utilized to treat recurrent or residual pituitary adenomas. However, fractionated radiation therapy has a prolonged latency for its desired effects (i.e. tumor control and hormonal normalization) and is associated with a significant risk for undesired effects (i.e. radiation-induced tumors, cerebral vasculopathy, necrosis, visual damage, and hypopituitarism). Stereotactic radiosurgery has been demonstrated to be a safe and effective treatment for patients with recurrent or residual pituitary adenomas. Radiosurgery affords effective growth control and hormonal normalization for patients with a generally shorter latency period than that of fractionated radiotherapy. This shorter latency period with radiosurgery can typically be managed with suppressive medications. Furthermore, radiosurgery is associated with fewer complications (e.g. radiation-induced neoplasia, cerebral vasculopathy, etc.) than radiotherapy. Radiosurgery may even serve as a primary treatment for those patients deemed unfit for microsurgical resection as a result of other co-morbidities or with demonstrable tumors in a surgically inaccessible location. Radiosurgery can frequently preserve and, at times, even restore neurological and hormonal function.

The introduction of the gamma knife automatic positioning system, incorporation of new neuroimaging technologies into dose planning, and improvements in the shielding techniques of radiosurgical units will likely result in improved conformity, steeper dose falloff, and better clinical and imaging outcomes [74, 75]. Neurosurgeons and endocrinologists will need to clarify the optimal timing for cessation of antisecretory medications with regard to the date of radiosurgery. At the time of surgical resection, the neurosurgeon should make efforts to create a persistent space between the optic pathways and the tumor. Additional neurological, neuroimaging, and endocrinological follow-up of patients must be performed to assess for delayed complications or tumor recurrence. Finally, physicians caring for pituitary patients should establish uniform endocrinological criteria and diagnostic testing for pre- and post-radiosurgical evaluations.

References

1 Laws ER, Ebersold MJ, Piepgras DG: The results of transsphenoidal surgery in specific clinical entities; in Laws ER, Randall RV, Kern EB, et al (eds): Management of Pituitary Adenomas and Related Lesions with Emphasis on Transsphenoidal Microsurgery. New York, Appleton-Century-Crofts, 1982, pp 277–305.

2 Laws ER, Vance ML: Radiosurgery for pituitary tumors and craniopharyngiomas. Neurosurg Clin North Am 1999;10:327–336.

3 Laws ER Jr, Fode NC, Redmond MJ: Transsphenoidal surgery following unsuccessful prior therapy. An assessment of benefits and risks in 158 patients. J Neurosurg 1985;63:823–829.

4 Sheehan JM, Lopes MB, Sheehan JP, Ellegala D, Webb KM, Laws ER Jr: Results of transsphenoidal surgery for Cushing's disease in patients with no histologically confirmed tumor. Neurosurgery 2000;47:33–36.

5 Sheehan JM, Vance ML, Sheehan JP, Ellegala DB, Laws ER Jr: Radiosurgery for Cushing's disease after failed transsphenoidal surgery. J Neurosurg 2000;93:738–742.
6 Milker-Zabel S, Debus J, Thilmann C, Schlegel W, Wannenmacher M: Fractionated stereotactically guided radiotherapy and radiosurgery in the treatment of functional and nonfunctional adenomas of the pituitary gland. Int J Rad Oncol Biol Phys 2001;50:1279–1286.
7 Meij BP, Lopes MB, Ellegala DB, Alden TD, Laws ER Jr: The long-term significance of microscopic dural invasion in 354 patients with pituitary adenomas treated with transsphenoidal surgery. J Neurosurg 2002;96:195–208.
8 Shaffi OM, Wrightson P: Dural invasion by pituitary tumours. NZ Med J 1975;81:386–390.
9 Chandler WF, Schteingard DE, Lloyd RV, McKeever PE, Ibarra-Perez G: Surgical treatment of Cushing's disease. J Neurosurg 1987;66:204–212.
10 Friedman RB, Oldfield EH, Nieman LK, Chrousos GP, Doppman JL, Cutler GB Jr, Loriaux DL: Repeat transsphenoidal surgery for Cushing's disease. J Neurosurg 1989;71:520–527.
11 Mampalam TJ, Tyrrell JB, Wilson CB: Transsphenoidal microsurgery for Cushing disease. Ann Intern Med 1988;109:487–493.
12 Leksell L: The stereotaxic method and radiosurgery of the brain. Acta Chir Scand 1951;102: 316–319.
13 Kondziolka D, Maitz AH, Niranjan A, Flickinger JC, Lunsford LD: An evaluation of the Model C gamma knife with automatic patient positioning. Neurosurgery 2002;50:429–432.
14 Friedman WA, Foote KD: Linear accelerator radiosurgery in the management of brain tumours. Ann Med 2000;32:64–80.
15 Lyman JT, Phillips MH, Frankel KA, Levy RP, Fabrikant JI: Radiation physics for particle beam radiosurgery. Neurosurg Clin North Am 1992;3:1–8.
16 Kondziolka D, Dempsey PK, Lunsford LD, Kestle JR, Dolan EJ, Kanal E, Tasker RR: A comparison between magnetic resonance imaging and computed tomography for stereotactic coordinate determination. Neurosurgery 1992;30:402–407.
17 Semple PL, Laws ER Jr: Complications in a contemporary series of patients who underwent transsphenoidal surgery for Cushing's disease. J Neurosurg 1999;91:175–179.
18 Shimon I, Ram Z, Cohen ZR, Hadani M: Transsphenoidal surgery for Cushing's disease: endocrinological follow-up monitoring of 82 patients. Neurosurgery 2002;51:57–62.
19 Attanasio R, Epaminonda P, Motti E, Giugni E, Ventrella L, Cozzi R, Farabola M, Loli P, Beck-Peccoz P, Arosio M: Gamma-knife radiosurgery in acromegaly: a 4-year follow-up study. J Clin Endocrinol Metab 2003;88:3105–3112.
20 Choi JY, Chang JH, Chang JW, Ha Y, Park YG, Chung SS: Radiological and hormonal responses of functioning pituitary adenomas after gamma knife radiosurgery. Yonsei Med J 2003;44: 602–607.
21 Feigl GC, Bonelli CM, Berghold A, Mokry M: Effects of gamma knife radiosurgery of pituitary adenomas on pituitary function. J Neurosurg 2002;97(suppl 5):415–421.
22 Fukuoka S, Ito T, Takanashi M, Hojo A, Nakamura H: Gamma knife radiosurgery for growth hormone-secreting pituitary adenomas invading the cavernous sinus. Stereotact Funct Neurosurg 2001;76:213–217.
23 Ganz JC, Backlund EO, Thorsen FA: The effects of gamma knife surgery of pituitary adenomas on tumor growth and endocrinopathies. Stereotact Funct Neurourg 1993;61(suppl 1):30–37.
24 Hayashi M, Izawa M, Hiyama H, Nakamura S, Atsuchi S, Sato H, Nakaya K, Sasaki K, Ochiai T, Kubo O, Hori T, Takakura K: Gamma knife radiosurgery for pituitary adenomas. Stereotact Funct Neurosurg 1999;72(suppl 1):111–118.
25 Hoybye C, Grenback E, Rahn T, Degerblad M, Thoren M, Hulting AL: Adrenocortcotrophic hormone-producing pituitary tumors: 12- to 22-year follow up after treatment with stereotactic radiosurgery. Neurosurgery 2001;49:284–292.
26 Ikeda H, Jokura H, Yoshimoto T: Transsphenoidal surgery and adjuvant gamma knife treatment for growth hormone-secreting pituitary adenoma. J Neurosurg 2001;95:285–291.
27 Inoue HK, Kohga H, Hirato M, Sasaki T, Ishihara J, Shibazaki T, Ohye C, Andou Y: Pituitary adenomas treated by microsurgery with or without gamma knife surgery: experience in 122 cases. Stereotact Funct Neurosurg 1999;72(suppl 1):125–131.

28 Izawa M, Hayashi M, Nakaya K, Satoh H, Ochiai T, Hori T, Takakura K: Gamma knife radiosurgery for pituitary adenomas. J Neurosurg 2000;93(suppl 3):19–22.
29 Kim SH, Huh R, Chang JW, Park YG, Chung SS: Gamma knife radiosurgery for functioning pituitary adenomas. Stereotact Funct Neurosurg 1999;72(suppl 1):101–110.
30 Kim MS, Lee SI, Sim JH: Gamma Knife radiosurgery for functioning pituitary microadenoma. Stereotact Funct Neurosurg 1999;72(suppl 1):119–124.
31 Kobayashi T, Kida Y, Mori Y: Gamma knife radiosurgery in the treatment of Cushing disease: long-term results. J Neurosurg 2002;97(suppl 5):422–428.
32 Landolt AM, Haller D, Lomax N, Scheib S, Schubiger O, Siegfried J, Wellis G: Stereotactic radiosurgery for recurrent surgically treated acromegaly: comparison with fractionated radiotherapy. J Neurosurg 1998;88:1002–1008.
33 Landolt AM, Lomax N: Gamma knife radiosurgery for prolactinomas. J Neurosurg 2000;93(suppl 3): 14–18.
34 Levy RP, Fabrikant JI, Frankel KA, Phillips MH, Lyman JT, Lawrence JH, Tobias CA: Heavy-charged-particle radiosurgery of the pituitary gland: clinical results of 840 patients. Stereotact Funct Neurosurg 1991;57:22–35.
35 Lim YL, Leem W, Kim TS, Rhee BA, Kim GK: Four years' experiences in the treatment of pituitary adenomas with gamma knife radiosurgery. Stereotact Funct Neurosurg 1998;70(suppl 1): 95–109.
36 Martinez R, Bravo G, Burzaco J, Rey G: Pituitary tumors and gamma knife surgery. Clinical experience with more than two years of follow-up. Stereotact Funct Neurosurg 1998;70 (suppl 1):110–118.
37 Mitsumori M, Chrieve DC, Alexander E 3rd, Kaiser UB, Richardson GE, Black PM, Loeffler JS: Initial clinical results of LINAC-based stereotactic radiosurgery and stereotactic radiotherapy for pituitary adenomas. Int J Radiat Oncol Biol Phys 1998;42:573–580.
38 Mokry M, Ramschak-Schwarzer S, Simbrunner J, Ganz JC, Pendl G: A six year experience with the postoperative radiosurgical management of pituitary adenomas. Stereotact Funct Neurosurg 1999;72(suppl 1):88–100.
39 Morange-Ramos I, Regis J, Dufour H, Andrieu JM, Grisoli F, Jaquet P, Peragut JC: Gamma-knife surgery for secreting pituitary adenomas. Acta Neurochir (Wien) 1998;140:437–443.
40 Muramatsu J, Yoshida M, Shioura H, Kawamura Y, Ito H, Takeuchi H, Kubota T, Maruyama I: Clinical results of LINAC-based stereotactic radiosurgery for pituitary adenoma (in Japanese). Nippon Igaku Hoshasen Gakkai Zasshi 2003;63:225–230.
41 Pan L, Zhang N, Wang EM, Wang BJ, Dai JZ, Cai PW: Gamma knife radiosurgery as a primary treatment for prolactinomas. J Neurosurg 2000;93(suppl 3):10–13.
42 Petrovich Z, Yu C, Giannotta SL, Zee CS, Apuzzo ML: Gamma knife radiosurgery for pituitary adenoma: early results. Neurosurgery 2003;53:51–59.
43 Pollock BE, Carpenter PC: Stereotactic radiosurgery as an alternative to fractionated radiotherapy for patients with recurrent or residual nonfunctioning pituitary adenomas. Neurosurgery 2003;53: 1086–1094.
44 Pollock BE, Nippoldt TB, Stafford SL, Foote RL, Abboud CF: Results of stereotactic radiosurgery in patients with hormone-producing pituitary adenomas: factors associated with endocrine normalization. J Neurosurg 2002;97:525–530.
45 Pollock BE, Young WF Jr: Stereotactic radiosurgery for patients with ACTH-producing pituitary adenomas after prior adrenalectomy. Int J Radiat Oncol Biol Phys 2002;54:839–841.
46 Sheehan JP, Kondziolka D, Flickinger J, Lunsford LD: Radiosurgery for residual or recurrent nonfunctioning pituitary adenoma. J Neurosurg 2002;97(suppl 5):408–414.
47 Shin M, Kurita H, Sasaki T, Tago M, Morita A, Ueki K, Kirino T: Stereotactic radiosurgery for pituitary adenoma invading the cavernous sinus. J Neurosurg 2000;93(suppl 3):2–5.
48 Witt TC, Kondziolka D, Flickinger JC, Lunsford LD: Gamma knife radiosurgery for pituitary tumors; in Lunsford LD, Kondziolka D, Flickinger JC (eds): Gamma Knife Brain Surgery. Prog Neurol Surg. Basel, Karger, 1998, vol 14, pp 114–127.
49 Wolffenbuttel BH, Kitz K, Beuls EM: Beneficial gamma-knife radiosurgery in a patient with Nelson's syndrome. Clin Neurol Neurosurg 1998;100:60–63.

50 Wowra B, Stummer W: Efficacy of gamma knife radiosurgery for nonfunctioning pituitary adenomas: a quantitative follow up with magnetic resonance imaging-based volumetric analysis. J Neurosurg 2002;97(suppl 5):429–432.
51 Yoon SC, Suh TS, Jang HS, Chung SM, Kim YS, Ryu MR, Choi KH, Son HY, Kim MC, Shinn KS: Clinical results of 24 pituitary macroadenomas with linac-based stereotactic radiosurgery. Int J Radiat Onc Biol Phys 1998;41:849–853.
52 Zhang N, Pan L, Wang EM, Dai JZ, Wang BJ, Cai PW: Radiosurgery for growth hormone-producing pituitary adenomas. J Neurosurg 2000;93(suppl 3):6–9.
53 Abe T, Yamamoto M, Taniyama M, Tanioka D, Izumiyama H, Matsumoto K: Early palliation of occulomotor nerve palsy following gamma knife radiosurgery for pituitary adenoma. Eur Neurol 2002;47:61–63.
54 Chen JC, Giannotta SL, Yu C, Petrovich Z, Levy ML, Apuzzo M: Radiosurgical management of benign cavernous sinus tumors: dose profiles and acute complications. Neurosurgery 2001;48: 1022–1032.
55 Losa M, Valle M, Mortini P, Franzin A, Da Passano CF, Cenzato M, Bianchi S, Picozzi P, Giovanelli M: Gamma knife surgery for treatment of residual nonfunctioning pituitary adenomas after surgical debulking. J Neurosurg 2004;100:438–444.
56 Lindholm J: Cushing's syndrome: historical aspects. Pituitary 2000;3:97–104.
57 Arnaldi G, Angeli A, Atkinson AB, Bertagna X, Cavagnini F, Chrousos GP, Fava GA, Findling JW, Gaillard RC, Grossman AB, Kola B, Lacroix A, Mancini T, Mantero F, Newell-Price J, Nieman LK, Sonino N, Vance ML, Giustina A, Boscaro M: Diagnosis and complications of Cushing's syndrome: a consensus statement. J Clin Endocrinol Metab 2003;88:5593–5602.
58 Giustina A, Barkan A, Casaneuva FF, Cavagnini F, Frohman L, Ho K, Veldhuis J, Wass J, Von Werder K, Melmed S: Criteria for cure of acromegaly: a consensus statement. J Clin Endocrinol Metab 2000;85:526–529.
59 Vance ML: Endocrinological evaluation of acromegaly. J Neurosurg 1998;89:499–500.
60 Landolt AM, Haller D, Lomax N, Scheib S, Schubiger O, Siegfried J, Wellis G: Octreotide may act as a radioprotective agent in acromegaly. J Clin Endocrinol Metab 2000;85:1287–1289.
61 Laws ER, Vance ML, Thapar K: Pituitary surgery for the management of acromegaly. Horm Res 2000;53(suppl 3):71–75.
62 Estrada J, Boronat M, Mielgo M, Alfaro J, Lucas T, Diez S, Salto L, Barcelo B: The complete normalization of the adrenocortical function as the criterion of cure after transsphenoidal surgery for Cushing's disease. J Clin Endocrinol Metab 2001;86:5695–5699.
63 Pan L, Zhang N, Wang E, Wang B, Xu W: Pituitary adenomas: the effect of gamma knife radiosurgery on tumor growth and endocrinopathies. Stereotact Funct Neurosurg 1998;70(suppl 1): 119–126.
64 Ove R, Kelman S, Amin PP, Chin LS: Preservation of visual fields after peri-sellar gamma knife radiosurgery. Int J Cancer 2000;90:343–350.
65 Stafford SL, Pollock BE, Leavitt JA, Foote RL, Brown PD, Link MJ, Gorman DA, Schomberg PJ: A study on the radiation tolerance of the optic nerves and chiasm after stereotactic radiosurgery. Int J Radiat Oncol Biol Phys 2003;55:1177–1181.
66 Girkin CA, Comey CH, Lunsford LD, Goodman ML, Kline LB: Radiation optic neuropathy after stereotactic radiosurgery. Ophthalmology 1997;104:1634–1643.
67 Tishler RB, Loeffler JS, Lunsford LD, Duma C, Alexander E 3rd, Kooy HM, Flickinger JC: Tolerance of cranial nerves of the cavernous sinus to radiosurgery. Int J Radiat Oncol Biol Phys 1993;27:215–221.
68 Leber KA, Bergloff J, Pendl G: Dose-response tolerance of the visual pathways and cranial nerves of the cavernous sinus to stereotactic radiosurgery. J Neurosurg 1998;88:43–50.
69 Lundstrom M, Frisen L: Atrophy of optic nerve fibres in compression of the chiasm. Degree and distribution of ophthalmoscopic changes. Acta Ophthalmol (Copenh) 1976;54:623–640.
70 Rodriguez O, Mateos B, de la Pedraja R, Villoria R, Hernando JI, Pastor A, Pomposo I, Aurrecoechea J: Postoperative follow-up of pituitary adenomas after trans-sphenoidal resection: MRI and clinical correlation. Neuroradiology 1996;38:747–754.

71 Muron T, Rocher FP, Sentenac I, Marquis I, Romestaing P, Gatignon D, Croisille M, Gerard JP: Stereotactic radiosurgery. Preliminary experience of a team of Lyon. Ann Med Interne (Paris) 1993;144:9–14.
72 Jane JA Jr, Vance ML, Woodburn CJ, Laws ER: Stereotactic radiosurgery for hypersecreting pituitary tumors: part of a multimodality approach. Neurosurg Focus 2003;14:e12.
73 Vladyka V, Liscak R, Novotny J Jr, Marek J, Jezkova J: Radiation tolerance of functioning pituitary tissue in gamma knife surgery for pituitary adenomas. Neurosurgery 2003;52:309–316.
74 Horstmann GA, Van Eck AT: Gamma knife model C with the automatic positioning system and its impact on the treatment of vestibular schwannomas. J Neurosurg 2002;97(suppl 5):450–455.
75 Regis J, Hayashi M, Porcheron D, Delsanti C, Muracciole X, Peragut JC: Impact of the model C and automatic positioning system on gamma knife radiosurgery: an evaluation in vestibular schwannomas. J Neurosurg 2002;97(suppl 5):588–591.

Jason P. Sheehan, MD, PhD
Department of Neurological Surgery, Health Sciences Center
University of Virginia, PO Box 800212
Charlottesville, VA 22908 (USA)
Tel. +1 434 924 8129, Fax +1 434 243 6726, E-Mail jps2f@virginia.edu

Laws ER Jr, Sheehan JP (eds): Pituitary Surgery – A Modern Approach.
Front Horm Res. Basel, Karger, 2006, vol 34, pp 206–235

Neuropathological Considerations of Pituitary Adenomas

Ashok Asthagiri, M. Beatriz S. Lopes

Department of Neurological Surgery and Division of Neuropathology, Department of Pathology, Health Sciences Center, University of Virginia, Charlottesville, Va., USA

Abstract
Pituitary tumors constitute around 15–20% of intracranial tumors. The understanding of the molecular mechanisms of tumorigenesis and the functional regulation of pituitary adenoma has greatly advanced in the last decade. The current WHO classification scheme of pituitary tumors reflects this progress on tumor biology knowledge, and embraces the most widely utilized diagnostic methods of evaluation of these lesions. The present chapter highlights the different aspects of the tumor diagnosis and reviews the classification of pituitary tumors.

Copyright © 2006 S. Karger AG, Basel

Introduction

Pituitary adenomas are clonal proliferations of adenohypophysial origin, and are in general considered benign neoplasms confined to the region of the sella turcica. Symptomatically, patients present with endocrinologic manifestations of pituitary dysfunction and/or mass effect on adjacent structures including the optic chiasm, neurovascular elements coursing through the cavernous sinus, dura mater investing the sella, or native pituitary gland. Even to the dedicated clinician, the insidious onset of systemic or local symptoms is at times difficult to discern. The proper diagnosis, treatment, and surveillance of pituitary disease require the expertise and coordination of a multidisciplinary team including endocrinologists, neurosurgeons, radiologists, and pathologists.

Historically, the prevalence of pituitary adenomas and the significance of pituitary 'incidentalomas' have been topics of debate [1]. Postmortem studies have reported an incidence rate varying from 1 to 35%, and reports of imaging studies displayed a similar variability in their incidence, reporting 10–40% [2–5]. The best estimate of the true prevalence of pituitary adenomas in the general population has been proposed to be 16.7%, through a meta-analysis of all existing English-language articles reporting on the incidence of pituitary adenomas [6]. Given the high prevalence of pituitary adenomas, it should be of no surprise that they account for approximately 10% of all symptomatic intracranial tumors [7].

Advances in laboratory evaluation with the advent of biochemical hormone assays, radiographic evaluation with magnetic resonance imaging and dynamic protocols, and the integration of these advances in procedures such as inferior petrosal sinus sampling have yielded the ability to make an earlier diagnosis with both higher sensitivity and specificity. With the diagnostic capabilities of localizing lesions improving and surgical techniques utilized in resection of symptomatic tumors expanding, the stimulus to provide more accurate interpretations of submitted specimens so as to help guide postoperative care and management has been focused upon pathologists specializing in this field.

The armamentarium of diagnostic modalities available to pathologists continues to grow, and by necessity more thorough paradigms of classification become proposed and employed. The latest World Health Organization (WHO) classification system of pituitary adenomas incorporates most of the major advances in evaluation of tissue specimens over the past century [8]. In this chapter, we will discuss neuropathologic considerations in pituitary surgery, encompassing the procurement, processing, evaluation, and classification of these lesions.

Neurosurgical Procurement of Tissue

Neurosurgical advances in accessing the sellar contents have centered upon the minimally invasive approach sweeping the surgical specialty as a whole. The minimally invasive, microscopic and endoscopic approaches now employed to resect a large number of these lesions provide another challenge to the interpretation of an already limited sample size. Pituitary tumor specimens obtained from such resections are submitted piecemeal due to the nature of the small operative window, microinstruments used to remove them, and the discohesive and semisolid nature of the tumors. Optimal tissue fixation and processing are essential to obtain reliable results in the analysis of pituitary specimens. Therefore, for the several morphological and specialized molecular and biochemical studies, the pathologist should receive fresh specimens from the operating room for adequate sampling (fig. 1).

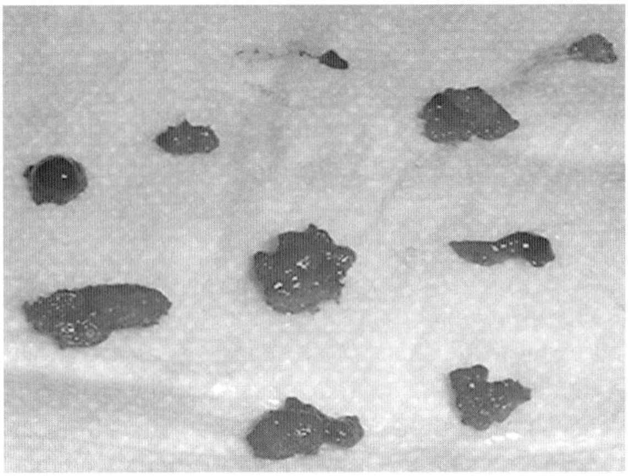

Fig. 1. Gross imaging of a pituitary adenoma. Typical sample submitted for pathologic evaluation. Note the small sample size, fragmented, and discohesive nature of the lesion.

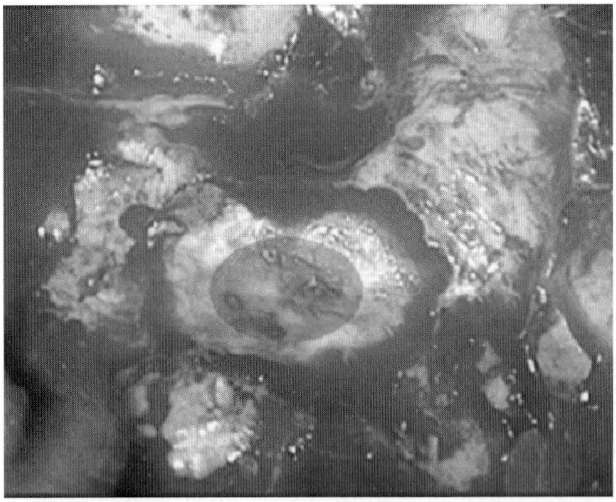

Fig. 2. Operative view of the dura mater along the inferior aspect of the sella turcica. Planned circumferential cautery along the border of the ellipse is planned, and resection of the dural specimen is performed.

Lesions presenting with radiologic findings of large size, macroadenomas, and recurrent lesions often display invasion into the dura mater along the floor of the sella. The microscopic evaluation of dural specimens obtained at the time of adenomectomy is routine in the majority of pituitary neurosurgical services (fig. 2). Dural microinvasion has been seen in 45.5–85% of cases [5, 9, 10].

Although correlation with recurrence after initial cure of pituitary disease is not consistent or significant, the persistence of residual tumor based on endocrinologic profile or mass effect was statistically greater in lesions displaying adjacent dural invasion [9]. Biopsy of the dura along the floor of the sella turcica is often complicated by the vascular nature of the dura and the juxtaposed vascular structures, namely the intercavernous and cavernous sinus. Cautery used to bring the periosteal and meningeal layers of the dura together prior to durotomy and biopsy may lead to artifact, which makes the identification of microinvasion ambiguous. The judicious use of circumferential cautery along the margin of the biopsy specimen has helped tremendously with both the preservation of dural specimens from heat artifact and minimizing hemorrhage [11]. Fresh specimens of dura are sent as separate tissue samples, and their size recorded. Tissues are fixed in 10% zinc formalin and normally processed for paraffin embedding. Serial sections stained with hematoxylin and eosin (H&E) are analyzed for microscopic evidence of tumor invasion, as represented by individual cell invasion or dissection of the dural planes by clusters of tumor cells [9].

After obtaining access to the intrasellar contents, neurosurgeons are met with the challenge of performing a selective adenomectomy. Both large macroadenomas, where the native pituitary gland may be compressed into a small multilayer pseudocapsule engulfing the mass, and microadenomas that are buried deep within the gland usually have a small portion of the adjacent native gland excised with the neoplastic tissue. Even in the instance of easily visualized microadenomas, peeling of the pseudocapsule and biopsy of the surrounding normal pituitary tissue is often performed [12]. This small sample of native pituitary tissue (fig. 3a) is important as an internal control while fixing and processing the tissue. Its presence validates the various methods used to interpret the pathologic specimen, including light microscopic and immunohistochemical evaluation. In addition, the presence of compressed anterior pituitary tissue may support the presence of a mass-occupying lesion, even if the submitted tissue does not contain the designated pathology. Likewise, if the diagnosis of Cushing's disease is not elucidated by the pathologic specimen, a systemic hypercortisolemic state may be affirmed by the presence of Crooke's hyaline changes within normal corticotroph cells of the compressed pituitary gland [13].

Processing and Evaluation of Specimen

Intraoperative Consultation

Upon submission of a specimen, accurate and rapid identification of an adenoma guides the immediate operative course when this finding is ambiguous to

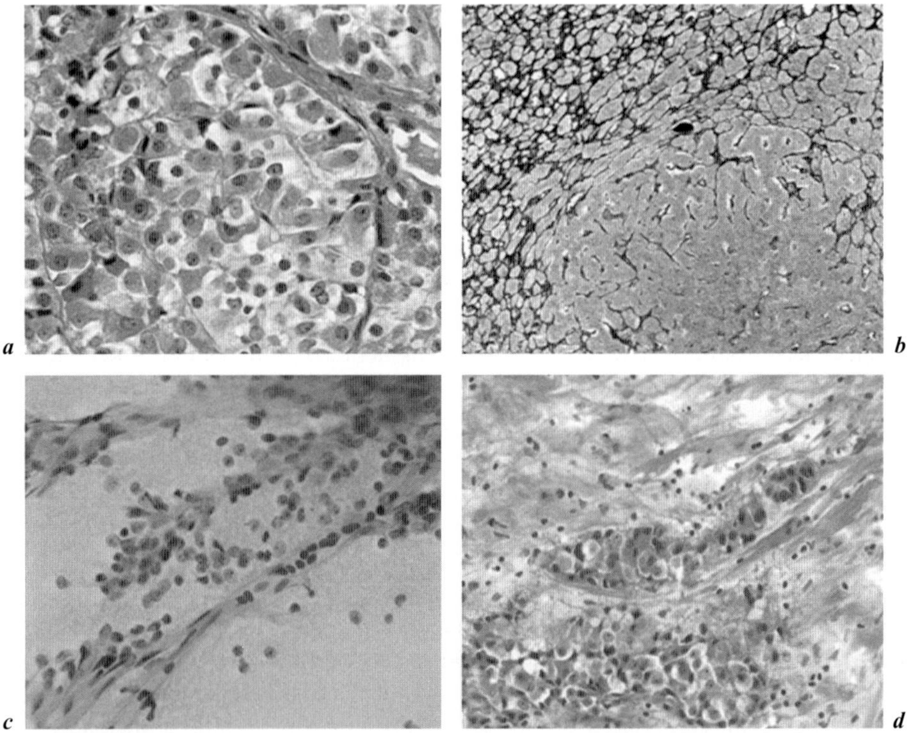

Fig. 3. ***a*** The normal anterior pituitary shows the multiple cell types of the gland. Basophilic, eosinophilic and chromophobic cells are intermixed in a single acinus. H&E stain. ***b*** The dissolution of the normal reticulin network in an adenoma (lower right) is seen in comparison with the compressed residual normal gland (upper left). Reticulin stain. ***c*** Intraoperative smear preparation of a pituitary adenoma shows homogeneous population of cells arranged in a papillary structure. Morris stain. ***d*** Dura biopsy displaying invasion by an adenoma. H&E stain.

the operating team based on preoperative imaging and intraoperative observation. The use of intraoperative consultation as an adjunct to the intraoperative course was described in the literature as early as 1965, although the staining methods were not so clearly delineated [14]. In the 1970s the use of H&E-stained frozen sectioned tissues became the standard for intraoperative evaluation of these tissues, although differentiation between tumor and normal gland was often unsatisfactory in small pieces of tissue removed.

Due to these difficulties with clear identification of adenomas by H&E staining which poorly highlighted the fibrovascular architecture, Velasco et al. [15] introduced the use of the reticulum stain for intraoperative frozen section diagnosis. The identification of sheet-like growth within the adenoma in contrast to the regular alveolar compartmentalization of native pituitary, in conjunction with a band-like compression of the native reticular framework rendered the diagnosis almost unmistakable [15]. The use of the reticulin stain on permanent sections is now a powerful tool in the identification of the smallest adenomas (fig. 3b). Reporting difficulties with the reproducibility of the reticulin stain in frozen sections, Adelman and Post [16] proposed the use of the Orange G-hematoxylin stains. With this modified technique, both basophils and chromophobes remained stained. They achieved 90% diagnostic accuracy, reported instances of improved resection beyond the gross margins, and excellent postoperative results possibly attributable to their novel intraoperative analysis techniques [16]. Other fast and simple frozen techniques, including the use of fluorescein-labeled *Ricinus communis* agglutinin 120 (RCA 120) staining of vessels and stroma with propidium iodide nuclear counter stain, provided alternative diagnostic methods for intraoperative consultation [17]. Still, drawbacks such as the ephemeral nature of fluorescence, time requirement and degradation of reagents used in silver-staining methods, and lack of fibrovascular differentiation with the Orange-G-hematoxylin stains limited their widespread use as the intraoperative diagnostic tool of choice.

Through the years, the advent of magnetic resonance imaging and improved markers for neuroendocrine function, have made the necessity for intraoperative diagnosis of functioning microadenomas within the submitted specimen less critical. These consultations may be helpful in positively identifying adenomatous tissue, but the evaluation of adenoma type, surgical margins and tumor invasion is often impractical. The use of intraoperative techniques is often limited to the differentiation of entities arising in the sellar location with similar radiologic appearance as pituitary adenomas.

The use of smear preparations in conjunction or not with frozen sections is now the standard approach to intraoperative evaluation of sellar contents and neurosurgical biopsies. Pituitary adenomas possess distinct cytologic features which are readily apparent on smear preparations such as epithelial cords, sheets with dyscohesive ends, and papillary formations that are important in intraoperative differential diagnoses from normal pituitary tissues (fig. 3c), and other tumor entities involving the sellar region such as germinomas, meningiomas, craniopharyngiomas and chordomas [18, 19].

Processing of the Specimen

Subsequent evaluation of pituitary adenomas has undergone an evolution that has seen the relative importance of light microscopy evaluation of paraffin-embedded specimens, ultrastructure analysis with electron microscopy, and immunohistochemical characterization fluctuate over the past two decades. As we approach a better understanding of the importance of these diagnostic tools, various other techniques of molecular and genomic profiling have arisen in conjunction with methods of isolating neoplastic tissue for this analysis. The ability to utilize these methods in delineating the origin, development, and relationship of the adenomas gives us better hope for the prevention and cure of adenomatous lesions of the pituitary. The proper preservation of tissue for subsequent thorough analysis requires an understanding of the purpose of each methodology.

Often in the case of microadenomas, a discernible neoplasm cannot be grossly identified and, in the majority of the cases, the entirety of the specimen is submitted for formalin fixation and paraffin embedding. In cases of macroadenoma where the neoplastic tissue is readily identified, fixation and preservation via different methodologies is appropriate. Appropriation for fixation using cross-linking solutions and snap-freezing techniques should be employed in all these specimens. 10% neutral buffered or zinc-enhanced formaldehyde solution, a cross-linking fixative, followed by preservation by paraffin processing is optimal for light microscopic and immunohistochemical evaluation. 2% buffered glutaraldehyde provides rapid cross-linking fixation, thus preserving cytoplasmic and nuclear detail, and it is optimal for electron microscopy evaluation.

The preservation of macromolecules, in contrast to tissue architecture, is critical in molecular profiling techniques such as in situ hybridization, complimentary genomic hybridization, reverse transcription-polymerase chain reaction, proteomics, and ribonucleic acid interference studies [20]. Macromolecule preservation is best accomplished with snap freezing of tissue with liquid nitrogen and subsequent storage in −80°C freezers. This method of preservation can also be utilized in storing cells for future tissue culture methods and research protocols.

Current standards of morphologic assessment mandate the use of immunohistochemical analysis to classify adenomatous lesions. Therefore, in addition to the preparation of an H&E-stained slide, consecutive sections should be analyzed for reticulin silver impregnation and immunohistochemical preparations for the pituitary hormones. A full spectrum of antibodies for pituitary hormones is usually applied including growth hormone (GH), prolactin (PRL), adrenocorticotropic hormone (ACTH), β-luteinizing hormone (β-LH), β-follicle-stimulating hormone (β-FSH), β-thyroid-stimulating hormone (β-TSH) and the α-subunit of glycoproteins (α-subunit). Due to economic restrictions, some laboratories may apply immunostains in a selective manner depending on the clinical setting. Although immunoreactivity corresponds to hormone storage, it does not necessarily correlate with levels of hormonal synthesis or function.

Classification of Pituitary Adenomas

Historical Overview

Pituitary adenoma pathology encompasses a broad spectrum of disease states ranging from incidental microadenomas found at necropsy to aggressive lesions that behave in a fulminant manner. The first lesions of the sellar region were approached surgically in the 1890s. As Harvey Cushing and Herbert Olivecrona amassed hundreds of cases of surgically treated adenomas it became readily apparent that certain subsets of these lesions behaved differently with respect to their clinical presentation, surgical management, and postoperative outcomes. Attempts to classify various adenomas centered on the tinctorial characteristics of these lesions with H&E staining and subsequent light microscopy evaluation. The division into acidophilic, basophilic, and chromophobic adenomas were based on the staining characteristics of the cytoplasm. Correlation of these findings with historical presentation led to the popularized schema that acidophilic adenomas produced excessive GH, thus resulting in acromegaly and gigantism. Basophilic adenomas were correlated with excess ACTH production and Cushing's disease, and chromophobe adenomas were hormonally inactive tumors presenting with mass effect.

This classification scheme persisted until its obvious shortcomings were highlighted by the discordant findings of 'fugitive acromegalics' and patients afflicted with Cushing's disease who were found to have chromophobe adenomas [21, 22]. This brought the notion of the inadequacy of the light microscopic evaluation of cytoplasmic staining to the forefront of debate. Through the 1960s and 1970s, the development of biological markers for testing serum hormone levels in conjunction with the development of electron microscopy and immunohistochemical methods, led to novel attempts at changing the classification of pituitary adenomas. At this time, clinicians began to stress the anatomic and functional classification schemes while pathologists attempted to incorporate newer technologies into the morphologic evaluation of these entities, thereby creating a chiasm in attempts for a universal scheme.

The functional nomenclature of pituitary tumors gained significant popularity, especially among endocrinologists. Adenomas were broadly categorized into those with signs of endocrine activity (clinically functioning adenomas), and those that did not display such activity (clinically nonfunctioning adenomas). Further differentiation of the nonfunctioning group relied on ultrastructural evaluation for the presence of secretory granules and oncocytic change. The so-called 'true' chromophobe adenomas were those with no signs of endocrinologic activity that did possess scant numbers of cytoplasmic secretory granules. Functional adenomas were classified based on the number of hormones that were found to be hypersecreted during endocrinological evaluation under steady-state conditions, diurnal variation studies, and with stimulation and inhibition tests. Single-hormone-secreting adenomas consisted of somatotroph adenomas, prolactinomas, corticotroph adenomas (associated with Cushing's and Nelson's disease), thyrotroph adenomas, and gonadotropic adenomas. Double-hormone-secreting adenomas were represented by GH-PRL, ACTH-PRL, TSH-PRL, and FSH-PRL adenomas. One case of a multiple-hormone-secreting adenoma with GH-ACTH-PRL activity warranted its own subclassification [23].

Realizing the oversimplification of the previous morphologic classification of pituitary adenomas with light microscopy evaluation, Kovacs and Horvath [24, 25] introduced the morphologic classification scheme that took into account structure-function relationships through the use of electron microscope differentiation of adenomas. Reporting that various types of chromophobe adenomas were ultrastructurally distinguishable, they set forth the first schema of ultrastructural classification of all pituitary adenomas.

Electron microscopy served the field of pituitary pathology by delineating specific structure-function correlations which proved pivotal in the development of light microscopic markers of tumor cell differentiation through the validation of immunohistochemical methods. As immunohistochemical methods of characterizing lesions expanded, the time-consuming and expensive method of ultrastructural evaluation of every pituitary adenoma became less significant. The diminishing role of electron microscopy as a primary tool in the classification of pituitary adenomas came with the refinement of monoclonal antibodies and polyclonal antisera. The reduction in cross-reactivity and false-positivity yielded more accurate and highly reproducible results [26]. Correlating the immunohistochemical profile of adenomas with their ultrastructural features rendered a vast majority of adenomas easily identified by the use of immunohistochemistry alone. The remainder of lesions exhibiting plurihormonality or lack of immunohistochemical reactivity could be characterized with the use of the more labor-intensive and expensive ultrastructural evaluation.

An assimilation of the entire scope of information that can be afforded with a through analysis of clinical history, biochemical evaluation, radiologic studies, and submitted specimen yields the most accurate anatomic, morphologic, functional, and clinically relevant diagnosis. The WHO's attempt to unify pituitary tumor classification schemes represents the maximal utility of ubiquitous tools available to physicians attempting to treat these disorders.

Table 1. WHO classification of tumors of the pituitary

Pituitary adenoma
Typical adenoma
Atypical adenoma
Pituitary carcinoma
Adenoma types
Growth hormone-producing adenomas
Densely granulated somatotroph adenomas
Sparsely granulated somatotroph adenomas
Mixed somatotroph-lactotroph adenomas
Mammosomatotroph adenomas
Acidophil stem cell adenomas
Plurihormonal GH producing adenomas
Prolactin-producing adenomas
Sparsely granulated lactotroph adenomas
Densely granulated lactotroph adenomas
Acidophil stem cell adenomas
TSH-producing adenomas
ACTH-producing adenomas
Silent corticotroph (subtype 1 and 2) adenomas
Gonadotopin-producing adenomas
Null cell adenomas and oncocytomas
Plurihormonal adenomas

Current WHO Classification of Pituitary Tumors

The integration of data from intraoperative analysis, radiologic evaluation, light microscopic examination of tinctorial properties, immunohistochemical staining, and ultrastructural evaluation with electron microscopy has culminated in a classification scheme that attempts to assimilate structure-function relationships, morphologic analysis, and multidisciplinary efforts in the proper diagnosis of pituitary adenomas [8]. In addition, the WHO classification recognizes progression of pituitary adenomas to more aggressive tumors including atypical adenomas and carcinomas (table 1).

Growth Hormone-Producing Adenomas (fig. 4)

Pituitary adenomas associated with the excess secretion of GH are associated with clinical manifestations of acromegaly and gigantism, depending on the age at which the disease process initiates [27–29]. Nonfunctioning GH-immunopositive adenomas are very rare [30]. The mean interval between disease onset and diagnosis of a GH adenoma causing acromegaly is approximately

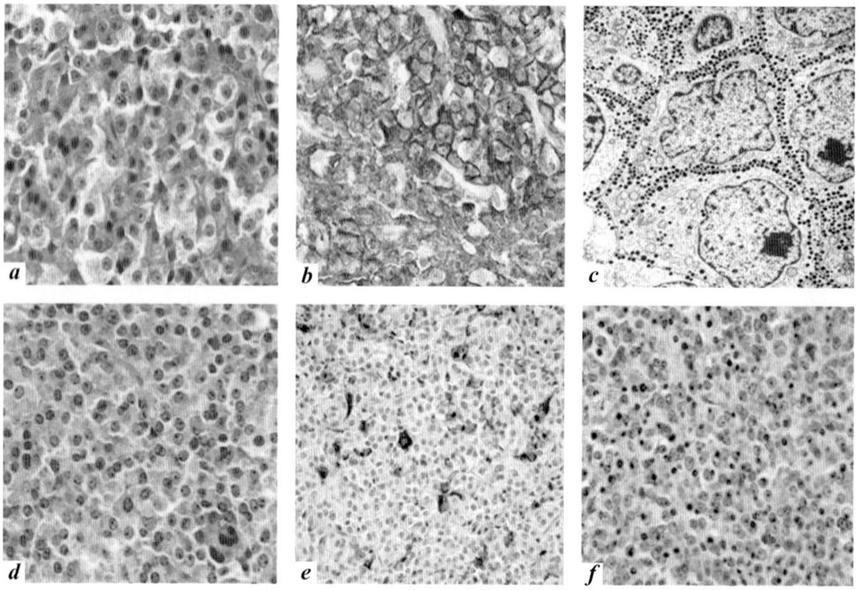

Fig. 4. Somatotroph adenomas. ***a–c*** Densely granulated GH adenoma shows cells with eosinophilic, granular cytoplasm (***a***), with strong immunoreactivity for GH (***b***), and the presence of large numbers of neurosecretory granules is seen by ultrastructural analysis (***c***). ***d–f*** In contrast, sparsely granulated GH adenomas are composed of cells with more chromophobic appearance (***d***), stain only focally for GH (***e***) and have a paranuclear 'fibrous body' demonstrated here by cytokeratin immunostain (***f***). ***a***, ***d*** H&E stain; ***b***, ***e*** GH immunostain; ***f*** cytokeratin immunostain.

8.7 years, and may be the cause for the relatively high proportion of these that present as macroadenomas (>60%) [31–33]. GH adenomas, though, are often confined to the anterior lobe of the pituitary gland, generally in the lateral wings where GH-producing cells predominate in the normal gland [34]. However, the majority of these tumors may present as macroadenomas with significant extrasellar extension, and have been thought to correlate with increased circulating GH levels [35, 36]. When encountered surgically, GH-producing adenomas are soft and loosely organized in texture, white to gray-red in color, and display varying degrees of invasiveness.

The histopathologic differentiation of GH adenomas began with the identification of acidophilic staining tumors removed from patients with acromegaly. Soon thereafter, conflicting findings of chromophobe adenomas among acromegalic patients led to the knowledge that classifying these tumors based on tinctorial properties alone was inadequate. Ultrastructural evaluation has confirmed the difference in density of secretory granules within these two distinct types of

GH-secreting adenomas. Likewise, immunohistochemistry has helped differentiate tumors based on their coexpression of other hormones. GH-producing adenomas are believed to derive from the acidophil stem line, a pluripotential stem cell under the influence of the transcription factor *Pit-1* that regulates the functional differentiation of the somatotrophs, lactotrophs and thyrotrophs [37]. It should come as no surprise that some of GH adenomas may possess an ability to secrete multiple hormones including PRL, TSH and α-subunit.

The admixture of varying morphologic appearance, histochemical profiles and ultrastructural findings have led to the division of GH-producing tumors into varying subtypes: densely granulated somatotroph adenomas; sparsely granulated somatotroph adenomas; mixed somatotroph-lactotroph adenomas; mammosomatotroph adenomas; acidophil stem cell adenomas, and plurihormonal GH-producing adenomas.

Densely Granulated Somatotroph Adenomas (fig. 4a–c)

These adenomas represent the classically strong acidophilic tumor associated with acromegaly. They display a diffuse growth pattern, with individual cells assuming a medium size and round or polyhedral shape. Immunoreactivity for GH is strong, densely granular, and uniform throughout the cytoplasm. A significant proportion of these tumors also show positivity for the α-subunit of the glycoprotein hormones. The most prominent ultrastructural finding is that of numerous, large, spherical, electron-dense secretory granules measuring 350–450 nm littered throughout the cytoplasm [24]. The ultrastructural features of these tumors resemble those of normal somatotrophs. They display a well-developed Golgi apparatus, rough endoplasmic reticulum (RER), spherical euchromatic nuclei with finely dispersed chromatin and distinct nucleoli.

Sparsely Granulated Somatotroph Adenomas (fig. 4d–f)

In contrast to the densely granulated variant, these chromophobic tumors assume a diffuse growth pattern and consist of small round cells with irregular nuclei that have conspicuous nucleoli. They display considerable nuclear and cellular pleomorphism, with interspersed bizarre cells seen frequently. Although these tumors may display a faster growth rate than their densely granulated counterpart, the atypia is not indicative of increased malignant potential [38, 39]. GH immunoreactivity is typically faint and focal. A diagnostic feature, which is highlighted by the intermediate filament cytokeratin immunoreactivity, is the presence of the juxtanuclear fibrous body [40]. Ultrastructurally, these neoplastic cells do not resemble those of the native somatotroph. The nuclei are often crescent-shaped with multiple indentations, and highly pleomorphic. Rough and smooth ER are abundant, and secretory granule size is small (100–250 nm) [24]. The hallmark feature is the presence of the globular fibrous body, located in the indented or concave side of the crescent-shaped nucleus, and composed of aggregates of intermediate filaments.

Mammosomatotroph Adenomas

These tumors, the most frequent cause of gigantism and frequently associated with acromegaly, are characterized by the production of both GH and PRL [38]. Light microscopic evaluation usually reveals strongly acidophilic, round to polyhedral cells with a round nucleus containing a conspicuous nucleolus. They display a solid or diffuse growth pattern. Immunohistochemical evaluation reveals the characteristic finding of intense cytoplasmic GH positivity and variable positivity for PRL within the same cells. Most adenomas also display immunohistochemical positivity for the α-subunit. Ultrastructural features of the mammosomatotroph adenoma are similar to that of the native densely granulated somatotroph cell. Notable exceptions include the pleomorphic dimensions of the secretory granules, up to 1,500 nm in size, and the presence of misplaced exocytosis, a feature indicative of lactotroph differentiation. Ultrastructural immunocytochemistry confirms the localization of both GH and PRL within the same secretory granules of a cell, and reverse hemolytic plaque assays have demonstrated the bihormonal secretion by individual tumor cells [39, 41].

Mixed Somatotroph-Lactotroph Cell Adenomas

The mixed adenoma consists of two distinct cell types, somatotrophs and lactotrophs. These tumors are in general, rare, but have invariably been associated with clinical manifestations of acromegaly and variable degrees of serum hyperprolactinemia [33]. The bimorphous nature of the tumor is visualized at the light microscopic level, where varying proportions of acidophilic (somatotrophs) and chromophobic (lactotrophs) neoplastic cells coexist. Immunohistochemistry clearly depicts the localization of GH and PRL reactivity in mutually exclusive cell types. Ultrastructural analysis typically reveals the presence of densely granulated somatotroph cells in association with sparsely granulated lactotroph cells, although the entire morphologic spectrum of somatotrophs and lactotrophs can be visualized in these adenomas [34].

Acidophil Stem Cell Adenomas

The acidophil stem cell adenoma is clinically a rare entity, accounting for less than 1% of all adenomas. These monomorphous tumors became a recognized entity on the basis of ultrastructural findings, and are assumed to be derived from the common precursor cell to somatotrophs and lactotrophs. Patients may present with minor symptoms of GH excess in addition to more commonly either hyperprolactinemia or mass effect from the rather invasive nature of these tumors (see also Prolactin Adenomas below). Light microscopic evaluation reveals a chromophobic adenoma with varying degrees of acidophilia, attributable to mitochondrial accumulation. Significant pleomorphism, coarse chromatin, and prominent nucleoli characterize the nuclear features of these tumors. The cells assume a diffuse growth pattern, and their cellular contents are noted for their sparsity in secretory granules. Large cytoplasmic vacuoles, sometimes reaching the size of the nucleus, provide for a characteristic honeycomb appearance on light microscopic evaluation, and represent the giant mitochondria visualized by electron microscopy. Immunohistochemistry displays PRL positivity, but not in the usual juxtanuclear, dot-like, 'Golgi' pattern that is characteristic of sparsely granulated PRL adenomas. In addition, GH immunoreactivity, if present, is generally faint at the light microscopic level. These tumors represent one of the rare entities that even after thorough light microscopic and immunohistochemical evaluation are completed, ultrastructural evaluation is required to confirm the diagnosis. Electron microscopy reveals the sparse and small (150–200 nm) secretory granules undergoing misplaced exocytosis at the lateral borders of the cell. The pathognomonic ultrastructural finding is that of accumulation of mitochondria (oncocytic change) mostly of giant proportions [34, 42].

Plurihormonal GH-Producing Adenomas

The plurihormonal nature of certain pituitary tumors was discovered through the methodical use of immunoperoxidase techniques and ultrastructural analysis, rather than through clinical association where these hormonal combinations are rarely relevant [38, 43]. Approximately half of all GH-producing adenomas exhibit plurihormonal features with PRL and α-subunit [33, 44]. The next most commonly reported combination is that of GH with TSH. This combination of hormone production has resulted in acromegaly or gigantism in association with hyperthyroidism [45, 46]. Nevertheless, these tumors for the most part, present with only one syndrome, the remainder accepting a silent role. The expression of any combination of GH, PRL, α-subunit, and TSH is indicative of the common precursor cell that gives rise to these mature functional lineages [37].

Prolactin-Producing Adenomas (fig. 5)

PRL-producing adenomas are the most common tumor of the adenohypophysis, accounting for up to half of all neoplasms in this location in both the pediatric and adult population [4, 47–50]. With the advent of primary medical management with dopamine agonists, the composition of surgical series has seen a precipitous decline in the ratio of prolactinomas [34, 38]. Adenomas that produce PRL include the sparsely granulated lactotroph adenoma and the densely granulated

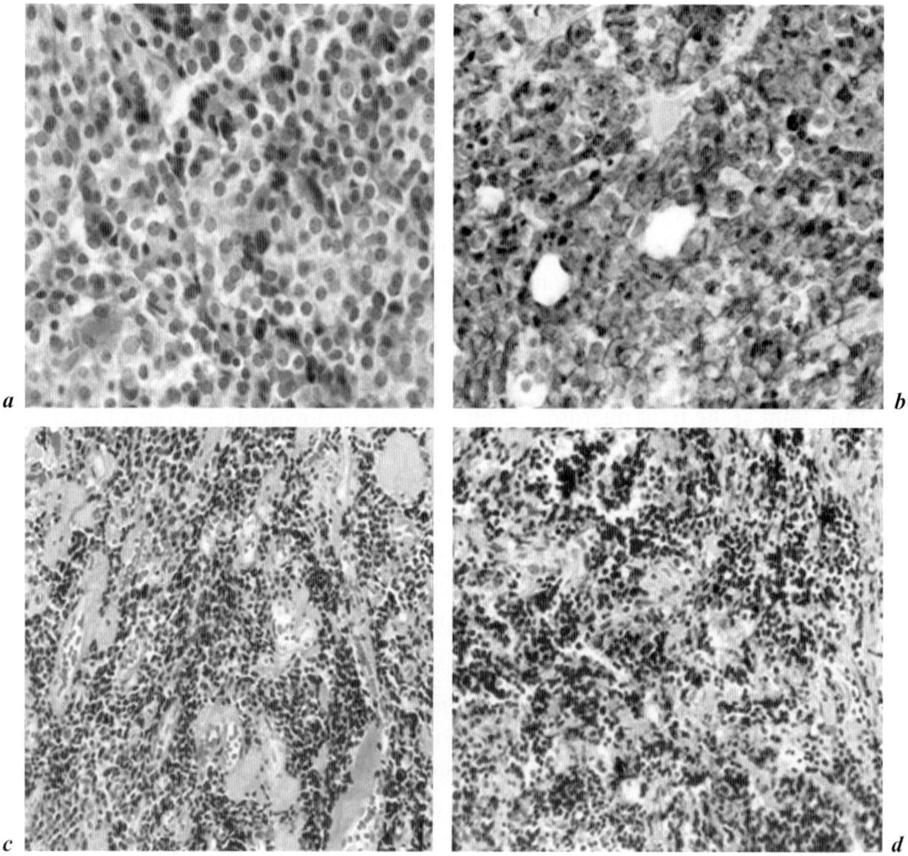

Fig. 5. Prolactinomas. ***a*** PRL-cell adenoma showing chromophobic cells with central nuclei with delicate chromatin. ***b*** PRL immunostain is typically seen in a paranuclear location ('Golgi' pattern). ***c***, ***d*** PRL-cell adenoma after medical treatment displaying shrinkage of the tumor cells and interstitial fibrosis (***c***), with only scanty PRL immunostain (***d***). ***a–c*** H&E stain; ***b–d*** PRL immunostain.

lactotroph adenoma, but also the acidophil stem cell adenoma, and the mixed somatotroph-lactotroph cell adenomas (both discussed above). The acidophil stem cell adenoma which biochemically and microscopically may masquerade as another type of prolactinoma, is an important clinicopathologic entity due to its relative resistance to bromocriptine therapy and rather aggressive behavior [51].

Sparsely Granulated Lactotroph Adenomas

Most PRL-producing adenomas are of the sparsely granulated variant. These tumors may display either a diffuse or papillary pattern of growth, with rare tumors exhibiting abundant connective tissue stroma. Calcification is common, and may be organized into calcospherites or psammoma bodies. If extensive, the tumor may appear as a 'pituitary stone' [52]. The tumor cells are of medium-size and the nuclei exhibit a salt and pepper pattern of chromatin arrangement. The tinctorial properties of these tumors are classically chromophobic, although slight basophilia associated with abundant RER and more commonly a small amount of acidophilia may be present.

Immunohistochemical evaluation with PRL reveals the characteristic juxtanuclear globular and granular staining referred to as the 'Golgi pattern'. The immunohistochemical profile of these tumors are generally devoid of reactivity for other adenohypophysial hormones, although rarely they may be positive for α-subunit [50]. Ultrastructural evaluation reveals abundant RER arranged in parallel rows and Nebenkerns (concentric whorls) and ample quantities of Golgi cisternae. Nuclei contain euchromatin with prominent large, dense nucleoli. Numerous immature secretory granules admix with mature granules with diameters ranging from 125 to 300 nm, the majority being 200–220 nm in size [38]. Extrusions of these granules along the lateral cell margins, into the extracellular space as opposed to the apical extrusion, are readily identified and termed 'misplaced exocytosis' [24].

Densely Granulated Lactotroph Adenomas

These tumors are rather rare in comparison to their sparsely granulated counterparts. Microscopic features are similar, but often the cytoplasm shows stronger stain of acidophilia. In sharp contrast to the 'Golgi pattern' of immunoreactivity found in sparsely granulated prolactinomas, the densely granulated lactotroph adenomas exhibit strong and diffuse PRL immunostaining. Electron microscopic evaluation reveals oval or oblong cells with oval or polyhedral nuclei. Well-developed Golgi complexes and moderately developed, well-organized RER can be found. Larger secretory granules (300–1000 nm) with average sizes between 500 and 600 nm are numerous [24, 38].

Dopamine Agonist Treatment and Prolactinomas

Currently, the majority of patients undergoing resection of prolactinomas have experienced some level of preoperative dopamine agonist treatment. Despite the efficacy of bromocriptine and its analogues in the treatment of prolactinomas, a subset of patients are unable to tolerate the side effects of medical therapy or harbor partially responsive or unresponsive tumors which may require surgical intervention. The effect of this treatment on tumor behavior, histology, and ultrastructure has been exhaustively examined. In the majority of prolactinomas, the cell cytoplasm shrinks and the nucleus displays hyperchromatic changes, resulting in an increase in the nuclear:cytoplasmic ratio [39, 53, 54].

Long-term therapy results in extensive perivascular and interstitial fibrosis. Ultrastructurally, the volume of RER and Golgi complexes are reduced, reflecting the downregulation of PRL synthesis and secretion [54]. Intuitively, prolonged exposure to these medical agents and the resultant fibrosis may make late surgery more difficult.

TSH-Producing Adenomas (fig. 6)

Thyrotropin-producing adenomas are a rare entity, accounting for less than 1% of all pituitary adenomas [55]. They are often associated with hypersecretion of TSH, resulting in goiter and secondary hyperthyroidism, or may present with subclinical hyperthyroidism discovered in hindsight and primary manifestations attributable to local mass effect [56, 57]. Although untreated primary hypothyroidism is typically associated with pituitary thyrotroph hyperplasia, focal neoplastic transformation has been rarely reported. In a patient with longstanding myxedema, protracted TRH stimulation has been suggested as a possible etiology for adenomatous formation [58].

The majority of tumors are macroadenomas exhibiting extensive invasion into parasellar and suprasellar locations. When evident symptomatology yields the diagnosis and discovery of a microadenoma, it may be localized to the mucoid wedge [59]. When encountered surgically, these lesions typically are more fibrous and firm, making tumors with significant extension rather difficult to obtain satisfactory results through operative intervention alone [57, 60].

The tumor cells are generally angular and elongate with indiscrete cell borders, and the cytoplasm assumes a chromophobic appearance with HE staining. Cells are generally arranged in a solid or sinusoidal pattern. Reflective of their consistency noted intraoperatively, these tumors on microscopic evaluation often exhibit stromal fibrosis. Scattered calcifications may occasionally form rare psammoma bodies [39]. Immunohistochemical analysis is positive for β-TSH and in the majority of cases for α-subunit as well. Electron microscopic evaluation reveals elongated cells with an eccentric oval nucleus, conferring a distinct component of polarity to the general organization of cellular contents. Abundant RER, prominent Golgi apparatus, and lysosomes populate the cytoplasm. Secretory granules are typically small (150–250 nm), vary in quantity, but have a unique localization in the plasmalemmar regions [34, 39].

ACTH-Producing Adenomas (fig. 7)

Adrenocorticotroph-producing adenomas of the pituitary gland are generally associated with Cushing's disease, but in a minority of patients the tumors may present mainly secondary to a mass effect and local invasion [61].

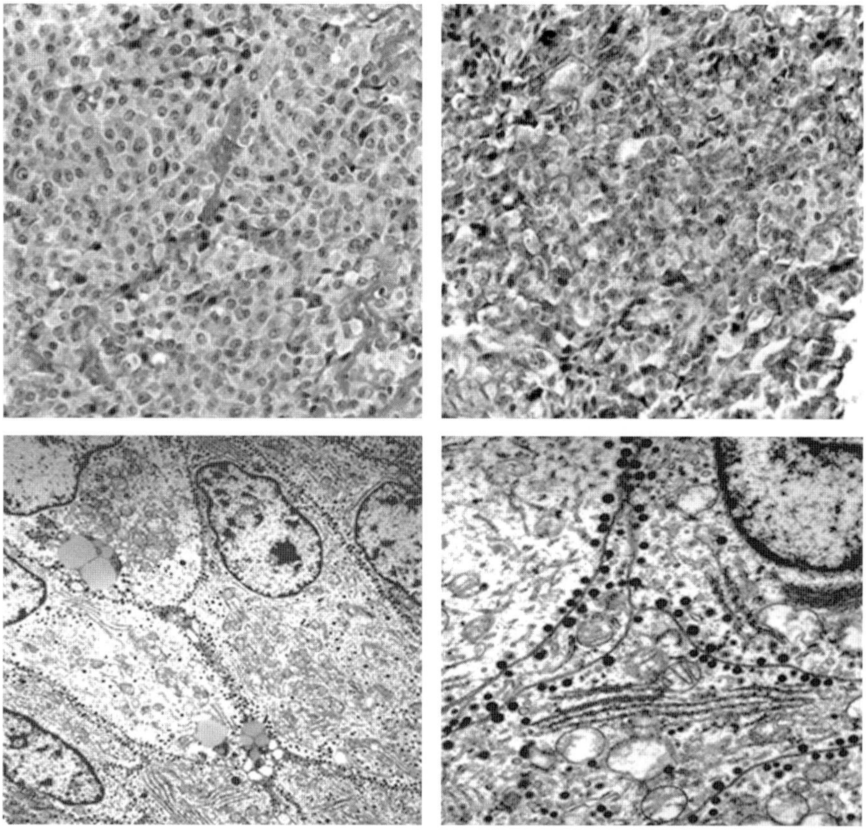

a b c d

Fig. 6. Thyrotroph adenomas. ***a*** Thyrotroph-cell adenomas are mostly composed of angulated cells with a central nucleus and prominent nucleoli. ***b*** TSH immunostain is relatively variable in the tumors, depending upon the differentiation of the cells. ***c***, ***d*** Ultrastructural analysis shows the angulated cells with prominent RER and numerous small neurosecretory granules preferentially located at the cell borders. ***a*** H&E stain; ***b*** β-TSH immunostain.

Cushing's disease encompasses the disease complex associated with anabolic and catabolic effects of hypercortisolism secondary to a pituitary neoplasm. Much less frequently, corticotroph adenomas arise in the setting of Nelson's syndrome which occurs in patients who undergo bilateral adrenalectomy. In general, the lack of end organ feedback inhibition presumably creates a trophic environment for the function and growth of an occult pituitary neoplasm [62]. Patients with Nelson's syndrome typically display an aggressive pituitary adenoma with an associated local mass effect in conjunction with hyperpigmentation

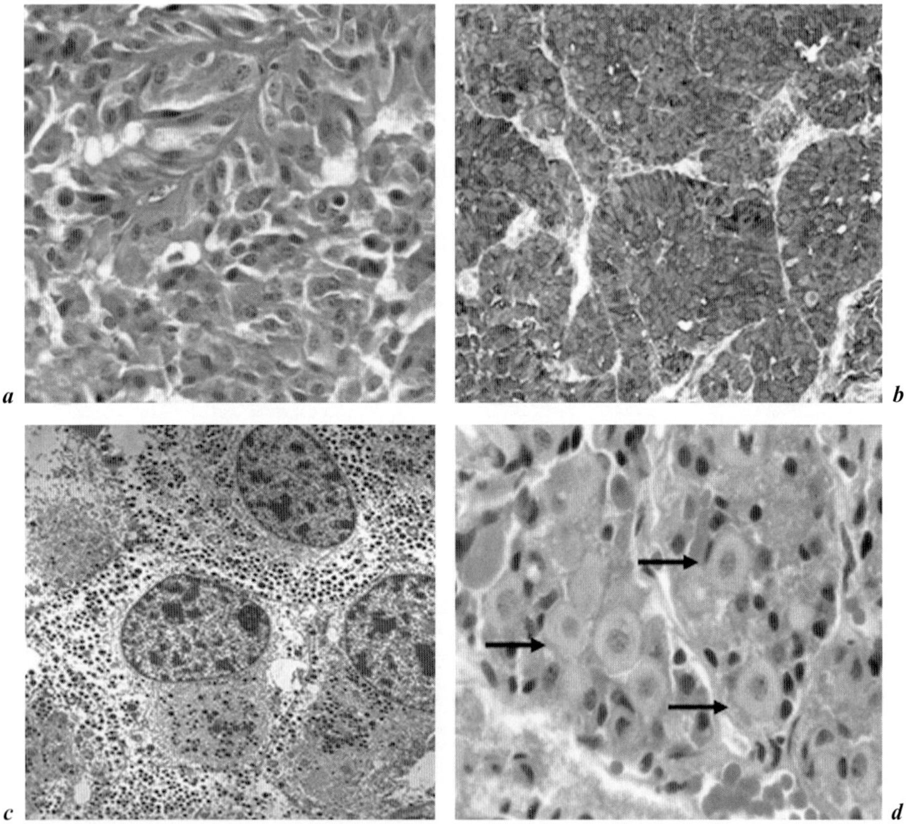

Fig. 7. Corticotroph adenomas. ***a*** A corticotroph-cell adenoma composed of large cells with angular, amphophilic cytoplasm within a papillary arrangement. ***b*** Intense ACTH immunoreactivity is present in the majority of the tumors reflecting the dense granular cytoplasm seen by ultrastructural analysis (***c***). ***d*** Crooke's cells are characterized by the accumulation of hyalin bundles in the cytoplasm (arrows) that represent accumulation of intermediate filament cytokeratin. ***a***, ***d*** H&E stain; ***b*** ACTH immunostain.

due to increased melanocyte-stimulating hormone production, a byproduct of increased ACTH production from division of the common precursor molecule, proopiomelanocortin (POMC).

Rarely, patients present without clinical or biologic evidence of hypercortisolism, but are found to have ACTH immunoreactive pituitary tumors [63]. These so-called 'silent' adenomas are distinct entities from functional adenomas. Typically found as macroadenomas, distinguishing these neoplasms and other types of nonfunctioning and null cell adenomas is of clinical importance since they behave in a much more aggressive manner [64, 65].

Histologically, the majority of functional tumors assume a sinusoidal architecture with a background of diffuse growth pattern. Staining is typically basophilic, but it is not uncommon to identify tumors with chromophobic tinctorial properties, especially among macroadenomas [25, 61]. A central nucleus with a discrete nucleolus is often encountered in neoplastic corticotrophs. Immunohistochemistry for ACTH and other POMC products (β-endorphin, melanocyte-stimulating hormone) are diffusely and strongly positive. Adjacent non-neoplastic corticotroph cells often display Crooke's hyaline change characterized by perinuclear accumulation of cytokeratin secondary to a chronic hypercortisolemic state [66]. Crooke's hyaline change can occasionally be found within neoplastic cells in addition to the suppressed non-tumorous corticotrophs. These tumors, classified as Crooke's cell adenomas, have been reported along a continuum of hormonal activity [67, 68].

Densely Granulated Corticotroph Adenomas

The vast majority of clinically functioning tumors share a common ultrastructural profile with normal corticotroph cells. The tumors are composed of medium-sized, angular cells with ovoid nuclei and a prominent nucleolus. The cytoplasm contains well-developed RER and moderately developed spherical Golgi complex. Dense secretory granules measuring 150–500 nm are numerous, and aggregate along the plasmalemma [39, 61]. The most striking feature is the perinuclear aggregates of intermediate filaments of cytokeratin [66]. These findings are helpful diagnostic markers, but are absent in patients with Nelson's disease [39].

Silent Corticotroph Adenomas (Silent Subtype-I and II Adenomas)

Silent subtype-I adenomas have similar histopathological characteristics to functional densely granulated adenomas with regard to light microscopy, immunohistochemistry and ultrastructural findings. Unlikely, the silent subtype-II adenomas do not share characteristics that are common to native corticotrophs. These tumors are composed of small, polyhedral cells that contain less well-developed membranous organelles, and secretory granules are fewer in number and smaller in size (150–300 nm). Intermediate filaments in perinuclear aggregates are notably absent [39, 61].

Gonadotropin-Producing Adenomas (fig. 8)

Gonadotropin-producing adenomas constitute a large number of nonfunctioning pituitary adenomas, and rarely are discovered secondary to their primary endocrine effects. This is chiefly because most tumors are hormonally inactive, and brought to clinical attention through symptoms secondary to mass effect, such as visual loss, hypopituitarism, and headaches [69]. The diagnosis

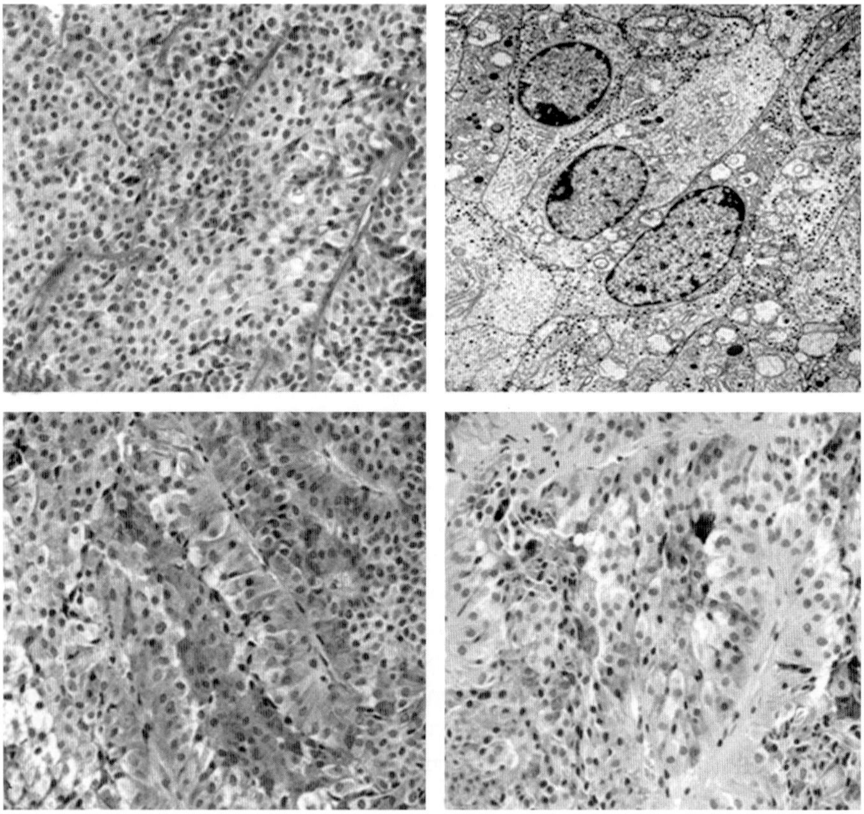

Fig. 8. Gonadotroph adenomas. ***a*** Gonadotropin-producing adenomas are mostly composed of chromophobic cells arranged in papillary-like formations. ***b*** Ultrastructural analysis shows elongate cells with small secretory granules and certain cellular polarity. ***c***, ***d*** Immunohistochemistry for the glycoprotein hormones is mostly reactive for β-FSH (***c***) and α-subunit (***d***). ***a*** H&E stain; ***c*** β-FSH immunostain; ***d*** α-subunit immunostain.

of gonadotropin-producing adenomas in these cases is by means of immunohistochemical and ultrastructural evaluation. Only a minority of patients harbor functional adenomas that cause dramatic increases in circulating levels of FSH, LH and/or α-subunit proteins [70, 71].

Due to the rather insidious onset of symptoms and limited systemic effects from gonadotropin-producing adenomas in the majority of patients, they often present as macroadenomas with extrasellar involvement. Gross evaluation reveals a well-vascularized lesion tan-brown in color, whose mucoid and dyscohesive properties aide intraoperative internal debulking and delineation of its borders from the compressed native pituitary glandular tissue, cavernous sinus walls, and diaphragma sella.

Light microscopic evaluation of tumors typically reveals elongated cells with polar features assuming a sinusoidal growth pattern, with pseudo-rosette formations around blood vessels [34, 39, 69]. Diffuse and papillary growth patterns may also be encountered [69]. The majority of cells are chromophobic, although moderate degrees of eosinophilia may be present. Immunohistochemical evaluation reveals positivity for β-FSH, β-LH, and α-subunit. Different regions within the same tumor may harbor varying growth patterns, which at times may correlate with regional differences in immunostaining profiles.

Ultrastructural evaluation reveals cells with uniform, ovoid euchromatic nuclei. Secretory granules measuring 50–150 nm in size aggregate along the plasmalemma and within long cytoplasmic processes. The cytoplasm harbors well-developed RER, and varying amounts of mitochondria. The Golgi complex shows marked differences among the sexes. In females, large, evenly dilated compartmentalization may give a pronounced honeycomb appearance, whereas males may lack this identifying feature [34].

Null Cell Adenomas (fig. 9)

Once encompassing all nonfunctioning chromophobe adenomas, these tumors have decreased in prevalence chiefly because of more stringent classification criteria as opposed to a true decrease in incidence. With the popularization of immunohistochemical techniques, it became readily apparent that a significant proportion of chromophobe adenomas, although nonfunctional endocrinologically, still expressed immunoreactivity for certain anterior pituitary hormones. Molecular and genomic analysis, reverse hemolytic plaque assays, and in vitro studies testing responses to stimulatory hormones have suggested that the vast majority of the remaining 'null cell' adenomas may truly represent nonfunctioning or very low functioning gonadotropin-producing tumors [72–74]. The addition of these techniques has shed significant doubt over the existence of null cell adenomas in general.

Null cell adenomas by definition have no endocrinologic, immunohistochemical, or ultrastructural features of specific adenohypophyseal cell differentiation. The tumors present essentially secondary to effect from direct invasion of adjacent structures or due to mass effect upon the native pituitary gland and stalk. In general, these tumors occur in adults, with a slight male preponderance. Biochemical evaluation targets evaluation of adenohypophyseal hypofunction and, if present, marginally elevated PRL levels secondary to 'stalk effect'. The majority of the tumors are macroadenomas with cystic and hemorrhagic regions. Cavernous sinus invasion, suprasellar extension, or sphenoid sinus extension are not uncommon.

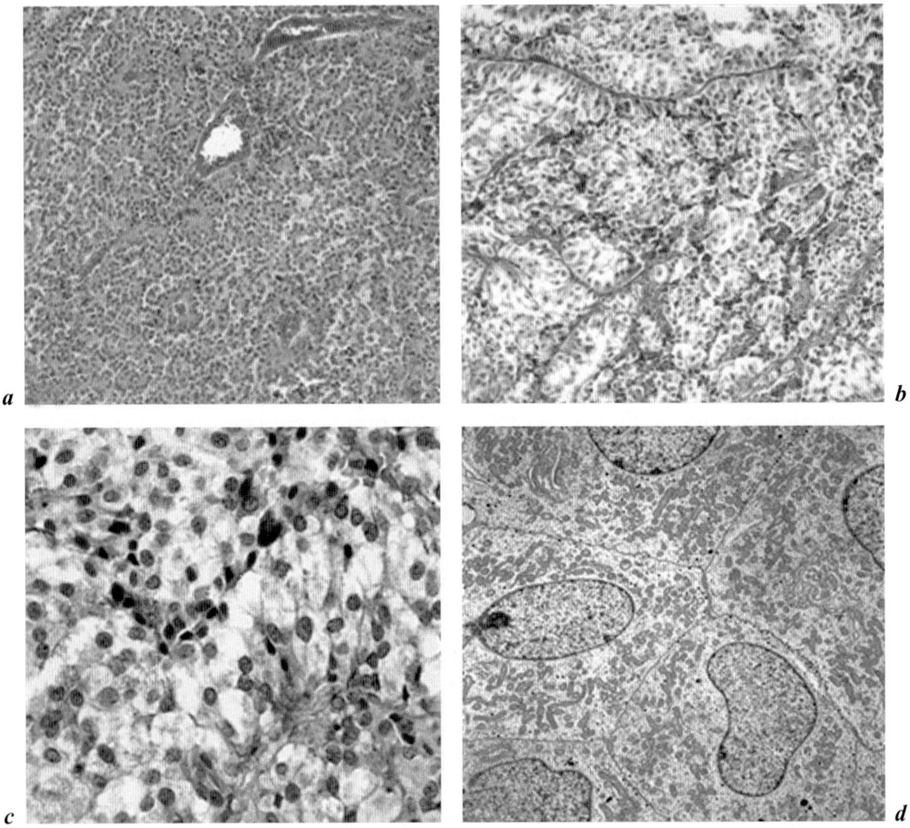

Fig. 9. Null-cell adenomas. ***a***, ***b*** Null-cell adenomas may have a number of histologic appearances including papillary formations (***a***) and nested patterns (***b***). ***c*** Immunohistochemistry may be weakly and focally positive for glycoprotein hormones. ***d*** The poor differentiation of the tumors is highlighted on the ultrastructure, and oncocytic changes characterized by numerous intracytoplasmic mitochondria may be seen. ***a***, ***b*** H&E stain; ***c*** α-subunit immunostain.

Light microscopic evaluation usually reveals relatively spherical cells in a diffuse pattern or polyhedral to oblong cells assuming a papillary or pseudopalisading arrangement. Tinctorial properties of these lesions are generally chromophobic, although eosinophilia may be quite prominent especially in cells with significant oncocytic change, which refers to the level of mitochondrial accumulation within the cytoplasm. When the neoplasm is constituted predominantly of cells harboring increased numbers and volume of mitochondria which constitute over 30–40% of their cell cytoplasmic volume, the lesion may be subclassified as an oncocytoma [34].

Null cell adenomas by definition lack prominent immunohistochemical reactivity and endocrinologic function. However, the identification of scattered cells with immunoreactivity for β-FSH, α-subunit, and less commonly β-LH is not uncommon [75]. Ultrastructural evaluation is reflective of the neoplasms' lack of protein synthesis for secretion. RER and Golgi complexes are poorly developed, and secretory granules are small, measuring 100–250 nm in size. The small secretory granules often display a halo effect, and localize to the plasmalemma, occasionally accumulating in cytoplasmic extensions [75].

Plurihormonal Adenomas

Plurihormonal adenomas arise from findings of immunohistochemical positivity for multiple hormones within the same neoplasm, not intuitively explained by normal cytodifferentiation of adenohypophyseal cells [76]. This does not include combinations of hormones which can be explained as the product of one cell lineage (GH-PRL-TSH, FSH-LH-α-subunit, ACTH-POMC derivatives). These tumors are generally rare, and when present, typically present secondary to mass effect. Hormone excess may occur, especially in the case of PRL, which may either be attributed to tumor hypersecretion or 'stalk effect'. Molecular and genomic evaluation may help clarify the origins of these lesions and predict their clinical behavior.

Atypical Pituitary Adenomas and Pituitary Carcinomas (fig. 10)

The mechanisms of progression of pituitary adenomas to more aggressive, invasive and recurrent tumors are not yet totally understood. A progressive continuum from typical adenoma to atypical adenoma and carcinoma has not been demonstrated in the great majority of the tumors. Most significant, the propensity of pituitary adenomas to locally infiltrate and invade adjacent structures seems disconnected to the histological features of the tumors. The WHO classification recognizes nonetheless that some adenomas have atypical morphologic features suggestive of aggressive behavior including invasive growth. Adenomas displaying features commonly associated with tumor anaplastic progression including pleomorphism, nuclear atypia, and elevated mitotic index are designated as atypical adenomas [8]. In addition, these adenomas have a Ki-67 (MIB-1) labeling index greater than 3%, as well as extensive nuclear immunoreactivity for the p53 protein [8].

Pituitary carcinomas are rare entities that have clinical presentations like their benign counterparts, typically with signs and symptoms of hormone excess in over 75% of patients, and in the remainder of patients present as nonfunctioning tumors with primary symptoms caused by mass effect. PRL and

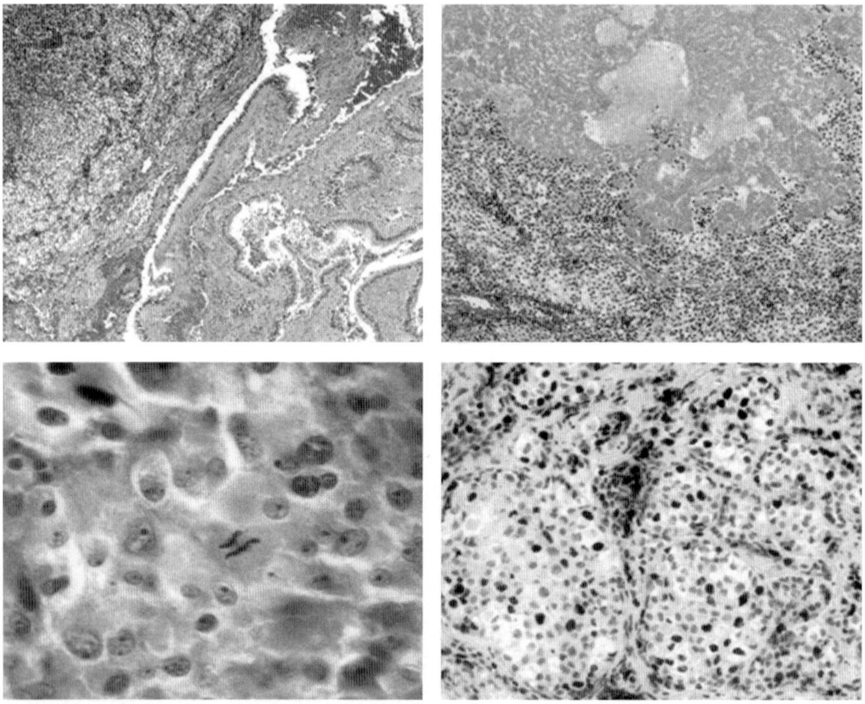

a *b* *c* *d*

Fig. 10. Progression of pituitary adenomas. ***a***, ***b*** Invasion of sinus mucosa and extensive areas of necrosis can be appreciated in this highly invasive null-cell adenoma. ***c***, ***d***. Atypical adenoma showing increased mitotic activity (***c***) and high labeling for the proliferative marker Ki-67 (MIB-1; ***d***). ***a–c*** H&E stain; ***d*** MIB-1 immunostain.

ACTH hypersecretion are most commonly found, followed much less frequently by GH, TSH, and gonadotropin production [77–79]. The hallmark of pituitary carcinoma is distant metastasis, whether manifested systemically or along the cerebrospinal pathways of the neuraxis. Pituitary tumors expressing significant tendencies toward malignant patterns of growth such as aggressive local invasion, increased microvascular density and brisk mitotic activity are not considered carcinomas regardless of their morphologic appearance without findings of distant metastasis. Trends toward increased microvascular density have been reported, but do not reach statistical significance, and thus are not a clear indicator and identifier of carcinoma [80]. Likewise, proliferative markers as reported by the immunohistochemical staining for Ki-67 (MIB-1), and histologic evaluation with mitotic figure counts have revealed significant differences among noninvasive adenomas (Ki-67 LI $<$1.37%), invasive adenomas (Ki-67 LI 1.7–4.66%; 2 mit/10 HPF), and pituitary carcinomas (Ki-67 LI 7.8–11.91%;

6 mit/10 HPF); however, overlaps exist in that some carcinomas have exhibited exceedingly low proliferative indices [77, 78, 81, 82].

Given this, diagnosis of pituitary carcinoma is a clinical and radiologic diagnosis, as opposed to one delineated by morphologic evaluation. Ultrastructural analysis tends to reveal less well-differentiated tumors, albeit relatively consistent with the immunophenotype of the composite cells [83]. Because disseminated disease is required for diagnosis, survival is generally poor, with mean survival of 2 years and an 80% mortality within 8 years from diagnosis [82]. Limited success has been achieved with surgery and adjunctive therapies, although occasional long-term survivors are reported [84].

Conclusion

The evaluation of pituitary pathology should not be restricted to a practice within a closed environment. Isolating the specimen from clinical presentation, biochemical assays, natural history of disease progression, and post-treatment course deprives us of important information required to make an expedited, meaningful, and helpful diagnosis. Any chance to identify relationships between pathologic diagnosis and clinical behavior must be captured and analyzed to improve our abilities to prognosticate in future cases.

The current WHO classification scheme is an example of an evaluation system that embraces most widely utilized diagnostic methods of evaluation. As our understanding of pituitary pathology grows, this system will likely become obsolete and reevaluation of current paradigms of classification will be mandatory. Morphologic differentiation of pituitary adenomas has reached its pinnacle with electron microscopy, and the focus of pathologists and researchers has turned to the comprehension of molecular mechanisms of tumorigenesis and functional regulation. It is through assimilation of these techniques into our classification systems that we can hope to continue to improve our ability to properly classify these lesions with respect to structure, morphology, function, and behavior.

References

1 Molitch ME, Russell EJ: The pituitary 'incidentaloma'. Ann Intern Med 1990;112:925–931.

2 Hall WA, Luciano MG, Doppman JL, Patronas NJ, Oldfield EH: Pituitary magnetic resonance imaging in normal human volunteers: occult adenomas in the general population. Ann Intern Med 1994;120:817–820.

3 Chambers EF, Turski PA, LaMasters D, Newton TH: Regions of low density in the contrast-enhanced pituitary gland: normal and pathologic processes. Radiology 1982;144:109–113.

4 Burrow GN, Wortzman G, Rewcastle NB, Holgate RC, Kovacs K: Microadenomas of the pituitary and abnormal sellar tomograms in an unselected autopsy series. N Engl J Med 1981;304:156–158.

5 Muhr C, Bergstrom K, Grimelius L, Larsson SG: A parallel study of the roentgen anatomy of the sella turcica and the histopathology of the pituitary gland in 205 autopsy specimens. Neuroradiology 1981;21:55–65.
6 Ezzat S, Asa SL, Couldwell WT, et al: The prevalence of pituitary adenomas: a systematic review. Cancer 2004;101:613–619.
7 CBTRUS: Statistical Report: Primary Brain Tumors in the United States, 1995–1999. Hinsdale, Central Brain Tumor Registry of the United States, 2002.
8 Lloyd RV, Kovacs K, Young WF Jr, et al: Pituitary tumours: introduction; in DeLellis RA, Lloyd RV, Heitz PU, Eng C (eds): World Health Organization Classification of Tumours. Pathology and Genetics of Tumours of Endocrine Organs. Lyon, IARC Press, 2004, pp 10–13.
9 Meij BP, Lopes MB, Ellegala DB, Alden TD, Laws ER Jr: The long-term significance of microscopic dural invasion in 354 patients with pituitary adenomas treated with transsphenoidal surgery. J Neurosurg 2002;96:195–208.
10 Selman WR, Laws ER Jr, Scheithauer BW, Carpenter SM: The occurrence of dural invasion in pituitary adenomas. J Neurosurg 1986;64:402–407.
11 Schmidek HH, Sweet WH: Schmidek and Sweet's Operative Neurosurgical Techniques: Indications, Methods, and Results, ed 4. Philadelphia, Saunders, 2000.
12 Hardy J, Mohr G: Prolactinoma: surgical aspects (in French). Neurochirurgie 1981;27(suppl 1): 41–60.
13 DeCicco FA, Dekker A, Yunis JE: Fine structure of Crooke's hyaline change in the human pituitary gland. Arch Pathol 1972;94:65–70.
14 Hardy J, Wigser SM: Transsphenoidal surgery of primary fossa tumors with televised radiofluoroscopic control. J Neurosurg 1965;23:612–619.
15 Velasco ME, Sindely SO, Roessmann U: Reticulum stain for frozen-section diagnosis of pituitary adenomas: technical note. J Neurosurg 1977;46:548–550.
16 Adelman LS, Post KD: Intra-operative frozen section technique for pituitary adenomas. Am J Surg Pathol 1979;3:173–175.
17 McKeever PE, Laverson S, Oldfield EH, Smith BH, Gadille D, Chandler WF: Stromal and nuclear markers for rapid identification of pituitary adenomas at biopsy. Arch Pathol Lab Med 1985;109:509–514.
18 Ng HK: Smears in the diagnosis of pituitary adenomas. Acta Cytol 1998;42:614–618.
19 Marshall LF, Adams H, Doyle D, Graham DI: The histological accuracy of the smear technique for neurosurgical biopsies. J Neurosurg 1973;39:82–88.
20 Komminoth P, Perren AA, Walch A, Werner M: Methods in cellular and molecular pathology; in Lloyd RV (ed): Endocrine Pathology – Differential Diagnosis and Molecular Advances. Totwa, Humana Press, 2003, pp 1–37.
21 Bailey P, Cushing H: Studies in acromegaly: VII. The microscopical structure of the adenomas in acromegalic dyspituitarism (fugitive acromegaly). Am J Pathol 1928;4:545–564.
22 Salassa RM, Kearns TP, Kernohan JW, Sprague RG, Maccarty CS: Pituitary tumors in patients with Cushing's syndrome. J Clin Endocrinol Metab 1959;19:1523–1539.
23 Scanarini M, Mingrino S: Functional classification of pituitary adenomas. Acta Neurochir (Wien) 1980;52:195–202.
24 Horvath E, Kovacs K: Ultrastructural classification of pituitary adenomas. Can J Neurol Sci 1976;3:9–21.
25 Kovacs K, Horvath E, Ezrin C: Pituitary adenomas. Pathol Annu 1977;12:341–382.
26 Labat-Moleur F, Trouillas J, Seret-Begue D, Kujas M, Delisle MB, Ronin C: Evaluation of 29 monoclonal and polyclonal antibodies used in the diagnosis of pituitary adenomas. A collaborative study from pathologists of the Club Français de l'Hypophyse. Pathol Res Pract 1991;187: 534–538.
27 Ezzat S, Melmed S: Acromegaly: etiology, diagnosis and management. Compr Ther 1991;17: 31–35.
28 Ezzat S, Strom C, Melmed S: Colon polyps in acromegaly. Ann Intern Med 1991;114:754–755.
29 Ezzat S, Melmed S: Clinical review 18: are patients with acromegaly at increased risk for neoplasia? J Clin Endocrinol Metab 1991;72:245–249.

30 Kovacs K, Lloyd R, Horvath E, et al: Silent somatotroph adenomas of the human pituitary. A morphologic study of three cases including immunocytochemistry, electron microscopy, in vitro examination, and in situ hybridization. Am J Pathol 1989;134:345–353.
31 Molitch ME: Clinical manifestations of acromegaly. Endocrinol Metab Clin North Am 1992;21:597–614.
32 Thapar K, Kovacs K, Muller PJ: Clinical-pathological correlations of pituitary tumours. Baillieres Clin Endocrinol Metab 1995;9:243–270.
33 Kreutzer J, Vance ML, Lopes MBS, Laws ER Jr: Surgical management of GH-secreting pituitary adenomas: an outcome study using modern remission criteria. J Clin Endocrinol Metab 2001;86: 4072–4077.
34 Kovacs K, Horvath E: Tumors of the Pituitary Gland. Atlas of Tumor Pathology. Washington, Armed Forces Institute of Pathology, 1986, series 2, fasc 21, 16–50.
35 Trouillas J, Girod C, Lheritier M, Claustrat B, Dubois MP: Morphological and biochemical relationships in 31 human pituitary adenomas with acromegaly. Virchows Arch A Pathol Anat Histol 1980;389:127–142.
36 Klijn JG, Lamberts SW, de Jong FH, van Dongen KJ, Birkenhager JC: Interrelationships between tumour size, age, plasma growth hormone and incidence of extrasellar extension in acromegalic patients. Acta Endocrinol (Copenh) 1980;95:289–297.
37 Scully KM, Rosenfeld MG: Pituitary development: regulatory codes in mammalian organogenesis. Science 2002;295:2231–2235.
38 Horvath E, Kovacs K: The adenohypophysis; in Kovacs K, Asa SL (eds): Functional Endocrine Pathology. Boston, Blackwell Scientific, 1991, pp 245–281.
39 Asa SL: Tumors of the Pituitary Gland, ed 3. Washington, Armed Forces Institute of Pathology, 1998.
40 Sano T, Ohshima T, Yamada S: Expression of glycoprotein hormones and intracytoplasmic distribution of cytokeratin in growth hormone-producing pituitary adenomas. Pathol Res Pract 1991;187:530–533.
41 Lloyd RV, Anagnostou D, Cano M, Barkan AL, Chandler WF: Analysis of mammosomatotropic cells in normal and neoplastic human pituitary tissues by the reverse hemolytic plaque assay and immunocytochemistry. J Clin Endocrinol Metab 1988;66:1103–1110.
42 Horvath E, Kovacs K, Singer W, Ezrin C, Kerenyi NA: Acidophil stem cell adenoma of the human pituitary. Arch Pathol Lab Med 1977;101:594–599.
43 Horvath E, Lloyd RV, Kovacs K, et al: Plurihormonal adenoma; in DeLellis RA, Lloyd RV, Heitz PU, Eng C (eds):World Health Organization Classification of Tumours. Pathology and Genetics of Tumours of Endocrine Organs. Lyon, IARC Press, 2004, p 35.
44 Osamura RY, Watanabe K: Immunohistochemical colocalization of growth hormone (GH) and alpha subunit in human GH secreting pituitary adenomas. Virchows Arch A Pathol Anat Histopathol 1987;411:323–330.
45 Beck-Peccoz P, Piscitelli G, Amr S, et al: Endocrine, biochemical, and morphological studies of a pituitary adenoma secreting growth hormone, thyrotropin (TSH), and alpha-subunit: evidence for secretion of TSH with increased bioactivity. J Clin Endocrinol Metab 1986;62:704–711.
46 Kovacs K, Horvath E, Ezrin C, Weiss MH: Adenoma of the human pituitary producing growth hormone and thyrotropin. A histologic, immunocytologic and fine-structural study. Virchows Arch A Pathol Anat Histol 1982;395:59–68.
47 Kovacs K, Ryan N, Horvath E, Singer W, Ezrin C: Pituitary adenomas in old age. J Gerontol 1980;35:16–22.
48 McComb DJ, Ryan N, Horvath E, Kovacs K: Subclinical adenomas of the human pituitary. New light on old problems. Arch Pathol Lab Med 1983;107:488–491.
49 Parent AD, Brown B, Smith EE: Incidental pituitary adenomas: a retrospective study. Surgery 1982;92:880–883.
50 Saeger W, Horvath E, Kovacs K, et al: Prolactin producing adenomas; in DeLellis RA, Lloyd RV, Heitz PU, Eng C (eds): World Health Organization Classification of Tumours. Pathology and Genetics of Tumours of Endocrine Organs. Lyon, International Agency for Research on Cancer, 2004, pp 20–23.

51 Asa SL, Kovacs K, Horvath E, Singer W, Smyth HS: Hormone secretion in vitro by plurihormonal pituitary adenomas of the acidophil cell line. J Clin Endocrinol Metab 1992;75:68–75.
52 von Westarp C, Weir BK, Shnitka TK: Characterization of a pituitary stone. Am J Med 1980;68:949–954.
53 Thorner MO, Martin WH, Rogol AD, et al: Rapid regression of pituitary prolactinomas during bromocriptine treatment. J Clin Endocrinol Metab 1980;51:438–445.
54 Tindall GT, Kovacs K, Horvath E, Thorner MO: Human prolactin-producing adenomas and bromocriptine: a histological, immunocytochemical, ultrastructural, and morphometric study. J Clin Endocrinol Metab 1982;55:1178–1183.
55 Bertholon-Gregoire M, Trouillas J, Guigard MP, Loras B, Tourniaire J: Mono- and plurihormonal thyrotropic pituitary adenomas: pathological, hormonal and clinical studies in 12 patients. Eur J Endocrinol 1999;140:519–527.
56 Smallridge RC: Thyrotropin-secreting pituitary tumors. Endocrinol Metab Clin North Am 1987;16:765–792.
57 Smallridge RC, Smith CE: Hyperthyroidism due to thyrotropin-secreting pituitary tumors. Diagnostic and therapeutic considerations. Arch Intern Med 1983;143:503–507.
58 Melnyk CS, Greer MA: Functional pituitary tumor in an adult possibly secondary to long-standing myxedema. J Clin Endocrinol Metab 1965;25:761–766.
59 Osamura, RY, Sano T, Ezzat S, et al: TSH producing adenomas; in DeLellis RA, Lloyd RV, Heitz PU, Eng C (eds): World Health Organization Classification of Tumours. Pathology and Genetics of Tumours of Endocrine Organs. Lyon, International Agency for Research on Cancer, 2004, pp 24–25.
60 Hill SA, Falko JM, Wilson CB, Hunt WE: Thyrotrophin-producing pituitary adenomas. J Neurosurg 1982;57:515–519.
61 Trouillas, J, Barkan AL, Watson RE Jr, et al: ACTH producing adenomas; in DeLellis RA, Lloyd RV, Heitz PU, Eng C (eds): World Health Organization Classification of Tumours. Pathology and Genetics of Tumours of Endocrine Organs. Lyon, International Agency for Research on Cancer, 2004, pp 26–29.
62 McNicol AM: Pituitary adenomas. Histopathology 1987;11:995–1011.
63 Horvath E, Kovacs K, Killinger DW, Smyth HS, Platts ME, Singer W: Silent corticotropic adenomas of the human pituitary gland: a histologic, immunocytologic, and ultrastructural study. Am J Pathol 1980;98:617–638.
64 Scheithauer BW, Jaap AJ, Horvath E, et al: Clinically silent corticotroph tumors of the pituitary gland. Neurosurgery 2000;47:723–730.
65 Webb KM, Laurent JL, Okonkwo DO, et al: Clinical characteristics of silent corticotrophic adenomas and creation of an internet-accessible database to facilitate their multi-institutional study. Neurosurgery 2003;53:1076–1085.
66 Felix IA, Horvath E, Kovacs K: Massive Crooke's hyalinization in corticotroph cell adenomas of the human pituitary. A histological, immunocytological, and electron microscopic study of three cases. Acta Neurochir (Wien) 1981;58:235–243.
67 Neumann PE, Horoupian DS, Goldman JE, Hess MA: Cytoplasmic filaments of Crooke's hyaline change belong to the cytokeratin class. An immunocytochemical and ultrastructural study. Am J Pathol 1984;116:214–222.
68 Horvath E, Kovacs K, Josse R: Pituitary corticotroph cell adenoma with marked abundance of microfilaments. Ultrastruct Pathol 1983;5:249–255.
69 Asa SL, Ezzat S, Watson RE Jr, et al: Gonadotropin producing adenoma; in DeLellis RA, Lloyd RV, Heitz PU, Eng C (eds): World Health Organization Classification of Tumours. Pathology and Genetics of Tumours of Endocrine Organs. Lyon, International Agency for Research on Cancer, 2004, pp 30–32.
70 Cook DM, Watkins S, Snyder PJ: Gonadotrophin-secreting pituitary adenomas masquerading as primary ovarian failure. Clin Endocrinol (Oxf) 1986;25:729–738.
71 Kovacs K, Horvath E, Rewcastle NB, Ezrin C: Gonadotroph cell adenoma of the pituitary in a women with long-standing hypogonadism. Arch Gynecol 1980;229:57–65.

72 Asa SL, Gerrie BM, Singer W, Horvath E, Kovacs K, Smyth HS: Gonadotropin secretion in vitro by human pituitary null cell adenomas and oncocytomas. J Clin Endocrinol Metab 1986;62: 1011–1019.
73 Jameson JL, Klibanski A, Black PM, et al: Glycoprotein hormone genes are expressed in clinically nonfunctioning pituitary adenomas. J Clin Invest 1987;80:1472–1478.
74 Asa SL, Bamberger AM, Cao B, Wong M, Parker KL, Ezzat S: The transcription activator steroidogenic factor-1 is preferentially expressed in the human pituitary gonadotroph. J Clin Endocrinol Metab 1996;81:2165–2170.
75 Sano T, Yamada S, Watson RE Jr, et al: Null cell adenoma; in DeLellis RA, Lloyd RV, Heitz PU, Eng C (eds): World Health Organization Classification of Tumours. Pathology and Genetics of Tumours of Endocrine Organs. Lyon, International Agency for Research on Cancer, 2004, pp 33–34.
76 Horvath E, Lloyd RV, Kovacs K, et al: Plurihormonal adenoma; in DeLellis RA, Lloyd RV, Heitz PU, Eng C (eds): World Health Organization Classification of Tumours. Pathology and Genetics of Tumours of Endocrine Organs. Lyon, International Agency for Research on Cancer, 2004, p 35.
77 Scheithauer BW, Kovacs K, Horvath E, et al: Pituitary carcinoma; in DeLellis RA, Lloyd RV, Heitz PU, Eng C (eds): World Health Organization Classification of Tumours. Pathology and Genetics of Tumours of Endocrine Organs. Lyon, International Agency for Research on Cancer, 2004, pp 36–39.
78 Ragel BT, Couldwell WT: Pituitary carcinoma: a review of the literature. Neurosurg Focus 2004;16:E7.
79 Kaltsas GA, Nomikos P, Kontogoergos G, et al: Diagnosis and management of pituitary carcinomas. J Clin Endocrinol Metab 2005;90:3089–3099.
80 Vidal S, Kovacs K, Horvath E, Scheithauer BW, Kuroki T, Lloyd RV: Microvessel density in pituitary adenomas and carcinomas. Virchows Arch 2001;438:595–602.
81 Thapar K, Kovacs K, Scheithauer BW, et al: Proliferative activity and invasiveness among pituitary adenomas and carcinomas: an analysis using the MIB-1 antibody. Neurosurgery 1996;38:99–107.
82 Pernicone PJ, Scheithauer BW, Sebo TJ, et al: Pituitary carcinoma: a clinicopathologic study of 15 cases. Cancer 1997;79:804–812.
83 Scheithauer BW, Fereidooni F, Horvath E, et al: Pituitary carcinoma: an ultrastructural study of eleven cases. Ultrastruct Pathol 2001;25:227–242.
84 Landman RE, Horwith M, Peterson RE, Khandji AG, Wardlaw SL: Long-term survival with ACTH-secreting carcinoma of the pituitary: a case report and review of the literature. J Clin Endocrinol Metab 2002;87:3084–3089.

M. Beatriz S. Lopes, MD
Division of Neuropathology, Department of Pathology, Health Sciences Center
University of Virginia, PO Box 800214
Charlottesville, VA 22908 (USA)
Tel. +1 434 924 9175, Fax +1 434 924 9177, E-Mail msl2e@virginia.edu

Laws ER Jr, Sheehan JP (eds): Pituitary Surgery – A Modern Approach.
Front Horm Res. Basel, Karger, 2006, vol 34, pp 236–255

Anesthetic and Critical Care Management of Patients Undergoing Pituitary Surgery

Catherine M. Burton, Edward C. Nemergut

Departments of Anesthesiology and Neurological Surgery,
Health Sciences Center, University of Virginia, Charlottesville, Va., USA

Abstract

Patients with tumors of the pituitary gland represent a heterogeneous yet commonly encountered neurosurgical population. Optimal anesthetic care requires an understanding of the complex pathophysiology secondary to each patient's endocrinological disease. Although patients presenting with Cushing's disease and acromegaly have unique manifestations of endocrine dysfunction, all patients with tumors of the pituitary gland require meticulous preoperative evaluation and screening. There are many acceptable strategies for optimal intraoperative anesthetic management; however, the selection of anesthetic agents should be tailored to facilitate surgical exposure, preserve cerebral perfusion and oxygenation, and provide for rapid emergence and neurological assessment. A rapid emergence from anesthesia is particularly important, as an early neurological assessment is necessary to evaluate cranial nerve integrity. In the postoperative period, careful monitoring of fluid balance and serum sodium is essential to the early diagnosis of diabetes insipidus (DI) and the syndrome of inappropriate anti-diuretic hormone (SIADH) secretion. DI is most often transient, but can require medical therapy. SIADH has a number of treatment options and decisions should be based upon the patient's status. A thorough understanding of the preoperative assessment, intraoperative management, and potential complications is fundamental to successful perioperative patient care and avoidance of morbidity and mortality.

Copyright © 2006 S. Karger AG, Basel

The multi-system nature of pituitary disease presents many challenges to the anesthesiologist. In addition, pituitary surgery and the resection of pituitary tumors have a unique set of possible perioperative complications. The successful anesthetic and critical care management of patients presenting for pituitary surgery requires a working understanding of the relevant pathophysiology and the possible implications of anesthesia and surgery.

Preoperative Assessment and Related Perioperative Concerns

Pituitary adenomas are commonly encountered in clinical practice and represent approximately 10% of diagnosed brain neoplasms. Various autopsy series suggest that as many as 20% of people may have a pituitary tumor on postmortem examination [1, 2]. Appropriate perioperative care of the patient undergoing pituitary surgery begins with preoperative assessment. Pituitary disease can present with a wide range of systemic manifestations and their recognition and diagnosis is critical to optimal patient care.

Although the overwhelming majority of pituitary adenomas are asymptomatic, most tumors present in three discrete ways: (1) hormonal hypersecretion; (2) local mass effects, or (3) tumors may be discovered incidentally during cranial imaging for an unrelated condition. Approximately 75% of pituitary tumors are 'functioning' and produce a single, predominant hormone. These patients typically present with the signs and symptoms of hormone excess. Specific symptomatology is directly related to the specific hormone produced in excess. Patients with acromegaly and Cushing's disease have unique anesthetic needs that will be discussed below.

The mass effects produced by pituitary tumors can be extensive and problematic given the location of the pituitary gland within the brain. Patients may present with varying degrees of hypopituitarism secondary to compression of normal anterior pituitary tissue by the expanding intrasellar mass. Indeed, 70–90% of patients with nonfunctioning pituitary macroadenomas exhibit deficiencies in at least one pituitary hormone with formal testing [3]. However, posterior pituitary dysfunction is unusual, even among patients with very large tumors.

In addition to compression of the pituitary gland, a pituitary tumor may affect the nearby cranial nerves. Visual loss, classically bitemporal hemianopsia, results from compression of the optic chiasm. Finally, like any patient with an intracranial mass, patients with a pituitary adenoma may present with the signs and symptoms of increased intracranial pressure (ICP). Although the most common presenting complaint of any patient with a pituitary tumor is headache [4], it is rarely associated with increased ICP.

All patients require thorough laboratory evaluation prior to surgery. Although transsphenoidal surgery is rarely associated with significant (>1,000 ml) blood loss, a complete blood count to determine a starting hematocrit/hemoglobin and other hematological abnormalities is indicated. It should be noted that men presenting with pituitary tumors and low testosterone have an increased incidence of preoperative anemia [5]. Coagulation studies including prothrombin time and partial thromboplastin time are not mandatory unless the patient has a history of bleeding. A metabolic panel to evaluate possible hyponatremia, hypercalcemia, hyperglycemia, and other metabolic abnormalities is indicated. Hyponatremia may indicate posterior pituitary dysfunction and the presence of diabetes insipidus (DI). Patients with Cushing's disease may present with a hypokalemic alkalosis. Patients with hypercalcemia are evaluated for the possible diagnosis of multiple endocrine neoplasia syndrome type 1. Hyperglycemia is indicative of impaired glucose tolerance and may be indicative of frank diabetes mellitus.

The endocrine evaluation of each patient should include a thyroid panel (thyroxine, thyroid-stimulating hormone), and serum levels of cortisol. Many patients will have hypothyroidism or low cortisol secondary to hypopituitarism and a mass effect of the tumor (as above). Overtly hypothyroid patients should have thyroid function normalized prior to surgery. Patients with adrenal suppression and low cortisol will require supplementation. Many patients will have a defective stress response to surgery and require perioperative 'stress dose' steroids. Patients with hypopituitarism may not effectively absorb orally administered corticosteroids in the perioperative period and parenteral administration should be considered [6].

Specific Perioperative Concerns in Acromegaly

Acromegaly results from the unregulated hypersecretion of growth hormone by the anterior pituitary. High levels of growth hormone result in the increased production of somatomedins by the liver, especially insulin-like growth factor-I. Approximately 98% of all acromegaly results from a pituitary adenoma.

Cardiac disease is the most important cause of morbidity in acromegalic patients [7, 8] and the most frequent cause of death in untreated acromegaly [9]. As many as 10% of newly diagnosed patients may have overt heart failure upon presentation [10] and 50% of untreated patients die before the age of 50 [9]. The most prominent feature of acromegalic cardiac disease is myocardial hypertrophy [7]. Echocardiography reveals increases in left ventricular mass, stroke volume, cardiac output, and isovolumic relaxation time [11]. Valvular disease is also common with as many as 20% of patients presenting with mitral or aortic valve abnormalities on formal imaging [12]. Valvular disease is closely related to the presence of left ventricular hypertrophy (LVH). Acromegalics frequently complain of heart palpitations and premature supraventricular and ventricular complexes are frequently observed [13]. Disorders of the conduction system, such as bundle branch blocks, can also occur [14, 15].

Even though cardiac disease is associated with the greatest morbidity and mortality among acromegalics, most physicians often first think of the obvious changes to the face and upper respiratory tract. High levels of growth hormone induce noticeable hypertrophy of facial bones. The mandible, in particular, becomes thicker and there is a generalized coarsening of facial features leading to the characteristic acromegalic facies. Growth hormone also induces changes in the upper airway. There is thickening of the laryngeal and pharyngeal soft tissues [16], hypertrophy of the periepiglottic folds, and calcinosis of the larynx [17]. Laryngeal stenosis [18] and abnormal vocal cord function may be present and patients may report hoarseness or changes in vocal tone, quality, or strength. These changes in upper airway anatomy can result in significant airway obstruction and respiratory disease.

Respiratory disease is the second most common cause of death in untreated acromegaly. Obstructive sleep apnea (OSA) can affect up to 70% of acromegalic patients [19] with a 3:1 male predominance [20]. Among acromegalics with history of OSA, a high risk of perioperative airway compromise has been clearly established [21]. Patients should be carefully questioned about symptoms for OSA including excessive daytime somnolence, snoring, or frank sleep apnea. The preoperative administration of sedative medications should be carefully considered, and only in the continuous presence of qualified personnel.

Specific Perioperative Concerns in Cushing's Disease

The unregulated hypersecretion of ACTH by a pituitary adenoma results in increased adrenal synthesis of cortisol and the clinical picture of Cushing's disease. The long-term exposure to excessive circulating glucocorticoids results in significant pathophysiology.

Systemic hypertension is frequently observed among patients with Cushing's disease. Indeed, as many as 80% of patients with Cushing's disease have systemic hypertension and 50% of untreated patients have severe hypertension with a diastolic blood pressure of >100 mm Hg [22]. Increased corticosteroids induce hypertension by a number of mechanisms including the increased expression of the angiotensinogen II (type 1) receptor [23], potentiation of inositol triphosphate production in vascular smooth muscle cells [24], increase in the hepatic production of angiotensinogens [25], and suppression of nitric oxide synthesis [26]. In addition, the mineralocorticoid effects of cortisol and hydrocortisone lead directly to sodium and water retention. The classic presentation of hypokalemic alkalosis is actually more common in Cushing's syndrome, especially with ectopic ACTH production. Regardless of the specific mechanism, patients with Cushing's disease exhibit an enhanced response to endogenous and exogenous catecholamines.

As might be anticipated among any group of hypertensive patients, the incidence of LVH is quite high. Using echocardiography, reduced midwall systolic performance with diastolic dysfunction can be observed in at least 40% of patients [27]. Disproportionate hypertrophy of the intraventricular septum has also been reported [28, 29]. On ECG, patients with Cushing's disease exhibit changes consistent with LVH. High-voltage QRS complexes and inverted T waves suggesting LVH and left ventricular strain have been described.

Despite resolution of many cardiovascular symptoms of disease upon successful resection of the adenoma, it is important to note that increases in cardiovascular morbidity and mortality persist for at least 5 years [30].

As in acromegaly, OSA is frequently observed among patients with Cushing's disease. The exact mechanism by which Cushing's disease causes OSA is a matter of some conjecture; however, a link between OSA and systemic hypertension has been well described [31]. Additionally, Cushing's disease induces characteristic fat depots over the cheeks and temporal regions, giving rise to the rounded 'moon-facies' appearance frequently observed. It is possible that these changes in head and upper airway anatomy also impact the incidence of OSA. Finally, centripetal obesity is commonly observed in Cushing's disease and a link between obesity and OSA has been well described. Regardless of the mechanism, patients with OSA are significantly more sensitive to sedative medications [32, 33], including benzodiazepines and narcotic analgesics. As such, narcotics and benzodiazepines should be used with great care and always during continuous monitoring by qualified personnel.

A link between endogenous and exogenous corticosteroids and insulin resistance has been well documented. It is estimated that up to one third of patients with Cushing's disease have overt diabetes mellitus and some investigators have argued that a high prevalence of occult Cushing's disease may exist among patients with diabetes mellitus type 2 [34]. The perioperative management of patients with diabetes mellitus has been well discussed in the literature, and will not be discussed further. Briefly, glucose should be carefully monitored and tested in the pre-, intra-, and postoperative periods. High blood sugar should be treated accordingly with insulin but one must always weigh the benefits of 'tight' intraoperative glucose control against the risk of severe, unintentional hypoglycemia in an anesthetized, unconscious patient.

Another manifestation of Cushing's disease is diffuse osteoporosis [35]. Pathologic fractures are common [36] and care should be taken when positioning patients intraoperatively. A myopathy of the proximal muscles of the lower limb and the shoulder girdle have also been described [36]; however, a change in the susceptibility to succinylcholine or nondepolarizing neuromuscular blockers has not been documented. Finally, hypercortisolism results in skin thinning [37] and the cannulation of superficial veins for intravenous access can be extremely difficult.

Intraoperative Anesthetic Management

The intraoperative management of patients with pituitary disease is based upon a thorough understanding of the disease processes as described above.

Anesthetic plans should be individualized, taking into consideration each patient's clinical disease and anesthetic history. Nevertheless, patients with pituitary disease may present unique challenges to the anesthesiologist. Cardiovascular and neurological monitoring may be indicated for some patients. In addition, airway management, especially in patients with acromegaly, may be particularly difficult. We will focus this discussion upon anesthesia for the transsphenoidal approach as it is much more commonly performed and has unique anesthetic considerations. Pituitary tumors may also be approached with a transcranial approach (classically, a bifrontal craniotomy); however, the anesthetic management does not significantly differ from that of other craniotomies.

Monitoring

The placement of invasive monitoring should always be based on each patient's preoperative assessment. Patients with acromegaly and Cushing's disease may present with significant cardiovascular disease and associated anesthetic risk. In addition, transsphenoidal surgery can be associated with significant intraoperative hemodynamic changes [38–40]. The combination of these two factors compels some anesthesiologists to routinely employ invasive arterial monitoring. Indeed, an arterial line provides for the early diagnosis and facilitates the rapid treatment of both hypo- and hypertensive episodes. Nevertheless, there is no evidence that excessive hemodynamic instability accompanies acromegaly in the absence of specific cardiovascular disease [41]. Consequently, the authors strongly believe that routine placement of invasive arterial monitors is not indicated. The authors reserve an arterial catheter for patients with poor exercise tolerance, patients with the signs and symptoms of congestive heart failure, or patients with documented cardiomyopathy. It should be noted that secondary to soft tissue overgrowth, blood flow through the ulnar artery may be compromised in up to 50% of acromegalic patients [42], especially in those with a history of carpal tunnel syndrome. In these patients, blood flow to the hand may be critically dependent upon the radial artery flow. Thus, radial artery catheterization may result in hand ischemia. Should an arterial line be needed in an acromegalic patient, the cannulation of alternative sites (e.g. femoral) for intra-arterial monitoring should be considered.

The placement of central intravenous access may be necessary in patients in whom adequate peripheral access is difficult or impossible. Nevertheless, the authors strongly believe that central intravenous access is almost never indicated for the sole purpose of central venous pressure (CVP) or pulmonary artery pressure (PAP) monitoring. Medical therapy is available to abrogate cardiovascular disease in most patients and should be initiated in any patient with cardiovascular disease significant enough to necessitate CVP or PAP monitoring. Should medical optimization be impossible secondary to the need for emergent surgery (increased ICP, pituitary apoplexy, etc.) or other medical comorbidities, it may be prudent to establish central monitoring prior to the induction of anesthesia. Although hemodynamic changes can occur at anytime during surgery, the induction of anesthesia and the preparation of the nasal mucosa by the topical application of vasoconstrictors often induces the most significant changes [38–40].

Airway Management

As noted above, airway management may be potentially difficult in patients with both acromegaly and Cushing's disease. Indeed, successful endotracheal intubation and management of the acromegalic airway can be particularly difficult [16, 43, 44]. Probably the most vexing aspect of acromegalic airway management relates to the unpredictability of difficult intubation [44]. Although, a high Mallampati classification (class III or IV) generally predicts a difficult intubation, a low Mallampati classification (class I or II) is still associated with a significant risk of difficulty [44]. Given that a difficult intubation may be impossible to predict, the authors strongly recommend the ready availability of secondary techniques should primary techniques fail. Awake techniques always offer the greatest margin of safety; however, it should be noted that flexible fiberoptic laryngoscopy can also be more difficult [45].

Airway management of patients with Cushing's disease and OSA may also prove challenging. Tracheal intubation may be more difficult [46, 47], especially in obese patients [48]. However, there are no data to suggest that a difficult intubation is any more unpredictable than it is in patients without Cushing's disease. Nevertheless, the prudent anesthesiologist should be prepared with secondary techniques available.

Patient Positioning and Preparation for Surgery

After the induction of anesthesia and tracheal intubation, the patient is positioned for surgery. Patients should be positioned in a semirecumbent 'beach-chair' position with the operative field above the heart to facilitate venous drainage and prevent venous engorgement. A degree of inclination of $>$25–30° is unnecessary. The neck is extended and the head is turned slightly to facilitate surgical access to both nares. Anytime the surgical field is placed above the heart, venous air embolism (VAE) is a theoretical risk. Although a 10% risk of VAE in the semi-seated position has been reported [49], a clinically significant VAE associated with significant morbidity or mortality has never been reported. As such, routine monitoring with capnography seems adequate.

Topical application or injection of local anesthetic and vasopressor solutions to the mucosal surfaces of the nose are commonly employed during surgical preparation. Cocaine may also be utilized [50], but most surgeons prefer lidocaine-epinephrine mixtures [51]. The resulting mucosal shrinkage facilitates surgical access and reduces blood loss from mucosal surfaces. Although the total systemic absorption of topical or submucosally injected vasopressors is relatively low, the routine use of relatively large quantities results in significant systemic effects [38–40]. Hypertension and cardiac dysrhythmias are the most frequently observed side effects. The profound systemic vasoconstriction that may result from the excessive use of vasoconstrictors can produce in significant increases in afterload. Myocardial ischemia has been reported in patients without coronary artery disease [40]. Hypertension is almost always transient and consequently patients should be treated with short-acting agents to avoid 'rebound' hypotension after the systemic effects of the vasopressors have worn off. Hypertension may be successfully treated with intravenous agents such nitroglycerin, nitroprusside, or phentolamine or by simply increasing the depth of anesthesia. The authors prefer to avoid Esmolol, especially in bradycardic patients, as the addition of a β-blocker in the presence of profound α-adrenergic stimulation can result in significant bradycardia and asystole.

All patients should have sequential compression devices placed during surgery. In addition to preventing venous pooling in the lower extremities that can complicate the semi-seated position, sequential compression devices also help to prevent deep venous thrombosis and pulmonary embolism. There are data to suggest that patients with Cushing's disease may have an increased perioperative risk of thromboembolism [52].

Anesthetic Technique

The selection of anesthetic agents should be tailored to facilitate surgical exposure, preserve cerebral perfusion and oxygenation, and provide for rapid emergence and neurological assessment. As always, anesthetic selection should also be based upon an understanding of the patient's anesthetic history, medical comorbidities, and neurological disease. Any anesthetic appropriate for intracranial surgery is acceptable for transsphenoidal surgery.

A rapid emergence from anesthesia is extremely important. The proximity of the pituitary to cranial nerves II–VI makes the assessment of cranial nerve integrity an early postoperative goal. Any patient with a change in cranial nerve function, especially changes in visual acuity, should be emergently re-explored or undergo intracranial imaging. The desire for rapid emergence makes techniques utilizing rapidly metabolized agents such as propofol and remifentanil, or inhalational agents with low blood solubility such as sevoflurane or desflurane, reasonable choices. Inhalational anesthesia supplemented with remifentanil may provide greater hemodynamic stability and an earlier neurological examination [53]. If remifentanil is utilized, it is important to provide transitional analgesia with a longer-acting opioid, otherwise emergence may be complicated by patient pain. Neuromuscular blockade should be maintained throughout the procedure as any patient movement during surgery could lead to significant patient injury.

Some surgeons will place an intrathecal catheter to add air or saline or remove cerebrospinal fluid (CSF) in order to manipulate CSF pressure and facilitate tumor resection. In patients harboring large tumors with suprasellar extension, many surgeons may inject intrathecal air to increase CSF pressure and outline the tumor for visualization with intraoperative fluoroscopy. If air is injected, it is important to discontinue the use of nitrous oxide to avoid an increase in ICP.

The intraoperative use of visual evoked potential (VEP) monitoring during transsphenoidal pituitary surgery has fallen out of favor. Although a small retrospective study indicated that patients with a preoperative visual field deficit who had intraoperative VEP monitoring have greater postoperative visual field improvements [54]; there has never been a study documenting the benefit of the routine utilization of VEP monitoring. Given the extraordinary sensitivity of VEPs to anesthetic technique and the lack of documented patient benefit, their use is both costly and unnecessary.

Transsphenoidal surgery is normally associated with minimal blood loss; however, the potential for catastrophic hemorrhage secondary to carotid injury always exists. Indeed, carotid artery injury is an infrequent but potentially fatal complication of transsphenoidal surgery [55]. Should arterial injury occur intraoperatively, deliberate hypotension might facilitate surgical repair of the injury. Large-bore intravenous access should be rapidly established and need for blood products should be continuously assessed. Often, postoperative angiography is essential to rule out pseudoaneurysm formation and to allow for endovascular techniques of hemostasis and repair. Nevertheless, arterial injury is a rare complication and venous ‘oozing’ from the cavernous sinus is a more common problem in clinical practice. Fluid restriction in order to reduce CVP and venous engorgement has not been shown to result in decreased blood loss. Tumor size and the presence of suprasellar extension seem to be the primary determinants of blood loss [56].

After successful resection of the tumor, a Valsalva maneuver may be utilized to test for a CSF leak. If a CSF leak is readily observed, most neurosurgeons will pack the sella with autologous fat before it is reconstructed. In addition, a lumbar drain (if placed before incision) may be used to control CSF pressure.

Acute Postoperative Care

The postoperative care after transsphenoidal surgery requires careful airway management as well as close neurological and endocrine assessment. Surgical complications following transsphenoidal surgery include bleeding, CSF leak, visual changes, and meningitis. Endocrine disorders including hypopituitarism and disorders of water balance (DI and the syndrome of inappropriate secretion of antidiuretic hormone (SIADH)) are commonly encountered. Each complication carries significant morbidity and vigilant postoperative screening is mandatory.

Airway

All patients are at an increased risk of airway obstruction after transsphenoidal surgery. Although uncommon, loss of airway patency can be associated with obvious morbidity and mortality. To tamponade mucosal bleeding, many neurosurgeons will leave nasal packs in place for variable periods of time after surgery. As any patient with nasal packs in place is an obligate mouth breather, care should be taken to assure oropharyngeal airway patency. Meticulous suctioning of the oropharynx for secretions and residual blood is critical. This can be especially important in acromegalic patients with a history of sleep apnea who have a high risk of respiratory obstruction [21]. Indeed, any patient with a history of OSA should be closely monitored. Patients who require nocturnal continuous positive airway pressure (CPAP) on a regular basis should have CPAP machines immediately available postoperatively; however, it should be noted that nasal packing may render CPAP ineffective [57].

Surgical Complications

Given the proximity of optic chiasm and cranial nerves (specifically II–VI) to the surgical field, a complete neurological examination, including visual fields testing and visual acuity should be performed postoperatively. Visual assessment is especially important when the transsphenoidal approach for resection of a tumor has been performed because it does not allow direct visualization of the optic chiasm, which could be directly injured from surgical manipulation or from heat injury [58]. Visual changes may also be the first sign of hematoma formation with compression of the optic chiasm. Any cranial nerve palsy or visual change should be immediately addressed with imaging or re-exploration. In addition, mental status changes should alert the care provider to the possibility of bleeding or hematoma formation. When complete resection of the tumor is not achieved, there is a possibility of residual tumor hemorrhage. This is more common after larger tumor resections. If it is known that the carotid artery was damaged during surgery, carotid angiography should be performed because of the risk of developing a pseudoaneurysm or carotid artery cavernous fistula. Additional vascular insults include carotid artery vasospasm, traumatic aneurysm, and subarachnoid hemorrhage [52, 58, 59].

Other postoperative complications include a CSF leak. If a CSF leak is present, patients will normally complain of postnasal drip, a salty taste in their mouth, or rhinorrhea. Often, symptoms do not become apparent until the nasal packings have been removed. If a CSF leak is suspected, symptoms can be provoked by asking the patient to flex the head forward. Suspicious nasal fluid can be evaluated for glucose or α,τ-transferrin (a protein found in CSF) [60, 61]. Patients with a CSF leak may have an associated 'spinal' headache similar to those following lumbar puncture. It is important to inquire about other associated symptoms such as fever, pain, and nuchal rigidity. Such symptoms are suggestive of meningitis and should not be overlooked. There have been rare case reports of a tension pneumocephalus after transsphenoidal surgery. This results from trapped intracranial air after surgical violation of the arachnoid membrane. Although uncommon, the diagnosis should be considered when headache or metal status changes are present [62].

Disorders of Water Balance

Disorders of water balance resulting from perturbations in secretion of antidiuretic hormone (ADH) are one of the most frequently encountered acute perioperative complications of transsphenoidal surgery [52, 58, 63–69]. Appropriate care of patients with DI or SIADH begins with an understanding of normal water balance and the control of ADH secretion.

ADH Secretion

ADH is synthesized in the supraoptic and paraventricular nuclei of the hypothalamus. After initial synthesis, the precursor hormone is transported down the axonal extensions into the posterior lobe of the pituitary where ADH undergoes final maturation to active hormone and is stored for future release [70]. Plasma osmolarity is the primarily stimulus for ADH secretion; however, other factors such as left atrial distention, circulating blood volume, exercise, and certain emotional states can also alter ADH release. Plasma osmolarity is chiefly dependent on the sodium concentration since it is the most abundant ion in the extracellular compartment. It should be noted that ADH is considerably more sensitive to small changes in osmolarity than to similar changes in blood volume. A 1–2% increase in osmolarity is sufficient to increase ADH secretion. Secretion is a rapid process with several-fold increases in hormone levels within minutes. Once ADH is released it binds to specialized V2 receptors on the renal collecting ducts and they become more permeable to water. This results in a significant increase in water reabsorption.

Diabetes Insipidus

The relative or absolute deficiency of ADH results in DI. After transsphenoidal surgery, DI can result from an interruption in the transport of ADH from the hypothalamus, from impairment of ADH release from the posterior pituitary, or from retrograde damage to the cell bodies in the hypothalamic nuclei. Thus, damage anywhere along the hypothalamus-pituitary axis can result in DI. When release of ADH is inadequate, the kidneys are no longer able to retain water leading to free water diuresis. DI has been reported to occur in up to 80% of patients after transsphenoidal surgery [52, 58, 63, 65, 67, 69–72]; however, it appears most cases are transient with only 0.5–1.5% of patients having persistent DI [52, 58, 61, 70–72]. Certain clinical diseases including a craniopharyngioma or a Rathke cleft cyst may be associated with higher incidences of long-term DI [73, 74].

In addition to simple transient and persistent DI, some patients will develop a 'triphasic' pattern of DI [75]. The triphasic pattern has often been described in the context of pituitary surgery [72, 76]. Initially, there is a transient phase that occurs within 24–48 h postoperatively consisting of the classic clinical symptoms of polyuria and polydipsia. Symptoms are due to inhibition of ADH release or secretion of a biologically inactive ADH-like peptide hormone. A restoration of normal urine output or even a picture of inappropriate antidiuresis representing an unregulated leak of ADH from degenerating neurons usually ends this first phase. This second phase of antidiuresis occurs about a week after surgery and can last for several days. Finally, there is a polyuric phase; this is thought to be due to axonal death and cessation of ADH production. Not every patient will experience this last stage, but, if encountered, it usually leads to permanent DI. Postsurgical DI typically manifests within 24–48 h postoperatively and should be suspected when there is a sudden onset of voluminous polyuria. If the patient is awake and alert, thirst will accompany the polyuria. For early detection of DI, it is recommended that urine output and specific gravity be measured routinely after pituitary surgery. Diagnostic features of DI are hypotonic urine (<300 mosm or a specific gravity of <1.005) and high urine output (as much as 4–18 liters/day). The plasma osmolarity or serum sodium can rise, but since the majority of patients have an intact thirst mechanism, they are often able to keep up with ongoing losses [77].

Confirmation of the diagnosis of DI is especially important in the perioperative period because of the ubiquitous clinical presentation. A variety of factors could be responsible for polyuria. Overzealous perioperative fluid administration may result in immediate postoperative polyuria. Osmotic diuresis, which could be due to mannitol administration, steroid administration, and hyperglycemia, can also result in polyuria and polydipsia. Indeed, patients with diabetes mellitus or functioning tumors associated with hyperglycemia such as Cushing's disease and acromegaly can have increased urine output from glycosuria [72, 78]. Patients with acromegaly can also demonstrate a robust physiological diuresis following successful tumor resection [79]. Finally, the administration of diuretics including furosemide and hydrochlorothiazide should be eliminated as a potential cause of

Table 1. Differential causes of postoperative polyuria

Cause	Comment
Iatrogenic perioperative fluid administration	Urine specific gravity typically >1.005
Diabetes insipidus	Urine specific gravity <1.005; rising serum sodium
Glycosuria	Elevated serum and urine glucose
Acromegalic diuresis	Urine specific gravity usually >1.005

polyuria. Knowing the patient's medication regimen, urine specific gravity, and plasma glucose level will help differentiate most causes of postoperative polyuria (table 1).

Once the diagnosis of DI is confirmed, granting the alert and oriented patient free access to fluid is the preferred initial therapy. Conservative management coupled with close electrolyte and urine monitoring is the most appropriate management strategy. When patients are unable to keep up with their fluid requirements or unrelenting urination is present (often interfering with sleep), specific pharmacologic treatment should be instituted [76]. Desmopressin acetate (DDAVP) is a synthetic analog of ADH that is available by multiple routes and is the pharmacologic agent of choice. It is almost entirely devoid of vasopressor activity and side effects are uncommon [77, 78]. Often only a single dose is needed. Additional administration of DDAVP should be determined by persisting symptoms. As noted above, DI is transient and self-limited in the overwhelming majority of cases; however, treatment with DDAVP may result in 'overshoot' hyponatremia that can be associated with significant morbidity such as confusion and seizures. As such, it is imperative that careful electrolyte monitoring is continued during treatment with DDAVP [68]. The development of permanent DI is rare and tends to be related to the site and extent of injury that occurs during surgery, reportedly resulting from more proximal damage to the pituitary stalk and cell bodies in the hypothalamic nuclei [72, 80]. Patients discharged on DDAVP should periodically (usually once a week for 3–4 months) withhold medication to determine if long-term treatment is required. When on a medication holiday, the patient should track the frequency of urination and if a patient can either sleep through the night or only urinate once during the night, treatment can be discontinued [60].

Syndrome of Inappropriate Secretion of Antidiuretic Hormone

SIADH has been reported in approximately 12–20% of patients undergoing transsphenoidal surgery and occurs when there is sustained release of ADH

Table 2. Potential causes of postoperative hyponatremia

Cause	Comment
Hypocortisolism	Check serum cortisol; blunted cosyntropin test
Hypothyroidism	Check serum free thyroxine
Diabetes mellitus	Elevated serum and urine glucose
SIADH	Low serum osmolarity and hyperosmolar urine; typically serum sodium <135 mEq/l
Cerebral salt wasting	Serum osmolarity increased or normal; decreased extracellular fluid

from the injured posterior pituitary regardless of plasma osmolarity [78]. In this scenario, free water intake exceeds free water excretion while the kidneys' ability to handle sodium remains intact. It is characterized by low serum sodium (<135 mEq/l), low serum osmolarity (<280 mosmol/l), and concentrated urine (greater than serum osmolarity) in the setting of euvolemia and normal renal, adrenal, and thyroid function.

When making the diagnosis of SIADH, it is important to distinguish other causes of hyponatremia, particularly those associated with pituitary surgery such as hypothyroidism, hypercortisolism, and diabetes mellitus (table 2). Another potential cause of hyponatremia is hypothyroidism, although this diagnosis is normally made with preoperative endocrine screening. Hypothyroid patients can manifest low serum sodium secondary to a decreased cardiac output that activates carotid baroreceptors, thereby increasing ADH secretion. At the same time, there is decreased clearance of ADH. Patients with a relative adrenocortical insufficiency can present with increased ADH secretion leading to impaired free water secretion. A random cortisol level can be drawn to determine if a deficiency is present. Diabetes mellitus, when poorly controlled, is another potential cause of hyponatremia. Hyperglycemia provides an osmotic load in the intravascular compartment that draws water from the intracellular space, leading to dilutional hyponatremia [81]. As noted previously, diabetes mellitus can be particularly prevalent among patients with Cushing's disease as well as acromegaly [60, 63, 78].

The diagnosis of SIADH cannot be made in the presence of severe pain, stress, or hypotension, all of which can stimulate ADH secretion regardless of plasma osmolarity [82, 83]. Pharmacological agents should also be reviewed as a culprit of hyponatremia. As discussed earlier, the treatment of DI with DDAVP can cause hyponatremia, as can other medications such as antipsychotics [70], narcotics [72], and NSAIDS [76]. Cerebral salt wasting, most often associated with subarachnoid hemorrhage [82–86], is a rare potential cause of hyponatremia following pituitary surgery [87, 88]. The key distinction to be made is that patients with cerebral salt wasting are clinically hypovolemic while patients with SIADH are always euvolemic (or slightly hypervolemic).

Perhaps the most helpful clue in distinguishing SIADH from other causes of hyponatremia is the time frame in which it occurs. SIADH typically manifests a week after surgery – generally much later than the other conditions described [67, 82]. Patients with SIADH may be clinically asymptomatic and hyponatremia may only be detected through the serum electrolyte panel. Others may have generalized neurological complaints, reflecting brain edema. Complaints can range from nonspecific symptoms such as nausea, headache, anorexia, and emesis to more severe manifestations such as lethargy, coma and seizures. Presentation is dependent upon the speed of serum sodium decrease and not necessarily upon the absolute sodium level; the level of serum sodium at which symptoms will appear cannot be predicted.

When making a treatment decision for the patient, one should consider the severity and duration of hyponatremia as well as the symptomatology. If SIADH is mild, then water restriction (800–1,000 ml/day) is an important first-line treatment and may be the only intervention necessary. If significant hyponatremia (<120 mEq/l) is encountered, treatment with hypertonic saline (1.8 or 3%) may be reasonable. It is essential to avoid rapid correction as pontine and extrapontine myelinolysis [57, 80] remains a potential complication. Reasonable correction rates are in the order of 1–2 mEq/l/h and should not exceed 25 mEq/l over 24 h. The addition of a loop diuretic can be considered an adjuvant in treatment, often enhancing the effects of hypertonic saline. Urea, which is also an osmotic diuretic, has also been shown to correct decreased serum sodium levels at a relatively fast rate [67]. Other pharmacologic options include demeclocycline. At doses of 600–1,200 mg/day demeclocycline decreases the sensitivity of the kidney to ADH, inducing a syndrome similar to nephrogenic DI.

Postoperative Hypopituitarism

Endocrine management in the postoperative period should consist of a team approach that includes both surgical and medical expertise. Following surgical decompression, recovery of nonfunctional as well as hypersecretory tumors is possible if normal pituitary tissue is still present. Very large or long-standing tumors may have limited recovery after intervention due to the fact that pituitary tissue has scarce regeneration potential.

As noted above, at least 70% of patients with nonfunctioning adenomas have deficiencies in at least one pituitary hormone [60]. It is critical to ensure an adequate amount of hormonal replacement for deficient patients. This typically involves glucocorticoid or thyroid hormone supplementation [89].

Outpatient follow-up is important for nonfunctioning tumors to determine the need for long-term pharmacological therapy. This is true for both the patient who was taking hormones prior to surgery and for those given supplementation after surgery. Approximately 27% of patients presenting with hypopituitarism experience postoperative normalization of hormone secretion [79].

In patients with functional pituitary tumors, neuroimaging and endocrine follow-up will determine if resection has been successful. Although it is ideal to consider the result of surgery in terms of cure, it may be more realistic to consider the outcome in terms of remission. This involves assessing hormone production by the specific tumor cell type. Surgery obtains remission in 60–70% of patients with acromegaly with success rates higher in resection of microadenomas than macroadenomas [79, 90, 91]. Patients who have prolactinomas resected can have normalized prolactin levels in up to 87% of the resected microadenomas and 56% of macroadenomas [79]. Optimal hormonal levels in patients with Cushing's disease have been achieved in 90% of resected microadenomas and 65% for macroadenomas [52, 79].

Patients with surgical resection of pituitary lesions need lifelong medical management and monitoring as indicated by clinical and endocrine findings. As noted, since there is a risk of tumor recurrence, pituitary function will need to be routinely evaluated even if normal hormonal levels are achieved.

Conclusion

Patients with tumors of the pituitary gland are commonly encountered in clinical practice. The complex nature of pituitary disease necessitates coordination between the endocrinologist, the neurosurgeon, and the anesthesiologist to optimize perioperative care. Many patients with pituitary disease will present with significant preoperative systemic manifestations, especially patients with Cushing's disease and acromegaly. Ideally, serious systemic disease secondary to pituitary dysfunction should be controlled prior to surgery. As much of intraoperative management is based upon preoperative assessment, it is critical that the anesthesiologist plays a role in the preoperative optimization of patients with pituitary disease. Successful intraoperative anesthetic management hinges upon the understanding of the patient's disease and the unique requirements of pituitary surgery. At the conclusion of surgery, rapid emergence from anesthesia is important, as early neurological assessment will facilitate diagnosis of the most common and most serious surgical complications. DI and SIADH are the most common postoperative endocrine complications among patients undergoing pituitary surgery. DDAVP may be useful in the treatment of DI; however, DI is transient and self-limited 99% of the time. Regardless, treatment of both disorders should be based upon a continuous assessment of patient status. All patients require long-term follow-up with an endocrinologist to assess for remission and the need for hormone supplementation.

References

1 Burrow GN, Wortzman G, Rewcastle NB, Holgate RC, Kovacs K: Microadenomas of the pituitary and abnormal sellar tomograms in an unselected autopsy series. N Engl J Med 1981;304:156–158.

2 Elster AD: Modern imaging of the pituitary. Radiology 1993;187:1–14.

3 Singer PA, Sevilla LJ: Postoperative endocrine management of pituitary tumors. Neurosurg Clin North Am 2003;14:123–138.

4 Vance ML: Treatment of patients with a pituitary adenoma: one clinician's experience. Neurosurg Focus 2004;16:1–6.

5 Ellegala DB, Alden TD, Couture DE, Vance ML, Maartens NF, Laws ER Jr: Anemia, testosterone, and pituitary adenoma in men. J Neurosurg 2003;98:974–977.

6 Jane JA Jr, Thapar K, Kaptain GJ, Maartens N, Laws ER Jr: Pituitary surgery: transsphenoidal approach. Neurosurgery 2002;51:435–442.

7 Matta MP, Caron P: Acromegalic cardiomyopathy: a review of the literature. Pituitary 2003;6: 203–207.

8 Colao A, Marzullo P, Di Somma C, Lombardi G: Growth hormone and the heart. Clin Endocrinol (Oxf) 2001;54:137–154.

9 Rajasoorya C, Holdaway IM, Wrightson P, Scott DJ, Ibbertson HK: Determinants of clinical outcome and survival in acromegaly. Clin Endocrinol (Oxf) 1994;41:95–102.

10 Damjanovic SS, Neskovic AN, Petakov MS, Popovic V, Vujisic B, Petrovic M, Nikolic-Djurovic M, Simic M, Pekic S, Marinkovic J: High output heart failure in patients with newly diagnosed acromegaly. Am J Med 2002;112:610–616.

11 Lopez-Velasco R, Escobar-Morreale HF, Vega B, Villa E, Sancho JM, Moya-Mur JL, Garcia-Robles R: Cardiac involvement in acromegaly: specific myocardiopathy or consequence of systemic hypertension? J Clin Endocrinol Metab 1997;82:1047–1053.

12 Lie JT: Pathology of the heart in acromegaly: anatomic findings in 27 autopsied patients. Am Heart J 1980;100:41–52.

13 Tachibana H, Yamaguchi H, Abe S, Sato T, Inoue S, Yamaki M, Kubota I: Improvement of ventricular arrhythmia by octreotide treatment in acromegalic cardiomyopathy. Jpn Heart J 2003;44: 1027–1031.

14 Kahaly G, Olshausen KV, Mohr-Kahaly S, Erbel R, Boor S, Beyer J, Meyer J: Arrhythmia profile in acromegaly. Eur Heart J 1992;13:51–56.

15 Rodrigues EA, Caruana MP, Lahiri A, Nabarro JD, Jacobs HS, Raftery EB: Subclinical cardiac dysfunction in acromegaly: evidence for a specific disease of heart muscle. Br Heart J 1989;62: 185–194.

16 Kitahata LM: Airway difficulties associated with anaesthesia in acromegaly. Three case reports. Br J Anaesth 1971;43:1187–1190.

17 Edge WG, Whitwam JG: Chondro-calcinosis and difficult intubation in acromegaly. Anaesthesia 1981;36:677–680.

18 Williams RG, Richards SH, Mills RG, Eccles R: Voice changes in acromegaly. Laryngoscope 1994;104:484–487.

19 Guilleminault C, van den Hoed J: Acromegaly and narcolepsy. Lancet 1979;2:750–751.

20 Fatti LM, Scacchi M, Pincelli AI, Lavezzi E, Cavagnini F: Prevalence and pathogenesis of sleep apnea and lung disease in acromegaly. Pituitary 2001;4:259–262.

21 Piper JG, Dirks BA, Traynelis VC, VanGilder JC: Perioperative management and surgical outcome of the acromegalic patient with sleep apnea. Neurosurgery 1995;36:70–75.

22 Ross EJ, Marshall-Jones P, Friedman M: Cushing's syndrome: diagnostic criteria. Q J Med 1966;35:149–192.

23 Sato A, Suzuki H, Murakami M, Nakazato Y, Iwaita Y, Saruta T: Glucocorticoid increases angiotensin II type 1 receptor and its gene expression. Hypertension 1994;23:25–30.
24 Sato A, Suzuki H, Iwaita Y, Nakazato Y, Kato H, Saruta T: Dexamethasone potentiates production of inositol trisphosphate evoked by endothelin-1 in vascular smooth muscle cells. J Cardiovasc Pharmacol 1992;20:290–295.
25 Mantero F, Boscaro M: Glucocorticoid-dependent hypertension. J Steroid Biochem Mol Biol 1992;43:409–413.
26 Kelly JJ, Tam SH, Williamson PM, Lawson J, Whitworth JA: The nitric oxide system and cortisol-induced hypertension in humans. Clin Exp Pharmacol Physiol 1998;25:945–946.
27 Muiesan ML, Lupia M, Salvetti M, Grigoletto C, Sonino N, Boscaro M, Rosei EA, Mantero F, Fallo F: Left ventricular structural and functional characteristics in Cushing's syndrome. J Am Coll Cardiol 2003;41:2275–2279.
28 Sugihara N, Shimizu M, Kita Y, Shimizu K, Ino H, Miyamori I, Nakabayashi H, Takeda R: Cardiac characteristics and postoperative courses in Cushing's syndrome. Am J Cardiol 1992;69: 1475–1480.
29 Sugihara N, Shimizu M, Shimizu K, Ino H, Miyamori I, Nakabayashi H, Takeda R: Disproportionate hypertrophy of the interventricular septum and its regression in Cushing's syndrome. Report of three cases. Intern Med 1992;31:407–413.
30 Colao A, Pivonello R, Spiezia S, Faggiano A, Ferone D, Filippella M, Marzullo P, Cerbone G, Siciliani M, Lombardi G: Persistence of increased cardiovascular risk in patients with Cushing's disease after five years of successful cure. J Clin Endocrinol Metab 1999;84:2664–2672.
31 Wolk R, Shamsuzzaman AS, Somers VK: Obesity, sleep apnea, and hypertension. Hypertension 2003;42:1067–1074.
32 Boushra NN: Anaesthetic management of patients with sleep apnoea syndrome. Can J Anaesth 1996;43:599–616.
33 Ostermeier AM, Roizen MF, Hautkappe M, Klock PA, Klafta JM: Three sudden postoperative respiratory arrests associated with epidural opioids in patients with sleep apnea. Anesth Analg 1997;85:452–460.
34 Catargi B, Rigalleau V, Poussin A, Ronci-Chaix N, Bex V, Vergnot V, Gin H, Roger P, Tabarin A: Occult Cushing's syndrome in type-2 diabetes. J Clin Endocrinol Metab 2003;88:5808–5813.
35 Kaltsas G, Manetti L, Grossman AB: Osteoporosis in Cushing's syndrome; in Giustina A, Angeli A, Canalis E, Manelli F (eds): Glucocoticoid-Induced Osteoporosis. Front Horm Res. Basel, Karger, 2002, vol 30, pp 60–72.
36 Ross EJ, Linch DC: Cushing's syndrome – killing disease: discriminatory value of signs and symptoms aiding early diagnosis. Lancet 1982;ii:646–649.
37 Ferguson JK, Donald RA, Weston TS, Espiner EA: Skin thickness in patients with acromegaly and Cushing's syndrome and response to treatment. Clin Endocrinol (Oxf) 1983;18:347–353.
38 Keegan MT, Atkinson JL, Kasperbauer JL, Lanier WL: Exaggerated hemodynamic responses to nasal injection and awakening from anesthesia in a Cushingoid patient having transsphenoidal hypophysectomy. J Neurosurg Anesthesiol 2000;12:225–229.
39 Pasternak J, Atkison J, Kasperbauer J, Lanier W: Hemodynamic responses to epinephrine-containing local anesthetic injection and to emergence from general anesthesia in transsphenoidal hypophysectomy patients. J Neurosurg Anesthesiol 2004;16:189–195.
40 Chelliah YR, Manninen PH: Hazards of epinephrine in transsphenoidal pituitary surgery. J Neurosurg Anesthesiol 2002;14:43–46.
41 Seidman PA, Kofke WA, Policare R, Young M: Anaesthetic complications of acromegaly. Br J Anaesth 2000;84:179–182.
42 Campkin TV: Radial artery cannulation. Potential hazard in patients with acromegaly. Anaesthesia 1980;35:1008–1009.
43 Messick JM Jr, Cucchiara RF, Faust RJ: Airway management in patients with acromegaly. Anesthesiology 1982;56:157.
44 Schmitt H, Buchfelder M, Radespiel-Troger M, Fahlbusch R: Difficult intubation in acromegalic patients: incidence and predictability. Anesthesiology 2000;93:110–114.
45 Hakala P, Randell T, Valli H: Laryngoscopy and fibreoptic intubation in acromegalic patients. Br J Anaesth 1998;80:345–347.

46 Siyam MA, Benhamou D: Difficult endotracheal intubation in patients with sleep apnea syndrome. Anesth Analg 2002;95:1098–1102.
47 Hiremath AS, Hillman DR, James AL, Noffsinger WJ, Platt PR, Singer SL: Relationship between difficult tracheal intubation and obstructive sleep apnoea. Br J Anaesth 1998;80:606–611.
48 Juvin P, Lavaut E, Dupont H, Lefevre P, Demetriou M, Dumoulin JL, Desmonts JM: Difficult tracheal intubation is more common in obese than in lean patients. Anesth Analg 2003;97: 595–600.
49 Newfield P, Albin MS, Chestnut JS, Maroon J: Air embolism during trans-sphenoidal pituitary operations. Neurosurgery 1978;2:39–42.
50 Fleming JA, Byck R, Barash PG: Pharmacology and therapeutic applications of cocaine. Anesthesiology 1990;73:518–531.
51 Kasemsuwan L, Griffiths MV: Lignocaine with adrenaline: is it as effective as cocaine in rhinological practice? Clin Otolaryngol Allied Sci 1996;21:127–129.
52 Semple PL, Laws ER Jr: Complications in a contemporary series of patients who underwent transsphenoidal surgery for Cushing's disease. J Neurosurg 1999;91:175–179.
53 Gemma M, Tommasino C, Cozzi S, Narcisi S, Mortini P, Losa M, Soldarini A: Remifentanil provides hemodynamic stability and faster awakening time in transsphenoidal surgery. Anesth Analg 2002;94:163–168.
54 Chacko AG, Babu KS, Chandy MJ: Value of visual evoked potential monitoring during transsphenoidal pituitary surgery. Br J Neurosurg 1996;10:275–278.
55 Fukushima T, Maroon JC: Repair of carotid artery perforations during transsphenoidal surgery. Surg Neurol 1998;50:174–177.
56 Lee HW, Caldwell JE, Wilson CB, Dodson B, Howley J: Venous bleeding during transsphenoidal surgery: its association with pre- and intraoperative factors and with cavernous sinus and central venous pressures. Anesth Analg 1997;84:545–550.
57 Smith M, Hirsch NP: Pituitary disease and anaesthesia. Br J Anaesth 2000;85:3–14.
58 Ciric I, Ragin A, Baumgartner C, Pierce D: Complications of transsphenoidal surgery: results of a national survey, review of the literature, and personal experience. Neurosurgery 1997;40: 225–237.
59 Ahuja A, Guterman L, Hopkines L: Carotid cavernous fistula and flase aneurysm of the cavernous carotid artery. Complications of transsphenoidal surgery. Neurosurgery 1992;31:774–779.
60 Vance ML: Perioperative managmenet of patients undergoing pituitary surgery. Endocrinol Metab Clin North Am 2003;32:355–365.
61 Black PM, Zervas NT Candia GL: Incidence and management of complications of transsphenoidal operation for pituitary adenomas. Neurosurgery 1987;20:920–924.
62 Sawka A, Aniszewski J, Young W, Nippoldt T, Yanez P, Ebersold M: Tension pneumocranium, a rare complication of transsphenoidal pituitary surgery: Mayo clinic experience 1976–1998. J Clin Endocrinol Metab 1999;84:4731–4734.
63 Olson BR, Gumowski J, Rubino D, Oldfield EH: Pathophysiology of hyponatremia after transsphenoidal pituitary surgery. J Neurosurg 1997;87:499–507.
64 Olson BR, Rubino D, Gumowski J, Oldfield EH: Isolated hyponatremia after transsphenoidal pituitary surgery. J Clin Endocrinol Metab 1995;80:85–91.
65 Sane T, Rantakari K, Poranen A, Tahtela R, Valimaki M, Pelkonen R: Hyponatremia after transsphenoidal surgery for pituitary tumors. J Clin Endocrinol Metab 1994;79:1395–1398.
66 Wei T, Zuyuan R, Changbao S, Renzhi W, Yi Y, Wenbin M: Hyponatremia after transspheniodal surgery of pituitary adenoma. Chin Med Sci J 2003;18:120–123.
67 Kelly DF, Laws ER Jr, Fossett D: Delayed hyponatremia after transsphenoidal surgery for pituitary adenoma. Report of nine cases. J Neurosurg 1995;83:363–367.
68 Seckl J, Dunger D: Postoperative diabetes insipidus. BMJ 1989;298:2–3.
69 Partington MD, Davis DH, Laws ER Jr, Scheithauer BW: Pituitary adenomas in childhood and adolescence. Results of transsphenoidal surgery. J Neurosurg 1994;80:209–216.
70 Singer PA, Sevilla LJ: Postoperative endocrine management of pituitary tumors. Neurosurg Clin North Am 2003;14:123–138.
71 Wilson CB, Dempsey LC: Transsphenoidal microsurgical removal of 250 pituitary adenomas. J Neurosurg 1978;48:13–22.

72 Hensen J, Henig A, Fahlbusch R, Meyer M, Boehnert M, Buchfelder M: Prevalence, predictors and patterns of postoperative polyuria and hyponatraemia in the immediate course after transsphenoidal surgery for pituitary adenomas. Clin Endocrinol (Oxf) 1999;50:431–439.
73 el-Mahdy W, Powell M: Transsphenoidal management of 28 symptomatic Rathke's cleft cysts, with special reference to visual and hormonal recovery. Neurosurgery 1998;42:7–16.
74 Lehrnbecher T, Muller-Scholden J, Danhauser-Leistner I, Sorensen N, von Stockhausen H-B: Perioperative fluid and electrolyte management in children undergoing surgery for craniopharyngioma. Childs Nerv Syst 1998;14:276–279.
75 Fisher C, Ingram WR: The effect of interruption of the supraoptico-hypophyseal tracts on the antidiuretic, pressor and oxytocic activity of the posterior lobe of the hypophysis. Endocrinology 1936;20:762–768.
76 Verbalis J: Management of disorders of water metabolism in patients with pituitary tumors. Pituitary 2002;5:119–132.
77 Cusick J, Hagen T, Findling J: Inappropriate secretion of antidiuretic hormone after transsphenoidal surgery for pituitary tumors. N Engl J Med 1984;311:36–38.
78 Singer I, Oster JR, Fishman LM: The management of diabetes insipidus in adults. Arch Intern Med 1997;157:1293–1301.
79 Jane JA Jr, Laws ER Jr: The surgical management of pituitary adenomas in a series of 3,093 patients. J Am Coll Surg 2001;193:651–659.
80 Cole C, Gottfried O, Liu J, Couldwell W: Hyponatremia in neurosurgical patient: diagnosis and management. Neurosurg Focus 2004;16:E9.
81 Hillier TA, Abbott RD, Barrett EJ: Hyponatremia: evaluating the correction factor for hyperglycemia. Am J Med 1999;106:399–403.
82 Harrigan MR: Cerebral salt wasting syndrome: a review. Neurosurgery 1996;38:152–160.
83 Harrigan MR: Cerebral salt wasting syndrome. Crit Care Clin 2001;17:125–138.
84 Gross PA, Pehrisch H, Rascher W, Schomig A, Hackenthal E, Ritz E: Pathogenesis of clinical hyponatremia: observations of vasopressin and fluid intake in 100 hyponatremic medical patients. Eur J Clin Invest 1987;17:123–129.
85 Wijdicks EF, Vermeulen M, Hijdra A, van Gijn J: Hyponatremia and cerebral infarction in patients with ruptured intracranial aneurysms: is fluid restriction harmful? Ann Neurol 1985;17:137–140.
86 Wijdicks EF, Ropper AH, Hunnicutt EJ, Richardson GS, Nathanson JA: Atrial natriuretic factor and salt wasting after aneurysmal subarachnoid hemorrhage. Stroke 1991;22:1519–1524.
87 Atkin SL, Coady AM, White MC, Mathew B: Hyponatraemia secondary to cerebral salt wasting syndrome following routine pituitary surgery. Eur J Endocrinol 1996;135:245–247.
88 Andrews BT, Fitzgerald PA, Tyrell JB, Wilson CB: Cerebral salt wasting after pituitary exploration and biopsy: case report. Neurosurgery 1986;18:469–471.
89 Warrick I, Hunt P: Glucocorticoid replacement in pituitary surgery: guidelines for perioperative assessment and management. J Clin Endocrinol Metab 2002;87:2745–2750.
90 Kreutzer J, Vance ML, Lopes MB, Laws ER Jr: Surgical management of GH-secreting pituitary adenomas: an outcome study using modern remission criteria. J Clin Endocrinol Metab 2001;86: 4072–4077.
91 Freda P, Wardlaw S, Post K: Long term follow-up evaluation in 115 patients who underwent transsphenoidal surgery for acromegaly. J Neurosurg 1998;89:353–358.

Edward C. Nemergut, MD
Department of Anesthesiology, Health Sciences Center
University of Virginia, PO Box 800710
Charlottesville, VA 22908–0710 (USA)
Tel. +1 434 924 2283, Fax +1 434 982 0019, E-Mail en3x@virginia.edu

Laws ER Jr, Sheehan JP (eds): Pituitary Surgery – A Modern Approach.
Front Horm Res. Basel, Karger, 2006, vol 34, pp 256–278

Vascular Injury and Transsphenoidal Surgery

Rod J. Oskouian[a], *Daniel F. Kelly*[b], *Edward R. Laws, Jr.*[a]

[a]Department of Neurological Surgery, Health Sciences Center, University of Virginia, Charlottesville, Va., and [b]Division of Neurosurgery, University of California School of Medicine, Los Angeles, Calif., USA

Abstract

Vascular complications can and do arise from transsphenoidal surgery and, when they occur, they have a high incidence of mortality and serious morbidity. The anatomic substrate for such complications is discussed, along with technical aspects of surgery and other methods for the avoidance of vascular complications.

Copyright © 2006 S. Karger AG, Basel

Introduction

The history of pituitary surgery is interesting in that the transsphenoidal approach to the sella turcica originated due to its safety. At the turn of the century when neurosurgeons first began to approach the pituitary area, a craniotomy was extraordinary difficult and had unacceptable mortality rates compared to the standards of today. The instruments, lighting, cautery, anesthesia, medications and the operating microscope, things that we take for granted today, were nonexistent, and therefore the transsphenoidal approach was significantly less dangerous for the patient than a craniotomy. The reemergence of transsphenoidal surgery began with Norman Dott who learned the technique from Harvey Cushing who then taught it to Guiot [1]. Guiot introduced the use of the radiofluoroscopy to visualize the sella and sphenoid sinus and then used this information to direct his trajectory, depth, and position of the instruments [1, 2]. Jules Hardy of Montreal learned the technique from Guiot and continued to refine and improve the procedure with the introduction of the operating microscope, and specialized instruments [2].

Iatrogenic injury to the internal carotid artery is one of the most feared complications associated with pituitary surgery. Historically, emergency surgical ligation was used to treat carotid injury during pituitary surgery when the carotid was injured. This treatment was associated with an unacceptable incidence of major complications. The ability to treat vascular injuries once they have occurred is crucial to obtaining a good outcome. Today, the neurosurgeon has the advantage of being able to use endovascular therapy to control bleeding, embolize carotid cavernous fistulas, stent pseudoaneurysms, and even use balloon occlusion if necessary. The endovascular approach has proved to be invaluable in the management of many of these complications. With improved technology, such as the use of intraoperative neuronavigation, real-time fluoroscopic guidance, computerized tomographic angiography and the use of the intraoperative microvascular Doppler, many of these complications can be prevented.

Despite our advancements in refining the techniques passed down from Cushing, the operative approach is still challenging and the incidence of carotid injury and vascular complications was thought to be uncommon. A current review of the literature and a recent survey suggest otherwise [3]. There are very few large series published and it is commonly believed that this complication occurs infrequently [4, 5]. Careful reviews of such studies reveal that carotid injury is not so uncommon, and recent responses to a national survey conducted suggest that the incidence of this complication is higher than previously thought, with 12% of neurosurgeons reporting that they have had a carotid injury occur during pituitary surgery [3].

Operative Approaches

The pioneering surgeons who used the transsphenoidal approach during the first decade of the 20th century had very few complications, and this continues to hold true in our modern era. The surgical approaches to the pituitary region have always been dependent upon a thorough knowledge of the surgical anatomy involved.

There are several approaches to reach the sphenoid sinus. The sublabial approach was originally very popular and is still used today. It involves making an incision under the lip and dissecting along the bony nasal septum. The endonasal transseptal approach avoids the oropharynx and is directed through a small incision in the nasal mucosa and dissection along one side of the septum. The direct endonasal approach enters one nostril, between the turbinates and the nasal septum and does not require an incision in the nose before reaching the face of the sphenoid. The direct endonasal approach, with or without the use of the endoscope, because of its minimally invasive characteristics is gaining more popularity and patients experience rapid recovery [6].

Regardless of the approach there is always a chance of vascular injury during pituitary surgery and when it does occur it can lead to permanent disability and even mortality. The boundaries of the sella turcica include the cavernous sinuses on either side. These vascular structures contain the carotid arteries, which, like the cavernous sinuses, are vulnerable to injury during the transsphenoidal approach. In many cases, the intracranial arteries and nerves lie just above the sella and are frequently in contact with the surface of the lesion where they may be subject to injury.

Technical Aspects of the Transsphenoidal Approach

The most common route for pituitary lesions used today is the endonasal transsphenoidal approach (fig. 1). There is a steep learning curve with pituitary surgery and like many surgical procedures it has its hazards and pitfalls which can be unanticipated even in experienced hands. Having a thorough understanding of the pituitary and its relationship to the cavernous sinus, internal carotid artery and circle of Willis is essential (fig. 2). The sella turcica lies in the center of the cranial base and surgical access to the pituitary is limited by the internal carotid artery, cavernous sinus, optic nerves, and the circle of Willis, as well as posteriorly by the brainstem and basilar artery. The sphenoid bone contains the carotid arteries with the carotid prominences on the lateral walls of the sphenoid sinus bilaterally.

The initial aspects of the transsphenoidal approach are through the mucous membranes of the nose or the undersurface of the lip. These membranes can often be quite vascular, with numerous small interconnecting vascular channels, and bleeding can be considerable if no attempt is made to produce decongestion and hemostasis. Rhinologic surgeons have traditionally used a number of techniques to avoid this type of bleeding, and currently the application of vasoconstrictors and the injection of a local anesthetic solution combine to produce excellent hemostasis within the mucous membranes during the approach. The paired sphenopalatine arteries, branches of the internal maxillary artery, supply the nasal structures; these are important vascular structures, which should be protected and avoided. Ordinarily, the midline approach will not disturb the main trunks of the sphenopalatine arteries and every attempt during the approach should be made to avoid injury to these vessels. The internal carotid, anterior choroidal, anterior cerebral, as well as the anterior and posterior communicating arteries also have perforating branches that reach the third ventricle that may be draped over suprasellar or posteriorly projecting tumors (fig. 3).

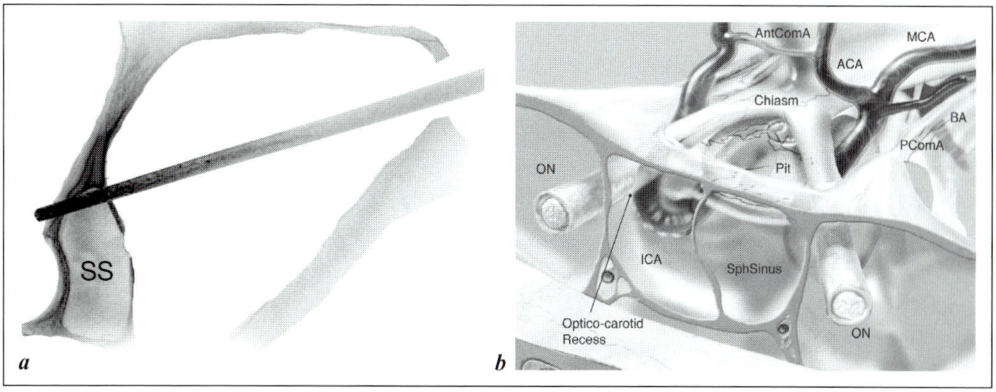

Fig. 1. The endonasal transsphenoidal approach demonstrating the trajectory from below (***a***) and the vascular structures shown from a suprasellar view (***b***). ACA = Anterior cerebral artery; AntComA = anterior communicating artery; BA = basilar artery; ICA = internal carotid artery; MCA = middle cerebral artery; ON = optic nerve; PComA = posterior communicating artery; SphSinus, SS = sphenoid sinus.

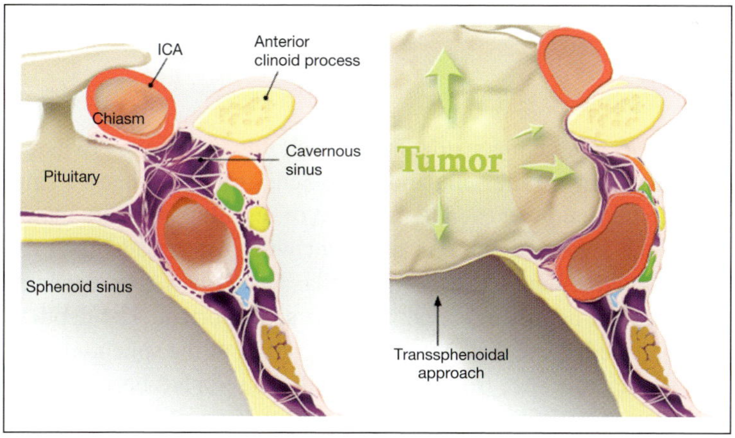

Fig. 2. Illustration demonstrating the intracranial structures at risk from a superior view and above the diaphragm: internal carotid, cavernous sinus and cranial nerves. ICA = Internal carotid artery.

Sphenoid Sinus

The sphenoid sinus lies anterior to the sella and separates the pituitary gland from the nasal cavity. The sphenoid sinus has tremendous variation in its degree of pneumatization, and in response to sellar pathology the sinus itself

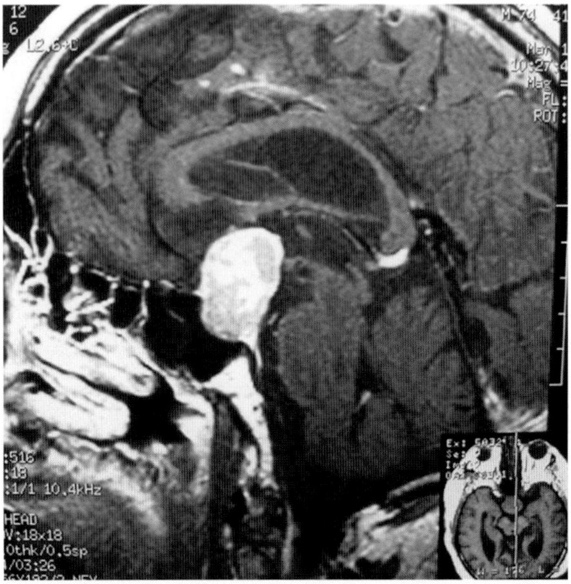

Fig. 3. Large macroadenoma with suprasellar extension projecting posteriorly and into the third ventricle.

can change in size. Very large macroadenomas or chordomas of the clivus can distort the normal anatomy of the sella and can extend into the sphenoid sinus with thinning of the normal bone even to the point of revealing the dura mater.

The depth of the sphenoid sinus in a patient with a macroadenoma can vary greatly due to enlargement of the normal sella. That is why a fundamental understanding of normal neurosurgical anatomy is so important. The depth of sphenoid sinus is defined as the distance from the ostium of the sphenoid sinus to the sella. This average distance from the ostium to the sella has been found to be around 15–17 (range 10–35) mm [7]. This is vital and important information for the pituitary surgeon since it provides a rough estimate of the length needed to reach the sella from the ostia. The nasal speculum that is most commonly used for the transsphenoidal route is 7–10 cm in length [8, 9]. The tip of the nasal speculum should be placed just anterior to the sphenoid sinus. Once inside the sphenoid sinus the floor of the sella turcica is easily appreciated, and the overall the distance is approximately 11–12 cm [7–9]. As a result, with macroadenomas or chordomas of the clivus we always suspect that there can be neural or vascular structures exposed directly within the sinus, above the diaphragma sellae, or within the sella itself and this is why we always use blunt rather than sharp ring curettes for microdissection in the sella and sphenoid sinus. The thickest part of the bone has been shown to be at the tuberculum sellae and clivus while the thinnest is along the anterior sellar wall [8]. The actual thickness of the bone of the anterior sella can be anywhere from 0.1 to 0.7 mm with an average thickness of about 0.5 mm [9].

When inside the sphenoid sinus one can see the carotid sulcus which houses the cavernous portion of the internal carotid artery and lies directly against the lateral surface of the sphenoid bone. The thickness of the bone separating the artery from the sphenoid sinus is thinnest over the anterior parts of the carotid prominence but it is actually very thin just below the tuberculum sellae (0.5–1.0 mm). Thus, once inside the sinus and facing the anterior wall of the sella or laterally on the bone covering the cavernous carotid artery the bone is not very thick and can easily be fractured. The relationship of the carotid artery to the sella is vital information to the pituitary surgeon, and the transverse diameter between the carotid prominences of each side has been measured in an elegant study by Fujii et al. [7]. They found that the shortest distance is usually located at the level of the tuberculum sellae but can vary significantly [7]. When removing the mucosa and the bone from the lateral walls of the sinus one can expose the dura covering the medial surface of the cavernous sinus and optic canals. In the process of removing bone one can inadvertently lacerate the dura and injure the carotid artery as well as the cavernous sinus and its contents. In some cases there may be no bony protection within the walls of the sinus therefore increasing the risk of cranial nerve deficits and carotid artery injury.

Sella Turcica

The diaphragma sellae covers the pituitary gland and forms the roof of the sella turcica. The diaphragma is thinner around the infundibulum and therefore represents a risk for injury of suprasellar structures especially in cases in which an extended transsphenoidal approach is used. The diaphragma has an aperture for the infundibulum and as a result part of the arachnoid from the suprasellar cistern can protrude into the sella turcica and is a potential source of postoperative cerebrospinal fluid leakage. The actual volume of the sella can be calculated by using the mathematical ellipsoid formula 0.5 (length $\times$ width $\times$ depth)/1,000 = volume (mm^3) with the upper limit of normal being around 1,000 mm^3 [7–9].

Carotid Artery

The most feared complication of pituitary surgery is injury to the carotid artery. During the approach to the sella and pituitary gland a perfectly midline trajectory needs to be taken since the carotid arteries lie on either side of the sphenoid sinus. The carotid artery can be quite tortuous and may project to the midline (fig. 3). Once inside the sella we always use blunt instruments for microdissection since there can often be little or no distance separating the medial portion of the carotid artery and the lateral surface of the pituitary gland. When dealing with microadenomas there is often a separation (0–9 mm) between the lateral surface of the gland and the carotid artery. While with macroadenomas the gland can lose its normal contour and incorporate the wall of the artery especially when there is invasion of the cavernous sinus. The lumen of the carotid can also be quite sclerotic and friable from hypertension and atherosclerosis particularly in patients with acromegaly or Cushing's disease. In microadenomas the carotid can and often does lie just behind the dura where it is prone to injury during the opening of the sella and exposure of the dura.

Important branches of the carotid artery that supply the sella arise from the meningohypophyseal trunk. The largest intracavernous arterial branch is the inferior hypophyseal artery, and runs medially to the posterior lobe. McConnell's capsular arteries usually are clinically insignificant and arise from the medial portion of the cavernous carotid artery. The cranial nerves that are within the wall of the cavernous sinus are, from superior to inferior: oculomotor nerve, trochlear, ophthalmic division of the trigeminal nerve, and abducens nerves. The abducens nerve courses within the sinus on the medial side of the ophthalmic division of the fifth nerve and is adherent to the carotid artery medially and the ophthalmic division laterally.

Venous Anatomy

Cerebral veins do not pose a formidable obstacle to operative approaches to the suprasellar area and lower part of the third ventricle as they do around the ventricular wall and third ventricle. The suprasellar area is drained by small branches of the basal veins. The internal cerebral veins course in the roof of the third ventricle and are rarely involved in pituitary adenomas.

The cavernous sinuses on either side of the sella are vascular structures filled with venous blood under venous pressure. The sinuses contain dural channels that can be injured during the opening of the dura. The intracranial dura consists of two layers and between these layers vascular channels proliferate, particularly in the normal-sized sella of most Cushing's disease patients. During the resection it is easy to directly enter the cavernous sinus which usually is of no clinical consequence but there is often profuse venous bleeding. More importantly it is vital to remember that in addition to the carotid artery the third, fourth, fifth and sixth cranial nerves are in the cavernous sinus. As with other venous structures in the brain, if the head of the patient is raised above the level of the heart, there is a potential for an air embolus into the interconnecting veins or directly into the cavernous sinus.

Venous sinuses that interconnect the paired cavernous sinuses may be found in the margins of the diaphragma. The venous channels are named on the basis of their anatomic relationship to the pituitary. For instance, the anterior intercavernous sinuses pass anterior to the hypophysis, and the posterior intercavernous sinuses pass behind. At times, the anterior intercavernous sinus may cover the entire anterior wall of the sella, and, if the anterior and posterior sinuses connect, the whole structure is often referred to as the circular sinus [9]. Entering the intercavernous sinuses may produce brisk bleeding which often resolves with temporary compression of the sinus or with a hemostatic agent, surgical clips or with light coagulation [4].

Circle of Willis

The vascular anatomy around in the suprasellar region is very complex and is frequently distorted by large tumors. The internal carotids, basilar artery and the circle of Willis with its major branches may be at risk of injury during pituitary surgery. Suprasellar tumors often extend into the anterior wall of the third ventricle where perforating vessels arise from the anterior portion of the circle of Willis (fig. 4). Our experience has been that in this region, the anterior cerebral arteries, and the anterior communicating artery are particularly at risk since they are often adherent to the tumor or enveloped by the tumor (fig. 5). The anterior cerebral artery branches off the internal carotid artery below the anterior perforated substance and projects anteromedially above the optic nerve and chiasm. The anterior communicating artery is usually located just above the chiasm. The anterior communicating and anterior cerebral arteries give off perforating branches that terminate in the hypothalamus, fornix, septum pellucidum, as well as the striatum. The recurrent branch of the anterior cerebral artery arises from the A_1 segment of the anterior cerebral artery and courses laterally above the bifurcation of the internal carotid artery.

The anterior choroidal artery is also at risk of injury during pituitary surgery since it comes off the posterior surface of the internal carotid artery just beyond the origin of the posterior communicating artery. It is directed posterolaterally below the optic tract and through the choroidal fissure to supply the choroid plexus in the temporal horn, optic tract, optic radiations, globus pallidus, internal capsule, midbrain, and thalamus.

The small branches that arise from the posterior communicating artery are at risk as well since the artery travels below the optic tract and the third

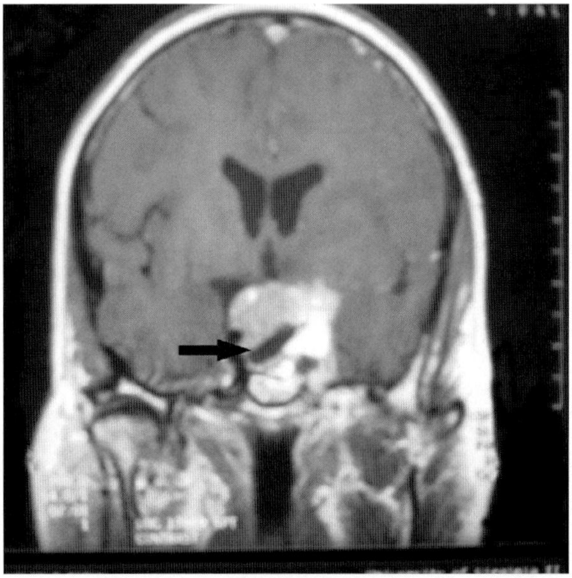

Fig. 4. Coronal T1-weighted magnetic resonance image demonstrating a tortuous carotid crossing the midline.

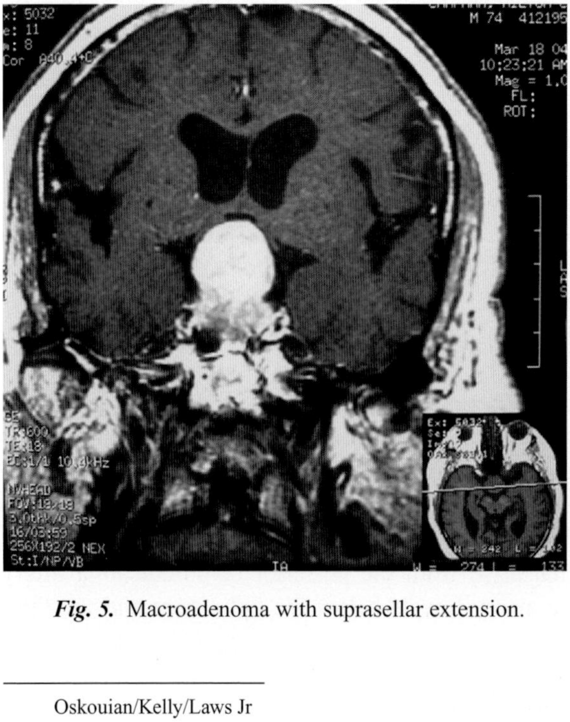

Fig. 5. Macroadenoma with suprasellar extension.

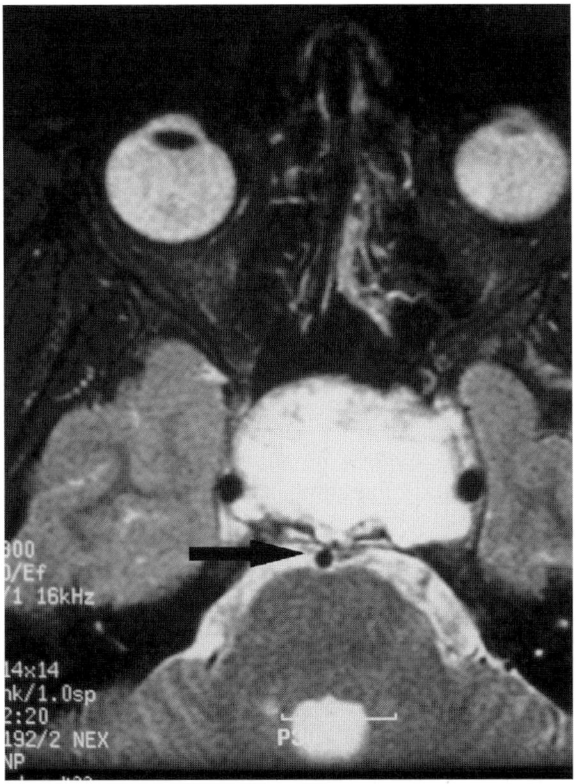

Fig. 6. T2-weighted magnetic resonance image demonstrating the proximity of the basilar artery posteriorly.

ventricle where branches reach the thalamus, hypothalamus, sub-thalamus, and internal capsule. Its posterior course often varies, depending on whether the artery provides the major supply to the distal posterior cerebral artery.

Basilar Artery Injury

Macroadenomas that extend posteriorly and chordomas of the clivus can erode the clivus and therefore can put the posterior circulation at risk for injury. Immediately posterior to the clivus and within millimeters of the clivus is the basilar artery and its perforators which irrigate the brainstem and thalamus (fig. 6). Keep in mind that a misdirected approach and one that is too low or posterior can injure these vital arteries.

Types of Vascular Complications

There are a number of vascular problems related to the approach whether it is by way of the endonasal approach or with the use of the traditional sublabial route [10, 11]. There can be significant bleeding from the vascular mucosal membranes. It is not uncommon to have excessive bleeding from injury to the sphenopalatine artery during the approach. Most often the bleeding may occur from the bone directly, from the venous diploic space or from the blood supply to stout bony structures, particularly in patients with acromegaly. Lesions within the sella may be inherently vascular. This is true of some pituitary tumors, but is also true of other unusual lesions such as hemangiopericytomas or hemangioblastomas where the surgeon may have difficulty in controlling bleeding from the tumor. Before the advent of modern imaging and magnetic resonance (MR) imaging it was not uncommon for some pituitary 'tumors' to be aneurysms that developed in the suprasellar compartment or within the sella turcica.

Cavernous Carotid Injury

Unfortunately, the most difficult vascular complication that a pituitary surgeon has to deal with is injury to the carotid artery. If direct surgical repair fails, which is often the case, then endovascular techniques need to be utilized, even though carotid occlusion carries the risk of cerebral ischemia and stroke. A direct midline approach is vital to minimize the risk of carotid injury. Anatomic variations in the sella and sphenoid sinus or even an absence of pneumatization, are well-known pitfalls of transsphenoidal surgery. Intraoperative bleeding is controlled initially by packing with muscle and hemostatic agents. Obtaining hemostasis may be difficult when there is limited access to the carotid due to limited exposure. Overpacking has its associated risks, with the possibility of causing complete carotid occlusion as well as postoperative ophthalmoplegia from cavernous sinus thrombosis.

Delayed epistaxis can also be a potentially devastating complication. Vascular injury may be unrecognized at the time of surgery and may not present in the immediate postoperative period. There can be a delay of hemorrhage that can range from days to months after the initial surgery and may occur as a result of rupture of carotid or sphenopalatine pseudoaneurysms. These delayed events illustrate the need to perform immediate angiography after transsphenoidal surgery that has been complicated by arterial injury or profuse bleeding, or has been followed by epistaxis. All patients with arterial injury must have postoperative angiography even if hemostasis is obtained intraoperatively. Carotid

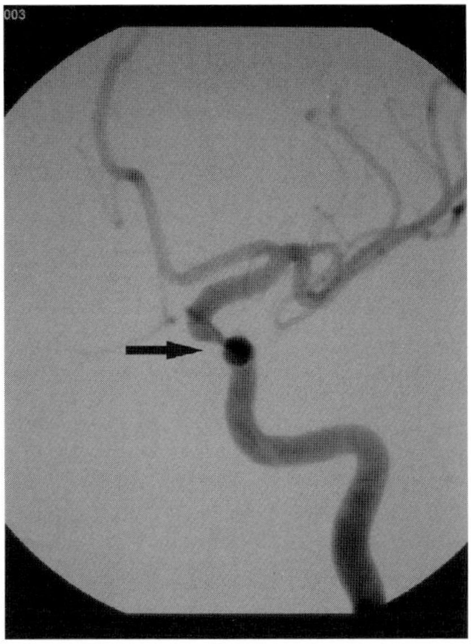

Fig. 7. Postoperative angiogram demonstrating focal cavernous carotid arterial spasm following direct injury and intrasellar repair with muscle.

occlusions, vasospasm, thromboembolism and stenosis of the vessel can be the result of overpacking, hematoma, dissection, or even partial thrombosis [10–15].

Perforation or laceration of the carotid arteries in the carotid canals or in the cavernous sinus represents a very serious complication in the transsphenoidal approach. In some cases, large invasive tumors that have eroded the skull base may actually surround the carotid arteries and, occasionally, may invade the adventitial wall of the vessel so that removal of the tumor can injure the integrity of the artery.

The intracranial vasculature can also develop vasospasm whether it is post-traumatic or related to hemorrhage around vessels or injury to them (fig. 7). Vasospasm can clearly cause arterial insufficiency and stroke (fig. 8). The dissection of tumor away from the carotid or displacement of the carotid arteries in the cavernous sinus during attempts at hemostasis can also lead to thrombosis of these vessels with vascular occlusion and distal emboli that can result in stroke.

Direct injury to the carotid artery will frequently result in a false aneurysm or pseudoaneurysm even if the artery appears to be packed to the point of maintaining its integrity without further bleeding (fig. 9). In our experience, virtually every direct injury to a carotid artery that is indirectly repaired during surgery results in a subsequent false aneurysm and its evolution can often be very subtle [16, 17]. Some patients, in addition to having tortuous carotids or atherosclerotic disease, may actually harbor an incidental unruptured aneurysm

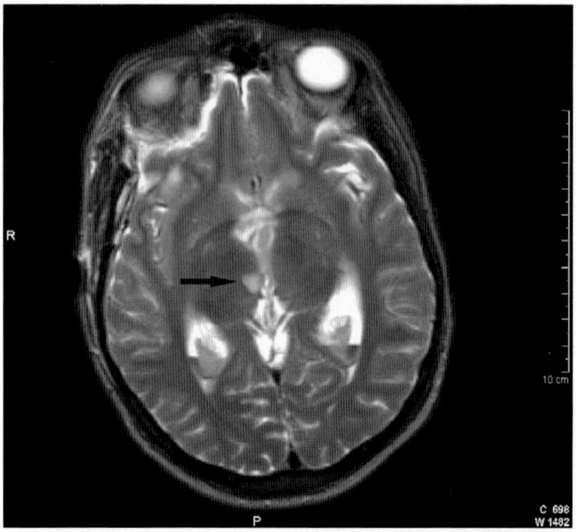

Fig. 8. Patient who developed cerebral vasospasm of the posterior circulation and a right thalamic stroke from vascular injury of the circle of Willis.

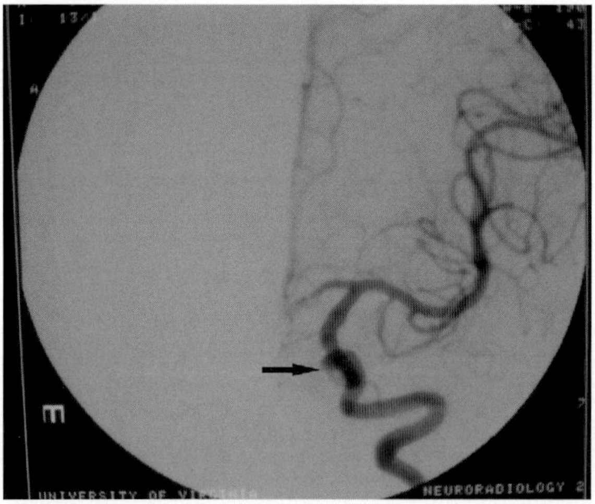

Fig. 9. Large pseudoaneurysm of the left cavernous carotid demonstrated on a postoperative angiogram.

of the cavernous carotid, the circle of Willis, or the basilar artery. We have had 3 patients with incidentally associated vascular lesions preoperatively: one arteriovenous malformation, a dural vascular malformation as well as intraoperative or perioperative rupture of a pre-existing basilar bifurcation aneurysm and

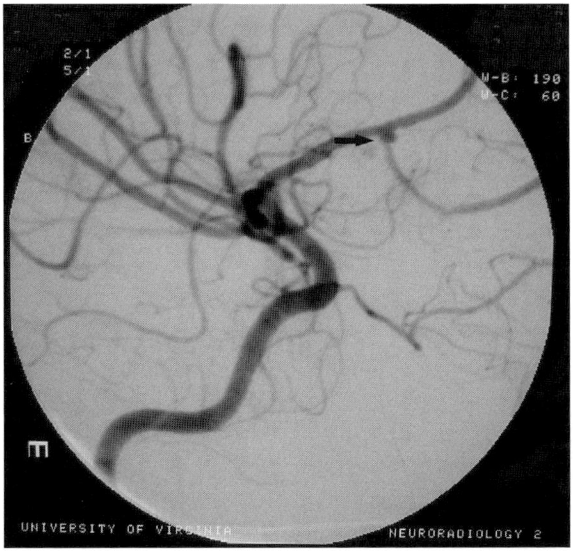

Fig. 10. Internal carotid injection demonstrating dye extravasation from a pericallosal artery aneurysm rupture perioperatively.

a pericallosal artery aneurysm (fig. 10) [18]. Another potential result of injury to the carotid artery is the subsequent development of a carotid cavernous fistula (fig. 11) [19–21].

Postoperative hemorrhage may occur from any aspect of the surgical approach or the sellar dissection. Ordinarily, hemorrhage of a significant degree once demanded immediate surgical re-exploration, but with angiography and embolization it is no longer required and is case-dependent.

Surgical dissection in the region of the cavernous sinus or the post-excision packing of the sella may extend to occlude the cavernous sinus and cause a symptomatic cavernous sinus thrombosis.

Management of Vascular Complications

During the approach, if there is excessive bleeding from the internal maxillary artery, it is occasionally necessary to isolate the vessel and to ligate it. This is a sizable vascular structure and cauterization alone may not be adequate to provide secure hemostasis. Its anatomic position is relatively constant, and the transsphenoidal surgeon should be familiar with methods for exposure and control of this important vessel, along with its implications for problems during the exposure, particularly of large and invasive tumors involving the skull base.

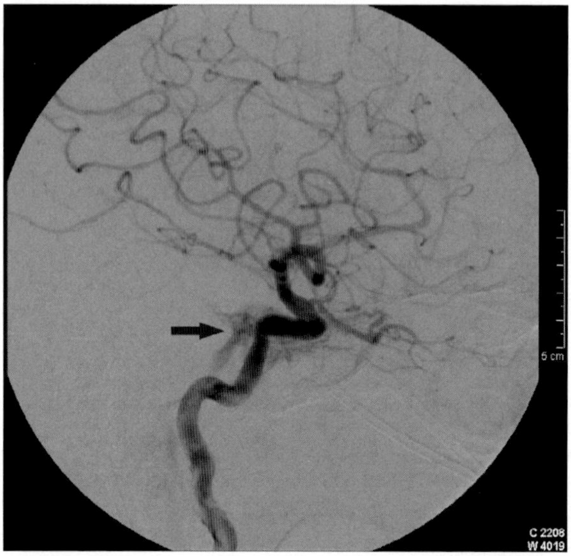

Fig. 11. Cavernous carotid fistula that developed in a patient who suffered a carotid injury.

When the carotid artery itself is injured, there are a number of options. Obviously, high-pressure arterial bleeding in a confined space visualized with the operating microscope or endoscope can represent a significant technical challenge. In some cases, if bleeding can be controlled adequately, the arterial injury can be directly sutured, and we have accomplished this successfully in a few cases. In other situations, particularly those where the arterial segment may be entirely surrounded by tumor, if the tumor has invaded the adventitia, there is a possibility that bleeding can be controlled and perfusion through the carotid maintained if one uses a Sundt-type clip graft; we accomplished this successfully in one case. More often, the area of bleeding must be packed with cottonoid patties, Gel foam, sometimes with Oxycel, as well as with muscle or fat. Placing muscle in an optimal position tends to be hemostatic and offers some opportunity for effective healing of the vessel. The muscle must be applied with just the right force; this can occasionally be accomplished using a suitably tailored bone plate or artificial material (acrylic, hydroxyapatite, miniplate, etc.) to provide enough support for the injury to prevent bleeding but not so much as to occlude the vessel. In some cases, the only feasible option is to perform occlusive packing of the damaged carotid artery and then to raise the blood pressure in the hopes that collateral circulation through the circle of Willis will prevent a stroke.

When a false aneurysm occurs after a carotid injury, there are just a few options for dealing with this potentially fatal complication. Direct coiling using

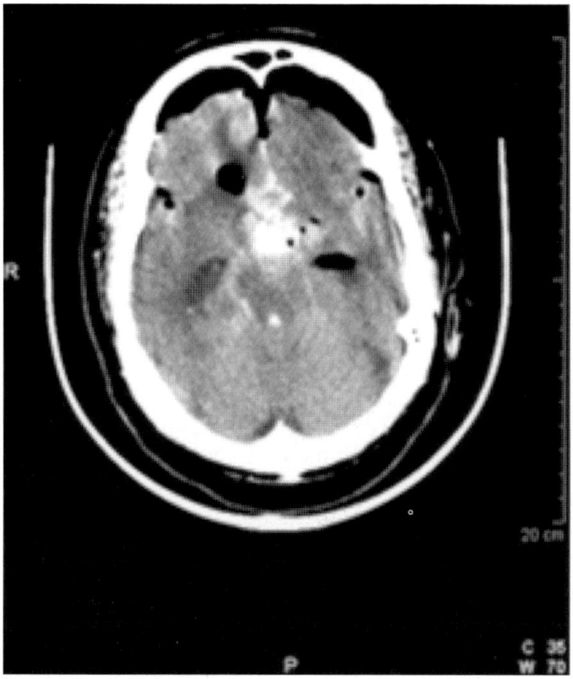

Fig. 12. Postoperative computerized tomography scan demonstrating subarachnoid and intraventricular hemorrhage following transsphenoidal surgery.

an endovascular approach is ordinarily not feasible for a false aneurysm as there is no aneurysmal wall to contain the coil. When faced with this situation, we have either done a craniotomy with direct entry into the cavernous sinus and direct repair of the injured vessel, maintaining patency, or endovascular balloon occlusion of the carotid artery trapping out the segment that contains the false aneurysm. In the case of intracranial hemorrhage, usually produced by bleeding from the tumor or from vessels associated with the dorsal aspect of the tumor itself, the diagnosis must be made as rapidly as possible, and at times it is necessary to do a craniotomy in order to remove hematoma, residual tumor and to achieve hemostasis.

In some cases, the intracranial hemorrhage is in the form of subarachnoid bleeding with intraventricular hemorrhage (fig. 12). We have had cases of neurologic deficit and even death from this form of subarachnoid hemorrhage. These patients are also at risk of developing vasospasm just like patients who harbor ruptured intracranial aneurysms. Obviously, if this occurs it should be treated with standard methods to deal with generalized vasospasm of the intracranial arterial tree. Ordinarily, maximizing medical therapy is the first line of therapy.

Angiography and the possibility of endovascular therapy with pharmacologic agents or with balloon angioplasty can be considered. In situations where major branches of the circle of Willis are injured intracranially from a transsphenoidal approach, there is often little choice but to attempt to sacrifice the branches with embolization. Ordinarily, the anterior communicating and the anterior cerebral arteries are the ones most at risk, and if one of these structures must be clipped, then induced hypertension is sometimes helpful in providing satisfactory collateral through the circle of Willis to avoid ischemic damage to the brain.

In circumstances where postoperative hemorrhage occurs, usually this is from the nasal structures and may merit repacking and cauterization of the bleeding points. This can be done in the otorhinological clinic setting and rarely does it involve taking the patient back to the operating theater where the full range of equipment and adjuncts is available. When cavernous sinus thrombosis occurs, it may be either immediate or delayed. Immediate cavernous sinus damage can result from over-vigorous packing of the cavernous sinus after removal of the tumor or attempts to control venous bleeding. If the surgeon is convinced that too much packing has been utilized, then it is prudent to reopen the wound, which can be done quite readily, and to repack with less pressure. Our custom is to pack these structures with Gel foam when there is no spinal fluid leak and to use fat taken from the abdomen when a spinal fluid leak has occurred intraoperatively. We ordinarily will coat the fat with Avitene powder, which may help in achieving the desired hemostasis. When cavernous sinus thrombosis occurs in a delayed fashion, it usually is from an expanding clot within the sinus and sometimes may be related to inflammatory changes in the packing material. Ordinarily, a delayed cavernous sinus syndrome has been treated conservatively with the use of increased doses of corticosteroid medication, and these problems with their associated neurologic deficits have resolved with this form of conservative management. Obviously, the appropriate diagnostic studies need to be done to rule out other sources of cavernous sinus problems such as pseudoaneurysm or the early development of a cavernous carotid fistula.

Immediate angiography should be performed in all patients with suspected vascular injuries and the studies should include bilateral selective internal maxillary injection. We recommend balloon occlusion of the carotid artery for carotid cavernous fistulas, and carotid false aneurysms, provided the patient can tolerate carotid test occlusion and has adequate collateral flow through the circle of Willis (fig. 13). Despite having postoperative angiographic findings that are normal, a repeat control study is recommend 1 week after the nasal packing is removed and before the patient is discharged. If the first postoperative angiogram shows incomplete occlusion of the vascular injury or pseudoaneurysm, permanent balloon occlusion may be performed. If balloon occlusion is not performed, an angiogram before discharge is recommended to establish a 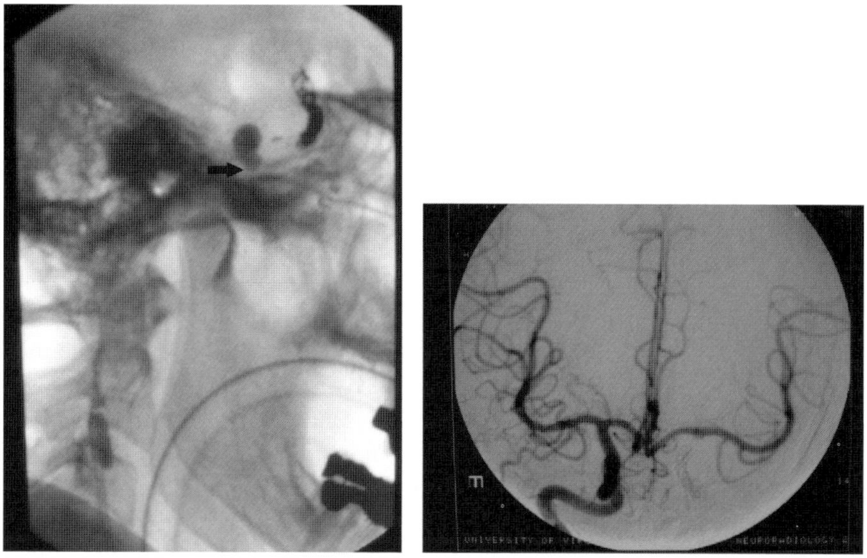 b

Fig. 13. ***a*** Left carotid injection demonstrating a large pseudoaneurysm just proximal to the coils before permanent balloon occlusion is performed. ***b*** Following balloon occlusion of the right carotid artery, excellent cross filling of the left cerebral circulation is demonstrated.

that the complete occlusion is still present. Patients who sustain vascular injuries need meticulous follow-up to detect the development of a pseudoaneurysm. Any delayed episode of significant or unusual epistaxis occurring after transsphenoidal surgery should be considered serious and selective angiography of both internal carotid and internal maxillary arteries should be performed without hesitation.

Our feeling is that endovascular carotid occlusion is the best treatment for carotid injury if the patient can tolerate the procedure since we have no long-term data on the efficacy of stents [22–24]. Most often there is no choice and the procedure is done on an emergency basis to prevent further hemorrhage and death. We do have the ability to use stents and grafts for carotid injuries but we feel that these techniques are best reserved for cavernous carotid fistulas since there is often a small channel or defect in the vascular wall itself. If the patient's ability to tolerate balloon occlusion after internal carotid artery injury is in doubt and his or her life is not in danger, then the stent-graft option represents a viable low-risk alternative that substantially reduces the risk of stroke. The main technical limitation associated with the placement of a stent within the carotid is limited longitudinal flexibility. Moreover, the long-term efficacy of stents for the treatment of iatrogenic internal carotid artery injury is still unknown. In addition, future technological advancements will most likely improve the current stent designs and offer more sophisticated delivery systems that will help solve the current limitations.

Pituitary Apoplexy

Pituitary apoplexy is an uncommon manifestation of a pituitary tumor. There are two basic mechanisms, the first of these is hemorrhage within a preexisting pituitary tumor. The second is infarction of the tumor with occlusion of its blood supply and subsequent swelling and necrosis of the lesion. The incidence of symptomatic pituitary apoplexy presenting as a medical emergency is approximately 1.0% of pituitary tumors. The 'subacute' or 'silent' presentation of pituitary apoplexy occurs much more commonly and there is evidence of prior minor hemorrhage present in between 20 and 22% of pituitary adenomas.

The differential diagnosis of acute pituitary apoplexy can be very confusing and patients are often misdiagnosed as having subarachnoid hemorrhage, stroke, myocardial infarction, sepsis or syncope. A number of precipitating factors have been postulated for pituitary apoplexy but, in fact, it is difficult to single out any of these as truly important because this event is so uncommon. Anticoagulation, hypertension or the use of bromocriptine and other medical agents have all been implicated in precipitating episodes of pituitary apoplexy, but there are no consistent patterns. Perhaps the most important general statement regarding pituitary apoplexy is the urgent need for steroid replacement therapy because these patients have acute adrenal insufficiency. Either operative or non-operative stress can readily result in collapse and even fatality. In virtually every instance, the correct procedure is to perform a rapid and effective decompression of the sella with removal of the lesion. In the setting of prolactin-secreting pituitary tumors in patients who are stable and not losing vision, there is a case to be made for medical therapy with dopamine agonists alone.

Complication Avoidance

Preoperative MR imaging can often demonstrate subtle anatomic variants such as sphenoidal septa and the position of the carotid arteries. Our experience has shown us that the risk of carotid injury is much higher in microadenomas than with large macroadenomas that often displace the carotids from their usual position and laterally from the midline (fig. 14). Microadenomas such as those in Cushing's disease can invade the cavernous sinus and may be in close proximity to the carotid artery. We have also seen complications occur in a subset of

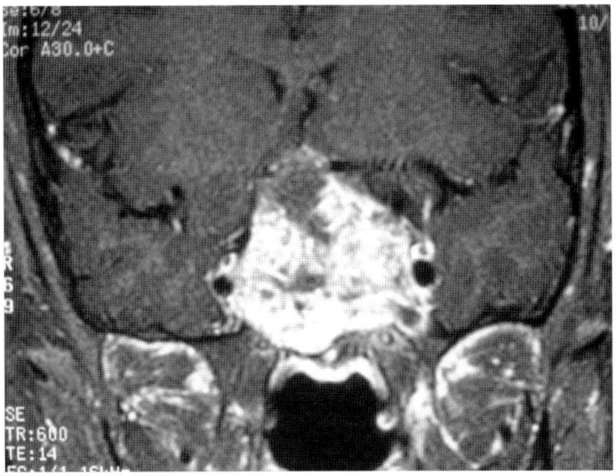

Fig. 14. Macroadenoma with suprasellar extension and invasion of the cavernous sinus that has displaced the carotids laterally.

another high-risk group of patients who had previous transsphenoidal surgery or radiation therapy.

Detailed information regarding the anatomy is the most reliable and effective way of avoiding complications of all kinds in transsphenoidal surgery, but particularly in the avoidance of vascular complications. Careful attention should be paid to the preoperative studies; high-quality MR imaging is the standard technique currently in use. Computerized tomography (CT) studies can often show the bony anatomy of the sphenoid more precisely than an MR study, but the ability of the MR images to show the vascular structures is an extremely important factor in making this modality the imaging procedure of choice. If there is any suspicion of a vascular anomaly or some unusual vascular feature of the lesion to be treated, then MR angiography, CT angiography or even standard angiography should be performed so that the entire vascular system in the region of the sella can be carefully evaluated. Obviously, judicious use of careful microsurgical technique is essential for the avoidance of complications. In removing bone, one should be careful that it is removed cleanly and not fractured, as ragged edges of fractured segments can easily tear the carotid artery either in the canal or in the cavernous sinus. Careful technique in removing tumor away from the region of the cavernous sinus and the carotid artery is also important, and the use of sharp curettes and other instruments with sharp edges should be assiduously avoided. Intraoperative image guidance can be based either on CT or MR data sets and in our hands have been able to provide accurate information with regard to the anatomic midline and have also allowed us to eliminate the use of intraoperative fluoroscopy in selected patients undergoing transsphenoidal surgery.

The use of the operative endoscope can also be a helpful adjunct in the avoidance of injuries to the carotid arteries, particularly during the initial exposure. The panoramic view provided by the endoscope can clearly delineate the position of the carotid canals when the sphenoid sinus is first entered. The use of angled endoscopes can allow one to visualize the carotid arteries in the walls of the sella and to evaluate the thoroughness of removal of cavernous sinus extensions. A microvascular Doppler sensor can also be used to probe for the carotids behind the exposed dura. Prior to making an incision we almost always use the microvascular Doppler to locate the position of the carotid bilaterally. We also rely heavily on intraoperative image guidance – an important adjunct for patients who had previous transsphenoidal surgery. More importantly, we always use the patient's own anatomic landmarks such as the vomer and the rostrum of the sphenoid, that give us good guidance to the midline. In patients who have had previous surgery, these anatomic guidelines may be missing or distorted, and unusual septations within the sphenoid sinus or lack of pneumatization of the sphenoid sinus can also be confounding factors in maintaining accurate operative position. The use of computerized stereotactic neuronavigational guidance can help determine accurate anatomic position.

Conclusions

Although experience, emerging technologies, and a thorough knowledge of the relevant anatomy can help prevent many potential complications of transsphenoidal surgery, the risk of arterial injury can never be eliminated. This is particularly true given the increasing number of such procedures performed and the increasing complexity of pathology treated. Despite the requisite thorough knowledge of microsurgical anatomy, arterial injuries can still occur. There is a trend in medicine and in neurosurgery toward more minimally invasive procedures, and this, in turn, has given rise to an increase in the popularity of the transsphenoidal approach and its variations for treating a myriad of pathologies that would often be difficult to reach through a standard craniotomy.

Vascular complications represent a serious hazard in performing transsphenoidal surgery for virtually any form of pathology. Immediate diagnosis and treatment is essential to prevent a fatal complication or a stroke. The most serious complication is injury to the internal carotid artery that can result in bleeding, pseudoaneurysm, carotid cavernous fistula, stroke and even death. These complications can occur at any time, are frequently devastating for the patient and for the surgeon, and they justify a consistent, careful and accurate surgical technique. In most cases, these complications can be avoided but, as with all others, it is important for the surgical team to anticipate the fact that such problems can develop and to make every effort to prevent them. Angiography is mandatory when these injuries occur and endovascular treatment has proven to be invaluable in the management of complications from arterial injuries due to transsphenoidal surgery.

References

1 Guiot G: Transsphenoidal approach in surgical treatment of pituitary adenomas: General principles and indications in non-functioning adenomas; in Kohler PO, Ross GT (eds): Diagnosis and Treatment of Pituitary Tumors: Proceedings of a Conference. International Congress Series. Amsterdam, Excerpta Medica, 1973, vol 303, pp 159–179.

2 Hardy J: Transsphenoidal hypophysectomy. J Neurosurg 1971;34:582–594.

3 Ciric I, Ragin A, Baumgartner C, Pierce D: Complications of transsphenoidal surgery: results of a national survey, review of the literature, and personal experience. Neurosurgery 1997;40:225–236.

4 Laws ER Jr: Vascular complications of transsphenoidal surgery. Pituitary 1999;2:163–170.

5 Raymond J, Hardy J, Czepko R, Roy D: Arterial injuries in transsphenoidal surgery for pituitary adenoma: the role of angiography and endovascular treatment. AJNR Am J Neuroradiol 1997;18: 655–665.

6 Zada G, Kelly DF, Cohan P, Wang C, Swerdloff R: Endonasal transsphenoidal approach for pituitary adenomas and other sellar lesions: an assessment of efficacy, safety, and patient impressions. J Neurosurg 2003;98:350–358.

7 Fujii K, Chambers SM, Rhoton AL: Neurovascular relationships of the sphenoid sinus. J Neurosurg 1979;50: 31–39.

8 Renn WH, Rhoton AL Jr: Microsurgical anatomy of the sellar region. J Neurosurg 1975;43: 288–298.

9 Rhoton AL Jr: The sellar region. Neurosurgery 2002;51(suppl 4):S335–S374.

10 Fahlbusch R, Buchfelder M: Surgical complications; in Landolt AM, Vance ML, Reilly PL (eds): Pituitary Adenomas. New York, Churchill Livingstone, 1996, pp 395–408.

11 Landolt AM: Transsphenoidal surgery of pituitary tumors: its pitfalls and complications. Prog Neurol Surg. Basel, Karger, 1990, vol 13, pp 1–30.

12 Laws ER Jr: Complications of transsphenoidal surgery. Clin Neurosurg 1976;23:401–416.

13 Laws ER Jr: Complications of transsphenoidal microsurgery for pituitary adenomas; in Brock M (ed): Modern Neurosurgery. Berlin, Springer, 1982, vol 1, pp 181–186.

14 Zervas NT: Surgical results in pituitary adenomas: results of an international survey; in Black PM, Zervas NT, Ridgway EC Jr, Martin JB (eds): Secretory Tumors of the Pituitary Gland. New York, Raven Press, 1979, vol 48, pp 13–22.

15 Camp PE, Paxton HD, Buchan GC, Gahbauer H: Vasospasm after transsphenoidal hypophysectomy. Neurosurgery 1980;7:382–386.

16 Paullus WS Jr, Norwood CW, Morgan HW: False aneurysm of the cavernous carotid artery and progressive external ophthalmoplegia after transsphenoidal hypophysectomy: case report. J Neurosurg 1979;51:707–709.

17 Reddy K, Lesiuk H, West M, Fewer D: False aneurysm of the cavernous carotid artery: a complication of transsphenoidal surgery. Surg Neurol 1990;33:142–145.

18 Wakai, S, Fukushima T, Furihata T, Sano K: Association of cerebral aneurysm with pituitary adenoma. Surg Neurol 1979;12:503–507.

19 Ahuja A, Guterman LR, Hopkins LN: Carotid cavernous fistula and false aneurysm of the cavernous carotid artery: complications of transsphenoidal surgery. Neurosurgery 1992;31:774–779.

20 Pigott TJD, Holland IM, Punt JAG: Carotico-cavernous fistula after transsphenoidal hypophysectomy. Br J Neurosurg 1989;3:613–616.
21 Takahashi M, Killeffer F, Wilson G: Iatrogenic carotid cavernous fistula: case report. J Neurosurg 1969;30:498–500.
22 Fox AJ, Vinuela F, Pelz DM, et al: Use of detachable balloons for proximal artery occlusion in the treatment of unclippable cerebral aneurysms. J Neurosurg 1987;66:40–46.
23 Higashida RT, Halbach VV, Dowd C, et al: Endovascular detachable balloon embolization therapy of cavernous carotid artery aneurysms: results in 87 cases. J Neurosurg 1990;72:857–863.
24 Vazquez Anon V, Aymard A, Gobin YP, et al: Balloon occlusion of the internal carotid artery in 40 cases of giant intracavernous aneurysm: Technical aspects, cerebral monitoring, and results. Neuroradiology 1992;34:245–251.

Edward R. Laws, Jr., MD, FACS
Department of Neurological Surgery, Health Sciences Center
University of Virginia, PO Box 800212
Charlottesville, VA 22908 (USA)
Tel. +1 434 924 2650, Fax +1 434 924 5894, E-Mail el5g@virginia.edu

Author Index

Subject Index